PSYCHIATRY/ NEUROLOGY

NOTICE

Medicine is an ever-changing science. As new research and clinical experience broaden our knowledge, changes in treatment and drug therapy are required. The editors and the publisher of this work have made every effort to ensure that the drug dosage schedules herein are accurate and in accord with the standards accepted at the time of publication. Readers are advised, however, to check the product information sheet included in the package of each drug they plan to administer to be certain that changes have not been made in the recommended dose or in the contraindications for administration. This recommendation is of particular importance in regard to new or infrequently used drugs.

PSYCHIATRY/ NEUROLOGY:

PreTest® Self-Assessment and Review

William DeMyer, M.D.

Professor of Child Neurology
Indiana University
School of Medicine
Indianapolis, Indiana

Marian K. DeMyer, M.D.

Professor of Psychiatry
Indiana University
School of Medicine
Indianapolis, Indiana

McGraw-Hill Book Company
Health Professions Division
PreTest Series

*New York St. Louis San Francisco
Auckland Bogotá Guatemala Hamburg
Johannesburg Lisbon London Madrid
Mexico Montreal New Delhi Panama
Paris São Paulo Singapore Sydney
Tokyo Toronto*

Library of Congress Cataloging in Publishing Data

DeMyer, William, 1924-
    Psychiatry/neurology: PreTest self-assessment
and review.

    Bibliography: p.
    1. Psychiatry—Examinations, questions, etc.
2. Neurology—Examinations, questions, etc.
3. Neuropsychiatry—Examinations, questions, etc.
I. DeMyer, Marian K. II. Title.
RC457.D45   616.8′0076   81-20712
                                       AACR2

ISBN 0-07-051660-X

Editor: *John H. Gilchrist*
Project Editor: *Wendy Green*
Editorial Assistant: *Donna Altieri*
Production: *Rosemary J. Pascale, Judith M. Raccio*
Designer: *Robert Tutsky*
Printer: *Hull Printing Company*

Contents

Introduction

Psychiatry/Neurology: PreTest Self-Assessment and Review has been designed to provide physicians with a comprehensive, relevant, and convenient instrument for self-evaluation and review within the broad areas of psychiatry and neurology. Although it should be particularly helpful to residents preparing for the American Board of Psychiatry and Neurology certification examination, it should also be useful for physicians in practice who are simply interested in maintaining a high level of competence in psychiatry or neurology. Study of this self-assessment and review book should help to (1) identify areas of relative weakness; (2) confirm areas of expertise; (3) assess knowledge of the sciences fundamental to psychiatry and neurology; (4) assess clinical judgment and problem-solving skills; and (5) introduce recent developments in psychiatry and neurology.

This book consists of 750 multiple-choice questions that parallel the format and degree of difficulty of the questions on the above-mentioned board exams. Each question is accompanied by an answer, a paragraph-length explanation, and a specific page reference to either *Principles of Neurology* by Adams and Victor, *Technique of the Neurologic Examination* by DeMyer, *Comprehensive Textbook of Psychiatry* by Kaplan, Freedman, and Sadock, or to more specialized textbooks and journal articles.

We have assumed that the time available to the reader is limited; as a result, this book can be used profitably a chapter at a time. By allowing no more than two and a half minutes to answer each question, you can simulate the time constraints of the actual board exams. When you finish answering all of the questions in a chapter, spend as much time as necessary verifying answers and carefully reading the accompanying explanations. If after reading the explanations for a given chapter, you feel a need for a more extensive and definitive discussion, consult the references listed.

Based on our testing experience, on most medical examinations, examinees who answer half the questions correctly would score around the 50th or 60th percentile. A score of 65 percent would place the examinee above the 80th percentile, while a score of 30 percent would rank him or her below the 15th percentile. In other words, if you answer fewer than 30 percent of the questions correctly, you are relatively weak in that area. A score of 50 percent would be approximately average, and 70 percent or higher would probably be honors.

We have used three basic question types in accordance with the format of the American Board of Psychiatry and Neurology certification and recertification exams. Considerable editorial time has been spent trying to ensure that each question is clearly stated and discriminates between those physicians who are well-prepared in a subject and those who are less knowledgeable.

This book is a teaching device that provides readers with the opportunity to objectively evaluate and update their clinical expertise, their ability to interpret data, and their ability to diagnose and solve clinical problems. We hope that you will find this book interesting, relevant, and challenging. The authors, as well as the PreTest staff, would be very happy to receive your comments and suggestions.

Preface

This text contains 750 questions and answers to test neurologists and psychiatrists preparing for Part I of their specialty Board examinations. Part I of the American Board of Psychiatry and Neurology tests the basic sciences pertinent to clinical practice. Part I does not purport to test clinical skills as such, which are tested on Part II. Candidates must pass Part I to become eligible to take Part II.

When taking Part I of the Board examination, the neurology candidates will answer approximately 270 questions in neurology and 90 in psychiatry, for a total of 360 questions. Psychiatry candidates will answer 250 questions in psychiatry and 90 in neurology, for a total of 340 questions. The actual proportion of questions devoted to each basic science in this text approximates the proportion that will appear on the Board examination.

The questions in this text are arranged according to subject matter. In this way candidates can readily score themselves in each field to determine the adequacy of their preparation. On the actual Board examination the questions will be arranged randomly rather than by subject matter. Within any given field in this text, as well as on the Board examination, the sequence of questions is meaningless. Do not look for any order or meaning in the sequence of questions.

William DeMyer, M.D.

Neurology

Neuroanatomy

DIRECTIONS: Each question below contains five suggested answers. Choose the **one best** response to each question.

1. Which of the following statements concerning pure interruption of the pyramidal tract in humans is true?

(A) It causes only a flaccid paralysis
(B) It causes only a spastic paralysis
(C) It causes spasticity only early in the course of the lesion
(D) It has an uncertain relationship to spasticity
(E) It has no effect on muscle tone

2. The cortical efferent pathway for volitional horizontal eye movements is best described by which of the following statements?

(A) The pathway does not decussate
(B) The pathway has equal numbers of decussating and nondecussating fibers
(C) The pathway decussates in the supraoptic commissure of Meynert
(D) The pathway decussates between the midcollicular and midpontine levels
(E) The pathway runs down to the medulla and returns to the pons without decussating

3. The taste buds on the anterior two-thirds of the tongue receive their innervation from cranial nerve

(A) V
(B) VII
(C) IX
(D) X
(E) XII

4. The term thalamic fasciculus is most closely synonymous with

(A) field H of Forel
(B) field H_1 of Forel
(C) field H_2 of Forel
(D) all three fields of Forel
(E) none of the above

5. The correct definition of the cerebrum is that portion of the central nervous system rostral to

(A) a plane through the pons-midbrain junction
(B) a plane through the midbrain-diencephalic junction
(C) the diencephalon
(D) the basal ganglia
(E) the optic chiasm

6. Use of horseradish peroxidase as a technique for identifying neuroanatomical pathways depends on

(A) retrograde transport along axons
(B) destruction of myelin sheaths
(C) Wallerian degeneration
(D) inhibition of oxidative metabolism
(E) inhibition of protein synthesis

3

7.   An elderly patient experiences a sudden onset of complete hemiplegia. Examination shows paralysis of mouth retraction on the hemiplegic side. The patient also exhibits moderate weakness of eyelid closure on that side. Which of the following statements about the weakness of eyelid closure is true?

(A) It suggests a brain stem localization of the hemiplegic lesion with a peripheral facial palsy
(B) It suggests a separate brain stem lesion
(C) It suggests an associated IIIrd nerve palsy
(D) It raises the question of another disease such as myasthenia gravis
(E) It is common in the acute stage of severe hemiplegia

8.   The reason that a patient with a herniated lumbar disk may feel severe pain in the hip or thigh rather than, or in addition to, pain in the foot is that

(A) the hip is often injured when the disk ruptures
(B) immobility of the leg causes a "frozen" hip joint as in the shoulder-hand syndrome
(C) the back spasm associated with disk pain alters the gait
(D) the pyriformis muscle goes into spasm, compressing the sciatic nerve
(E) the same somites contribute dermatomes to the feet and sclerotomes to the femur

9.   In respect to clinical testing, the gag reflex involves which of the following cranial nerve pathways?

(A) VIIth nerve afferent and VIIth nerve efferent
(B) IXth nerve afferent and IXth nerve efferent
(C) IXth nerve afferent and Xth nerve efferent
(D) Xth nerve afferent and Xth nerve efferent
(E) IXth nerve afferent and XIIth nerve efferent

10. Assuming that the other cranial nerves remain intact, interruption of the IIIrd nerve causes the eyeball to be rotated

(A) medially and up
(B) medially and down
(C) laterally and up
(D) laterally and down
(E) upward in the midline

11. A patient complaints of diplopia only when looking up and to the right. The diplopia most probably represents weakness of

(A) the right superior rectus or left inferior oblique muscle
(B) the right superior oblique or left inferior rectus muscle
(C) the right lateral rectus or left medial rectus muscle
(D) the right inferior oblique or left superior rectus muscle
(E) none of the above

12. A patient feels a sudden pop in his back while shovelling. The next day he awakens with severe pain and numbness of the big toe on the right foot. It is most likely that the patient has a herniated intervertebral disk at the interspace of

(A) L3-L4
(B) L4-L5
(C) L5-S1
(D) S1-S2
(E) S2-S3

13. The two cranial nerves that differ radically from the typical histology of peripheral nerves are

(A) I and II
(B) III and IV
(C) V and VI
(D) VII and VIII
(E) IX-XII

DIRECTIONS: Each question below contains four suggested answers of which **one** or **more** is correct. Choose the answer

A	if	1, 2, and 3	are correct
B	if	1 and 3	are correct
C	if	2 and 4	are correct
D	if	4	is correct
E	if	1, 2, 3, and 4	are correct

14. The IVth cranial nerve may correctly be described as

(1) the only cranial nerve to attach to the dorsal aspect of the brain stem
(2) having the smallest diameter of all of the cranial motor nerves
(3) undergoing complete internal decussation
(4) containing no myelinated fibers

15. The striatum receives significant afferent fibers from the

(1) cerebral cortex
(2) nucleus medialis dorsalis of the thalamus
(3) nucleus centromedianum
(4) subthalamic nucleus

16. Well-established striatal efferent connections run to the

(1) red nucleus
(2) globus pallidus
(3) nucleus pulvinaris of the thalamus
(4) substantia nigra

17. Correct statements concerning the perikarya of the norepinephrinergic neurons include which of the following?

(1) They are concentrated in largest number in the pontomedullary tegmentum
(2) They produce essentially small, unmyelinated axons with tremendous numbers of collaterals
(3) They were discovered only after the development of fluorescence microscopy
(4) They do not all group neatly into the previous cytoarchitectural subdivisions of the reticular formation

18. A lesion that occupies the shaded area in the figure shown below would cause which of the following signs?

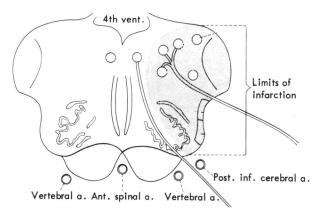

Used with permission of Macmillan Publishing Company, from *Medical Neurology* (p 546), by Gilroy J and Meyer JS, © 1975.

(1) Contralateral loss of the corneal reflex
(2) Contralateral paralysis of the arm and leg, sparing the facial movements
(3) Contralateral dystaxia
(4) Contralateral loss of pain and temperature of body and extremities

19. The clinical deficits resulting from a hemisection of the spinal cord would include which of the following?

(1) Ipsilateral ataxia
(2) Contralateral loss of pain and temperature sensation
(3) Ipsilateral analgesia for light touch
(4) Ipsilateral ptosis and pupilloconstriction

SUMMARY OF DIRECTIONS

A	B	C	D	E
1, 2, 3 only	1, 3 only	2, 4 only	4 only	All are correct

20. In the figure shown below, correct statements include which of the following?

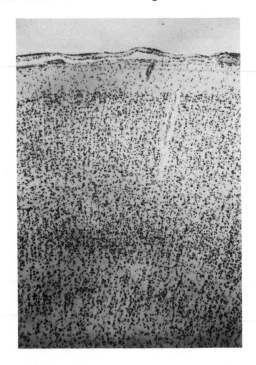

(1) Large neurons appear in the molecular (plexiform) layer
(2) The internal granular layer is strongly developed
(3) The section is most likely motor cortex
(4) A myelin stain would show well-developed laminations

21. The term striatum includes the

(1) caudate nucleus
(2) globus pallidus
(3) putamen
(4) claustrum

22. Major, well-established components of the thalamic fasciculus include the

(1) medial lemniscus
(2) dentatorubrothalamic tract
(3) pallidal efferent fibers
(4) corticothalamic fibers

23. A lesion of the nerve shown by the arrow in the figure below would produce which of the following clinical signs?

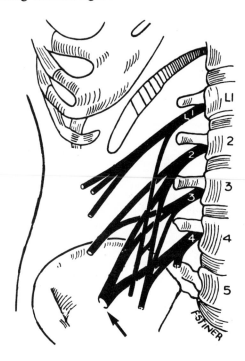

Used with permission of McGraw-Hill Book Company, from *Principles of Neurology* (p 449), by Adams RD and Victor M, © 1977 McGraw-Hill Inc.

(1) Absence of the quadriceps muscle stretch reflex
(2) Atrophy of the posterior muscles of the calf
(3) Reduction in the circumference of the thigh
(4) Loss of sensation over the posterior aspect of the thigh

24. Electron microscopy characteristically shows which of the following structural features at synapses?

(1) Small round vesicles
(2) Endoplasmic reticulum
(3) Electron-dense material along the pre- and post-synaptic membranes
(4) No mitochondria

25. The dopaminergic neurons of the midbrain are characterized by

(1) having their strongest concentration in the ventral part of the midbrain tegmentum
(2) having small, obscure perikarya that are difficult to distinguish from glia
(3) sending their main axonal connections to structures rostral to the location of their perikarya
(4) lacking conformity to any previously known cytoarchitectural subdivisions of the brain stem

26. A node of Ranvier has which of the following characteristics?

(1) It marks the site of apposition of two adjacent Schwann cells or oligodendroglial cells
(2) It is presumed to be the site of ionic flux in the theory of saltatory conduction of the nerve impulse
(3) It is visible in both electron and light microscopy
(4) It is a site of discontinuity of the endoneurium

27. Pallidothalamic fibers terminate in significant numbers on which of the following nuclei?

(1) Ventralis posterolateralis
(2) Ventralis lateralis
(3) Medialis dorsalis
(4) Ventralis anterior

DIRECTIONS: The groups of questions below consist of lettered choices followed by several numbered items. For each numbered item select the **one** lettered choice with which it is **most** closely associated. Each lettered choice may be used once, more than once, or not at all.

Questions 28-31

For each source of afferent fibers listed below, select the part of the cerebellum to which it most strongly projects.

(A) Cerebellar hemisphere
(B) Rostral vermis and paravermian area
(C) Caudal vermis
(D) Flocculonodular lobe
(E) All parts of the cerebellum equally

28. Spinocerebellar tracts

29. Pontocerebellar projection (from pontine nuclei of basis pontis)

30. Principal inferior olivary nuclei, lateral part

31. Vestibular nerve and nuclei

Questions 32-36

For each of the cortical connections or projections listed below, select the thalamic nucleus to which it most closely relates.

(A) Lateral geniculate body
(B) Nucleus medial dorsalis
(C) Nucleus pulvinaris
(D) Nucleus anterior and lateralis dorsalis
(E) Nucleus ventralis lateralis

32. Projects visual impulses to the calcarine cortex

33. Connects with frontal lobe anterior to the motor cortex (prefrontal cortex)

34. Projects to the nonstriate areas (eulaminate isocortex) of the parieto-occipito-temporal lobes

35. Projects to the motor cortex

36. Connects with the limbic cortex of the cingulate gyrus

Questions 37-40

For each of the fibers listed below, select the cerebellar cell type for which it provides a strong source of afferent impulses.

(A) Granule cells
(B) Purkinje cells only
(C) Purkinje cells and the other intrinsic cerebellar neurons
(D) Purkinje cells, inner and outer stellate cells, and stellate neurons of Golgi
(E) Bargmann cells

37. Climbing fibers (main branches and collaterals)

38. Mossy fibers

39. Basket fibers

40. Parallel fibers

Questions 41-45

For each lesion listed below, match the visual field defect to which it is most closely related.

(A) Partial contralateral superior homonymous quadrantanopia
(B) Superior altitudinal hemianopia of both eyes
(C) Partial contralateral inferior homonymous quadrantanopia
(D) Complete contralateral homonymous hemianopia without macular sparing
(E) Does not cause field defect

41. Complete destruction of the calcarine cortex of one occipital lobe

42. Destruction of the anterior part of the temporal lobe

43. Bilateral destruction of the inferior bank of the calcarine fissure

44. Unilateral destruction of the inferior part of the parietal lobe

45. Destruction of the splenium of the corpus callosum

Neuroanatomy Answers

1. The answer is D. *(Adams, ed 2. pp 39-40.)* The relation of pyramidal tract interruption to muscle tone in humans has not been clearly established. Although most patients with an upper motor neuron lesion have some degree of spasticity, at least in the later stages of the lesion, the final state of tonus in the muscle may depend on associated interruption of other pathways. The relatively few pure pyramidal tract lesions reported in humans leave the question in some doubt, but affected patients do have hyperactive reflexes, some hypertonus, and extensor toe signs. The notion that pyramidal tract interruption causes only flaccid paralysis is derived from experiments in lower animals in which the pyramidal tract is less advanced phylogenetically than in humans and has less importance in the organization of the motor system. These animal experiments, while widely quoted, do not necessarily apply to the state of affairs in humans.

2. The answer is D. *(DeMyer, ed 3. p 134.)* Although the exact corticobulbar pathway for horizontal conjugate eye movement has yet to be precisely identified, it is thought to decussate somewhere between the midcollicular level of the midbrain and midpontine levels. Interruption of the fibers at pontine levels after decussation impairs lateral conjugate gaze **ipsi**lateral to the lesion. Interruption of the fibers rostral to the decussation impairs gaze **contra**lateral to the lesion. The decussation of the optomotor fibers occurs in the tegmentum. These fibers do not enter the basis of the midbrain or pons. Thus, lesions of the basis may spare these fibers but interrupt the other cortical efferent fibers that occupy the basis.

3. The answer is B. *(DeMyer, ed 3. pp 272-276.)* The VIIth cranial nerve innervates the taste buds on the anterior two-thirds of the tongue. The IXth and Xth cranial nerves innervate the remaining taste buds. The major clinical indication for taste testing is the suspected presence of a VIIth nerve lesion. Taste testing of the posterior part of the tongue and pillars innervated by the IXth and Xth nerves lacks practical clinical value. The testing of taste is an unsatisfactory method for evaluation of brain stem function. No discrete brain stem lesions regularly occur that abolish taste, and the actual central pathway in humans remains in some doubt.

4. The answer is B. *(Carpenter, ed 2. p 246.)* Field H_1 of Forel is the lamina of myelinated fibers between the zona incerta and the thalamus. This lamina of fibers is also termed the thalamic fasciculus. It receives fibers from fields H and H_2, but is most nearly synonymous with field H_1. This field conveys sensory fibers from the lemnisical systems and motor fibers of cerebellar and pallidal origin. Therefore, it is not a unitary tract with a single unitary function. The thalamic fasciculus forms a shell of myelinated fibers around the ventral surface of the thalamus and becomes continuous with the shell of myelinated fibers around the lateral aspect of the thalamus, known as the external medullary lamina. The myelinated capsule extends continuously across the dorsum of the thalamus, where it is designated the stratum zonale. The medial border of the thalamus, which forms the boundary of the third ventricle, contains few myelinated fibers. Thus, the thalamus is surrounded by myelinated fibers that form a capsule ventrally, laterally, and dorsally, but not medially.

5.   The answer is A. *(DeMyer, ed 3. p 69.)*   The cerebrum is that part of the central nervous system rostral to a plane through the pons-midbrain junction. Thus, by definition, the midbrain belongs with the cerebrum. It is for this reason that parts of the midbrain—the cerebral peduncles, or cerebral aqueduct—receive their names as cerebral components, rather than being called the midbrain peduncles or midbrain aqueduct. The entire midbrain, having a smaller diameter than the pons, is called the cerebral isthmus. The mistake is often made of equating the brain and the cerebrum. The brain includes the pons, medulla, and the cerebellum in addition to the components of the cerebrum.

6.   The answer is A. *(Cooper, ed 3. pp 12-13.)*   Use of horseradish peroxidase to exhibit neuroanatomical connections depends on retrograde transport of the material along axons. Horseradish peroxidase, a glycoprotein of relatively low molecular weight (43,000 Daltons), enters axons or axonal endings by pinocytosis after injection into the central nervous system. The axon then transports the material to the perikaryon where it can be displayed by the appropriate chemical reactions, thus identifying the cell of origin of the axon. If given intravenously, horseradish peroxidase passes the muscle capillaries but fails to penetrate the blood-brain barrier. If it did penetrate the barrier, horseradish would lack usefulness as a tracer because the perikarya would take it up indiscriminately. This relatively new technique supplements the older techniques of tracing axonal pathways by degeneration methods, but is impractical for use in the human brain because it requires direct injection and sacrifice of the animal.

7.   The answer is E. *(DeMyer, ed 3. p 153.)*   In some patients with acute hemiplegia, the orbicularis oculi muscle may display obvious weakness, while in others the weakness affects only the lower part of the face. Occasionally, the orbicularis oculi muscle is so weak that it raises the question of a peripheral VIIth nerve palsy and a brain stem localization for the lesion. However, in the classical brain stem lesion, the peripheral facial palsy is on one side and the hemiplegia on the other, so-called hemiplegia alternans. In the patient presented in the question, the best explanation is a single lesion interrupting the cortical motor fibers to the brain stem, with participation of the orbicularis oculi in the hemiplegia. In such patients, presumably the facial nucleus receives mostly crossed fibers from the motor cortex for the orbicularis oculi muscle.

8.   The answer is E. *(DeMyer, ed 3. p 69.)*   Each somite produces derivatives that become skin, bone, and muscle. The dermatomes, sclerotomes, and myotomes so produced retain the motor and sensory nerve supply of their original somite. The sclerotomes of the L5 and S1 roots contribute to the proximal end of the femur, while their dermatomes and myotomes extend to the leg and foot. Depending on the particular root fibers affected by the herniated disk, the maximum expression of the pain may be in the dermatome, sclerotome, or muscle, or may be felt in all three. In some instances, the hip or thigh pain will exist with little or no pain in the dermatome, which suggests a false localization of the disease in the hip.

9.   The answer is C. *(DeMyer, ed 3. p 164.)*   The IXth cranial nerve conveys the afferent arc of the gag reflex and the Xth nerve, the efferent. Of the several nerves that innervate the mouth and pharyngeal cavity, the Vth innervates somatic sensation; the IXth and Xth innervate pharyngeal sensation and muscles; the XIIth innervates the tongue muscle; the VIIth, IXth, and Xth nerves innervate taste buds; and the Vth and Xth innervate the muscles of the palate. The tensor palatini muscle, innervated by the Vth cranial nerve, has little importance in comparison to the levator palatini muscle innervated by the Xth cranial nerve. Therefore, in respect to clinical testing, the gag reflex involves the IXth and Xth cranial nerves.

10.   The answer is D.   *(Adams, ed 2. p 181.)*   After interruption of the IIIrd nerve (with the other cranial nerves intact), the eyeball turns down and out. This position is dictated by the unopposed pull of both the intact lateral rectus, which turns the eyeball out, and the intact superior oblique, which turns the eyeball down as one of its actions and also intorts it. The eyeball is actively pulled into the down and out position by these intact muscles because the ocular muscles, unlike all other skeletal muscles, maintain some tonus even when the eye is not moving. Thus, the tone in these two muscles, unopposed by the paralyzed antagonistic muscles, actively deviates the eye in their direction of action.

11.   The answer is A.   *(DeMyer, ed 3. pp 54-55.)*   A patient who has diplopia on looking up and to one side most likely has weakness of either the superior rectus muscle of the **ab**ducting eye or the inferior oblique muscle of the **ad**ducting eye. With the eye abducted, the superior rectus muscle elevates the eye. With the eye adducted, the inferior oblique muscle elevates the eye. These muscles of the two eyes are yoked together by a central regulating mechanism. A patient who has weakness of the medial or lateral recti would experience diplopia on lateral gaze, not just when looking laterally and up. If a patient with a superior rectus palsy looks laterally and up with the eye, the superior rectus muscle is the only elevator, and the muscle has its strongest action as an elevator with the eye in that position. If that eye looks medially and up, the action of the superior rectus muscle converts to adduction and intorsion. Under these circumstances, the inferior oblique muscle of that eye becomes the strongest—and only—elevator muscle, when the eye rotates medially and up.

12.   The answer is B.   *(DeMyer, ed 3. p 304.)*   A patient with pain and numbness radiating into the right great toe most likely has an L4-L5 intervertebral disk herniation. Herniation of a lumbar disk is likely to affect the nerve root of the next lower segment. Thus an L4-L5 herniation affects L5 and an L5-S1 herniation affects S1. The L5 root innervates the large toe and dorsum of the foot in most individuals, and the S1 root innervates the lateral aspect of the foot and small toe. Compression of these roots causes sensory complaints in the corresponding regions of the foot. The sacral vertebrae fuse into a single mass and lack intervertebral disks.

13.   The answer is A.   *(DeMyer, ed 3. p 79.)*   Cranial nerves I and II do not have a histological pattern like the other cranial nerves. Cranial nerve I contains only small, unmyelinated afferent axons. Cranial nerve II, rather than being a peripheral nerve, is part of the central nervous system, and has oligodendroglial rather than Schwann cell myelin. Thus, nerves I and II fail to display the same pathological reactions as the nerves with the typical peripheral histological structure. The olfactory neurons arise from the ectodermal olfactory epithelium. The nerve cell bodies lie in the nasal mucosa. Their tiny, unmyelinated axons perforate the cribriform plate to synapse on the olfactory bulb. These axons may have the slowest conduction velocity of any nerves in the body. The so-called optic nerves represent the stalk of diverticuli that grow out from the ventral part of the diencephalon to produce the retina. Axons from the ganglion cell layer of the retina grow back through this stalk, constituting the optic nerve; but the stalk begins as central, rather than peripheral, nervous system and remains histologically as central nervous system.

14. The answer is A (1, 2, 3). *(Carpenter, ed 2. p 144. DeMyer, ed 3. p 81.)* The IVth cranial nerve is the only nerve to exit from the dorsal surface of the brain stem. It has the smallest diameter of any cranial nerve. It undergoes a complete internal decussation before exiting at the junction of the superior medullary velum with the inferior colliculus. It conveys myelinated motor axons to the superior oblique muscle. After exiting from the dorsal aspect of the brain stem, the IVth nerve runs between the posterior cerebral artery and the superior cerebellar, as does the IIIrd nerve. The IVth nerve runs through the lateral wall of the cavernous sinus before entering the orbit through the superior orbital fissure. Interruption of the IVth cranial nerve at any site along its course causes paralysis of only one ocular rotatory muscle — the superior oblique muscle — the only muscle that the nerve supplies. The patient has diplopia on looking downward and inward with the affected eye.

15. The answer is B (1, 3). *(Adams, ed 2. pp 49-50.)* In addition to the projection from the substantia nigra, significant projections to the striatum come from the cerebral cortex and certain thalamic nuclei including the centromedianum. The striatum thus belongs to the wider group of circuits that interconnect the thalamus, basal ganglia, and cortex in the control of motor activity. Thalamic axons probably also run from the ventrolateral and ventral anterior nuclei of the thalamus to the striatum. These thalamic nuclei receive axons from the dentato-rubrothalamic tract and the globus pallidus, making them a "crossroads" for motor input of diverse origin, with the striatum being only one of many nuclei contributing to the intricate, interlinking circuitry.

16. The answer is C (2, 4). *(Adams, ed 2. pp 49-50.)* The best established efferent pathways from the striatum run to the globus pallidus and substantia nigra. These pathways belong to the complicated extrapyramidal circuitry of the deep gray matter of the cerebrum. Although the red nucleus also belongs to the extrapyramidal circuits, it is not known to receive any significant projections from the striatum. The striatum connects with some thalamic nuclei, but not with nuclei like the pulvinaris, which have mainly neocortical connections. The efferent fibers from the striatum to the globus pallidus sweep down ventromedially from the hilus of the striatum directly into the globus pallidus, while those for the substantia nigra pass via the internal capsule to the pars compacta of the substantia nigra.

17. The answer is E (all). *(Cooper, ed 3. pp 167-169.)* The norepinephrinergic perikarya are concentrated in the pontomedullary tegmentum, in contrast to the dopaminergic perikarya, which occupy the midbrain tegmentum. Axons of catecholaminergic perikarya tend to be small and unmyelinated and were undetected before the advent of fluorescence microscopy. The catecholaminergic perikarya in some instances are grouped into previously recognized cytoarchitectural subdivisions of the brain stem, but in other instances are not. Two of these nuclei, the nucleus locus ceruleus and the substantia nigra, are grossly visible in the unstained human brain of mature individuals. These nuclei accumulate melanin as an end product of catecholamine metabolism and become grossly evident as the brain of the young child matures. The norepinephrinergic neurons of the locus ceruleus disperse their axons more widely over the CNS than any other known nuclei.

18. The answer is D (4). *(Adams, ed 2. pp 114, 938.)* The shaded area in the figure accompanying the question shows the area usually involved in the lateral medullary syndrome of Wallenberg. This area receives its blood supply from the posterior inferior cerebellar artery (PICA) and is most often affected by an infarct. The occlusive arterial lesion is frequently in the vertebral artery rather than the PICA. The lesion may be limited to the lateral medullary area or to the cerebellar hemisphere, which the PICA also irrigates with blood, or it may involve both the medulla and cerebellum. The signs of a lesion usually include contralateral loss of pain and temperature sensation due to interruption of the crossed spinothalamic tract, and loss of pain and temperature sensation on the ipsilateral face from interruption of the descending root of the Vth cranial nerve. The corneal reflex may be reduced ipsilaterally, but more often it remains intact. Involvement of the spinocerebellar tracts or cerebellar hemisphere itself results in ipsilateral ataxia. An ipsilateral Horner's syndrome indicates that the descending fibers for the thoracicolumbar autonomic system run through the lateral reticular formation of the medulla, the site of the infarct. Affected patients also usually have vertigo, sometimes nystagmus, and frequently nausea and vomiting. Such patients lack paralysis and pyramidal signs because the pyramids do not receive their blood supply from the PICA. Consciousness is preserved if the lesion is confined to the medulla.

19.   The answer is C (2, 4).   *(Carpenter, ed 2. pp 66-67.)*   The classical Brown-Séquard syndrome consists of ipsilateral paralysis of voluntary movements caudal to the lesion (from interruption of the corticospinal tract), contralateral loss of pain and temperature sensation caudal to the lesion (from interruption of the ascending spinothalamic tract), ipsilateral loss of vibration and position sense (from interruption of dorsal columns), and sometimes some hypalgesia (but not anesthesia) for light touch. Touch may be mediated by crossed and uncrossed pathways. Therefore, cord hemisection fails to abolish touch completely. If the hemisection is in the high cervical region, as shown in the figure accompanying the question, the patient will also have an ipsilateral Horner's syndrome from interruption of the autonomic fibers that descend to the T1 level, ultimately to synapse in the paravertebral chain and innervate the superior tarsal and pupillodilator muscles. Paralysis of the pupillodilator muscle allows the pupilloconstrictor muscle to act unopposed, resulting in a small pupil. Although the spinal cord hemisection interrupts spinocerebellar pathways, little clinical deficit results and, moreover, the paralysis of the limbs precludes demonstration of ataxia even though it might theoretically occur.

20.   The answer is C (2, 4).   *(Carpenter, ed 2. p 219.)*   The figure accompanying the question is a Nissl-stained section of cerebral cortex from the calcarine fissure. Thus, it is the visual receptive area, area 17 of Brodmann, which receives the geniculocalcarine tract. Area 17 typifies the specialization of cortical cytoarchitecture in sensory receptive cortex. All sensory receptive cortex—visual, auditory, and somatosensory—shares the common characteristics of having well-developed lamination in Nissl as well as myelin stains. In Nissl stain, primary sensory receptive cortex shows few or no neurons in the molecular (plexiform) layer, well-developed laminae of neurons of increasing size in layers II and III, and a strongly developed internal granular layer. The myelinated fiber laminae are so conspicuous in sensory receptive cortex that one can see them with the unaided eye. The most conspicuous laminae of myelinated fibers occupy layer IV and the deeper part of layer III, where they are called the line of Baillarger or of Vicq d'Azyr.

21.   The answer is B (1, 3).   *(Adams, ed 2. p 49.)*   By definition, the striatum (sometimes called by the phylogenetically inaccurate term neostriatum) includes only the caudate and putamen. The justification for the term is that it acknowledges that the caudate and putamen form a single nucleus that is partially cleft as the internal capsule slices through the striatum to divide it into two separate parts. The caudate-putamen do retain their original continuity around the anteroventral edge of the anterior limb of the internal capsule. The interdigitation of the white capsular fibers with the edges of the adjacent gray caudate-putamen give a striate appearance; thus, the name "the striatum."

22.   The answer is A (1, 2, 3). *(Carpenter, ed 2. p 245.)*   The thalamic fasciculus consists of the lamina of myelinated fibers that runs along the ventral or inferior aspect of the thalamus, between it and the zona incerta. It conveys those axons that synapse in the thalamus from the lemnisci, dentatorubral system, and globus pallidus. It lacks corticothalamic axons, which approach the thalamus from other directions via the thalamic peduncles, rather than the thalamic fasciculus. Thus, the thalamic fasciculus serves to connect the thalamus with infracortical structures rather than with the cerebral cortex. A synonym for the thalamic fasciculus is field H_1 of Forel.

23.   The answer is B (1, 3). *(Adams, ed 2. pp 924-925.)*   In the figure accompanying the question, the arrow indicates the femoral nerve, a major branch of the lumbosacral plexus. The femoral nerve arises from lumbar roots 2, 3, and 4. It supplies motor fibers to the quadriceps femoris muscle, composed of the rectus femoris, vastus lateralis, vastus medialis, and vastus intermedius muscles. These muscles occupy the anterior compartment of the thigh and extend the leg at the knee. A lesion of the femoral nerve would cause weakness of knee extension and atrophy of the quadriceps muscle, with a reduction in the circumference of the thigh and absence of the quadriceps femoris muscle stretch reflex. An affected patient would lose sensation over the anteromedial aspect of the thigh. The lateral femoral cutaneous nerve mediates sensation on the anterolateral aspect of the thigh. One of the commonest causes of femoral neuropathy is diabetes mellitus.

24.   The answer is B (1, 3). *(Cooper, ed 3. pp 13-15.)*   Electron microscopy shows that synapses contain small round structures called synaptic vesicles that are presumed to contain neurotransmitter. Synapses have electron-dense material called synaptic bars along the membrane of the pre- and post-synaptic cell. The synapses contain many mitochondria, but, as a rule they show few microtubules. Microtubules are numerous along the axon and in the perikaryon and dendrites. Endoplasmic reticulum is abundant in the perikaryon but lacking in the axon and synapse.

25.   The answer is B (1, 3). *(Cooper, ed 3. pp 167-169.)*   The dopaminergic neurons of the CNS are concentrated in the ventral part of the midbrain tegmentum (but also occur in the retina and hypothalamus). They have conspicuous perikarya that do in many instances conform to previously recognized cytoarchitectural subdivisions such as the substantia nigra and other midbrain nuclei, although this is not true of all groupings of catecholaminergic neurons. Their axons mainly project to rostral structures—the striatum, rhinencephalon, and limbic cortex. Catecholaminergic axons enter the cerebellum and a few descend, particularly into the spinal cord, but most project rostrally.

26.   The answer is A (1, 2, 3). *(Cooper, ed 3. pp 16-17.)*   A node of Ranvier is the site of apposition of two adjacent Schwann cells or oligodendroglial cells. The axolemma at the node lacks a myelin sheath and represents a site at which ionic flux might occur to permit saltatory conduction of the nerve impulse at a more rapid rate than in the unmyelinated axons. The nodes of Ranvier are visible both in light and electron microscopy. The endoneurium continues unbroken across the node and does not dip in or become interrupted at the node. The internodal distance is the length occupied by one Schwann or oligodendroglial cell. The nodes are much more evident in the peripheral nervous system than in the central, where their very existence has been disputed.

27.   The answer is C (2, 4). *(Adams, ed 2. pp 49-51.)*   The pallidothalamic fibers project to the ventral intermediate and anterior parts of the thalamus, where they end in nucleus ventralis lateralis and nucleus ventralis anterior. These connections help to bring the thalamus into the extrapyramidal motor circuits. The most posterior nucleus of the ventral tier is a sensory relay nucleus. The pallidothalamic fibers loop under the internal capsule as the ansa lenticularis, or run directly across the capsule as the fasciculus lenticularis. The fibers of the two fasciculi curve upward into the thalamus by joining the thalamic fasciculus, from which they enter the ventral tier of thalamic nuclei. These ventral tier nuclei then distribute to the motor cortex of the frontal lobe to form a link between the pyramidal and extrapyramidal circuits.

28-31.   The answers are: 28-B, 29-A, 30-A, 31-D. *(Carpenter, ed 2. p 95. DeMyer, ed 3. pp 245-247.)*   The different afferent fibers to the cerebellum end in different regions. The spino-cerebellar tracts end mainly in the rostral vermis and paravermian area (anterior lobe of *Larsell's* nomenclature). The pontocerebellar fibers project most strongly to the contralateral cerebellar hemisphere. The inferior olivary complex has a distinct topographic relation to the cerebellum, with the medial part of the principal complex projecting to the vermis and the lateral part to the hemispheres. The vestibular system has its strongest connections with the flocculonodular lobe. The vestibular nerve is unique in sending some axons directly to the cerebellum. The other afferent systems have at least one synapse intervening between the periphery and the cerebellum.

Although the cerebellum receives many other afferent fibers than those listed here, no clinical use can be made of knowledge of these connections at the present time. The projection of auditory and visual impulses on the declive, folium, and tuber is one such interesting pathway of unknown clinical significance.

In spite of the fact that different parts of the cerebellum receive different afferent fibers, in structure the cerebellar cortex is virtually identical from place to place. In the cerebral cortex, the situation is quite different. There, the cortex differs from place to place, giving rise to a whole science of cytoarchitecture aimed at mapping these differences. A map based solely on the histological architecture of the cerebellum would show little or no gradation in the intrinsic appearance of the cerebellar cortex.

32-36.   The answers are: 32-A, 33-B, 34-C, 35-E, 36-D. *(Carpenter, ed 2. pp 186-203.)*   The thalamic nuclei have particular connections with the cerebral cortex. The calcarine cortex of the occipital lobe receives the projections from the lateral geniculate body. The medial and lateral geniculate bodies constitute the metathalamus. The nucleus ventralis posterior is the other major specific sensory relay nucleus of the thalamus. It relays somatic sensation to the parietal cortex.

The frontal lobe anterior to the motor cortex, the prefrontal cortex, has strong thalamocortical and corticothalamic connections with nucleus medialis dorsalis. The psychosurgical operation called prefrontal lobotomy severs these connections. Bilateral damage to these connections results in apathy and indifference to pain. At one time, such surgery was in vogue for a variety of psychiatric disorders, including schizophrenia. Its use is now limited to some patients with intractable pain, obsessive-compulsive neuroses, and selected patients who are unresponsive to less radical therapies.

The nonstriate (eulaminate isocortical) areas of the parieto-occipito-temporal lobes have connections with the nucleus pulvinaris. This nucleus belongs to the dorsal tier of thalamic nuclei that lack a direct sensory relay function. Nucleus pulvinaris belongs with the association nuclei of the thalamus, which include the nucleus medialis dorsalis and the nucleus lateralis posterior. These nuclei connect with the parts of the cerebral cortex not directly devoted to the sensorimotor systems.

The motor cortex receives projections from the nucleus ventralis lateralis and the nucleus ventralis anterior. The nucleus ventralis lateralis constitutes the thalamic relay nucleus for the efferent system issuing from the cerebellum via the dentatorubrothalamic pathway. Along with the nucleus ventralis anterior, it also has connections with the globus pallidus. Thus these nuclei, which occupy anterior positions in the ventral tier of thalamic nuclei, have a prominent role in linking the extrapyramidal circuits with the pyramidal.

The limbic cortex has connections with the nucleus ventralis anterior and the nucleus dorsalis lateralis. The nucleus ventralis anterior projects to the anterior cingulate cortex, area 24 of Brodmann, while the nucleus lateralis dorsalis projects to the posterior cingulate cortex, area 23 of Brodmann. Thus, these are limbic nuclei of the thalamus.

37-40.   The answers are: 37-C, 38-A, 39-B, 40-D.   *(Carpenter, ed 2. pp 166-167.)*   In the cerebellar cortex, the main climbing fibers end on Purkinje cells and stellate neurons of Golgi. The mossy fibers end on granule cells. Basket fibers come from the inner stellate neurons of Golgi and end principally on the Purkinje cells. The parallel fibers, formed by the axons of the granule cells, end on the dendrites of Purkinje cells, inner and outer stellate neurons, and the stellate neurons of Golgi. Thus, the parallel fibers contact all other intrinsic neurons of the cerebellar cortex. The Bargmann cells are glia.

The granule cells are the smallest of the intrinsic neurons of the cerebellar cortex. They produce short, highly branched dendrites that enter into the formation of glomeruli. Each glomerulus receives dendritic tufts from several granule cells. Terminals of Golgi cell axons and the proximal parts of Golgi cell dendrites also contribute to the glomerulus, the core of which is a mossy fiber rosette. The climbing fibers, on the other hand, climb along the Purkinje cell dendrites. Climbing fibers also send collaterals to the other neurons of the cerebellar cortex. The various entering fibers of the cerebellum lose their myelin sheaths before reaching their synapses, but they are well myelinated as they pass through the medullary core of the cerebellum. Parallel fibers lack myelin sheaths.

41-45.   The answers are: 41-D, 42-A, 43-B, 44-C, 45-E.   *(Adams, ed 2. pp 174-175. DeMyer, ed 3. pp 106-117.)*   Complete destruction of the calcarine cortex of one occipital lobe causes a complete contralateral homonymous hemianopia without macular sparing. This cortex receives the pathway originating in the temporal half of the ipsilateral eye and nasal half of the contralateral eye.

Destruction of the anterior part of the temporal lobe destroys the portion of the geniculocalcarine tract that loops around the temporal ventricle (Adolf Meyer's loop). These fibers convey the pathway originating in the inferior temporal quadrant of the ipsilateral retina and the inferior nasal quadrant of the contralateral retina, causing a contralateral superior field defect. The quadrantic field defect is usually incomplete but fairly homonymous.

Bilateral destruction of the inferior bank of the calcarine fissure causes a superior altitudinal visual field defect in both eyes. The inferior bank of each calcarine fissure receives the pathway that originates in the inferior temporal quadrant of the ipsilateral retina and the inferior nasal quadrant of the contralateral retina. Joining the two superior quadrantic field defects gives a superior altitudinal hemianopia.

Bilateral destruction of the inferior part of the parietal lobe causes a partial contralateral inferior homonymous quadrantanopia. The lesion destroys the superior fibers of the geniculocalcarine radiation. These fibers mediate the inferior homonymous fields contralaterally.

Interruption of the corpus callosum fails to cause, per se, a visual field defect. The lesion might, however, also encroach on the calcarine cortex located posterior to the splenium of the corpus callosum and cause a field defect in this way. A lesion extending laterally from the corpus callosum, such as a butterfly glioblastoma, would be very unlikely to cause a field defect because the geniculocalcarine tract, which conveys optic impulses, passes lateral to the wall of the lateral ventricle, separating it a considerable distance from the splenium.

Neuropathology

DIRECTIONS: Each question below contains five suggested answers. Choose the **one best** response to each question.

46. The usual organisms cultured from brain abscesses are

(A) streptococci, staphylococci, and pneumococci
(B) staphylococci, *H. influenzae*, and *C. botulinum*
(C) streptococci, *Nocardia asteroides*, and *Amoeba*
(D) pneumococci, *Pseudomonas*, and *H. influenzae*
(E) *Pseudomonas*, *Nocardia asteroides*, and *C. botulinum*

47. Brain abscesses in association with congenital heart disease usually are

(A) solitary
(B) multiple
(C) frontal in location
(D) occipital in location
(E) cerebellar in location

48. In tuberous sclerosis, the periventricular nodules characteristically occur in which of the following locations?

(A) The frontal horns
(B) The occipital horns
(C) The ventricular roof
(D) Mainly in the third ventricle
(E) Along the thalamocaudate seam

49. An alcoholic patient shows severe dystaxia of gait with little involvement of the arms and no dysarthria or nystagmus. These findings result from which of the following lesions?

(A) Degeneration of the spinocerebellar tracts
(B) Degeneration of the flocculonodular lobe
(C) Atrophy of the anterior vermis
(D) Diffuse Purkinje cell loss in the entire cerebellum
(E) Diffuse granule cell loss in the entire cerebellum

50. A muscle biopsy of a patient suspected of having polymyositis shows moderate amounts of inflammatory cells, recent necrosis, some regenerative changes in the fibers, and also some grouped atrophy of muscle fibers suggesting denervation atrophy. In this context, the significance of the denervation atrophy is that it

(A) invalidates the diagnosis of polymyositis
(B) establishes neurogenic atrophy as the correct diagnosis
(C) suggests that the patient has two diseases
(D) suggests that the patient has a toxic neuropathy
(E) suggests a vasculitis of the vasa nervorum

51. In distinguishing polymyositis from muscular dystrophy, a single muscle biopsy

(A) excludes muscular dystrophy if inflammatory cells are present
(B) establishes dystrophy if a haphazard mixture of atrophic and hypertrophic fibers is present
(C) establishes polymyositis if regenerating muscle fibers are present
(D) establishes dystrophy if an admixture of atrophic and normal groups of muscle fibers is present
(E) frequently provides insufficient evidence to separate the two disorders

52. The pathogenesis of arthrogryposis multiplex congenita is best described as being

(A) overwhelmingly acknowledged as an expression of myelodysplasia
(B) overwhelmingly acknowledged as myopathic
(C) related to a defect in connective tissue
(D) a congenital peripheral neuropathy
(E) a symptom complex of varied causes

18

53. A muscle biopsy of a patient affected by the Kearns-Sayre syndrome of ophthalmoplegia with retinitis pigmentosa is likely to show

(A) giant mitochondria with excessive quantities of lipids
(B) dense central portions of muscle fibers that stain positively with the periodic acid-Schiff reaction
(C) bacillus-like rods in the muscle fibers
(D) ragged red Type I fibers in the Gomori stain
(E) central nuclei

54. The best current theory of the pathogenesis of myasthenia gravis is that the disorder involves

(A) a disturbance of protein contractility
(B) a myopathy with a disturbance in binding of calcium to muscle membranes
(C) an autoimmune process with antibodies against cholinergic receptor sites in skeletal muscle
(D) a metabolic block in the release of acetylcholine at the presynaptic nerve endings to skeletal muscle
(E) an endocrinopathy with a deficiency of circulating acetylcholine

55. In patients with brain abscess, the characteristic cell count (per mm^3) in the cerebrospinal fluid is

(A) less than 10
(B) 10-100
(C) 100-300
(D) 300-500
(E) over 500

56. The lesion pictured below is best described as

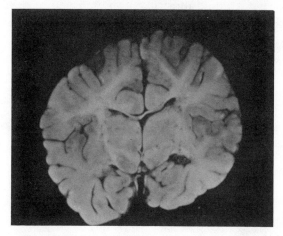

(A) hypertrophy of the caudate nuclei
(B) absence of the cingulate gyri
(C) active leukodystrophy
(D) hypoplasia of the corpus callosum
(E) pseudolaminar anoxic destruction of the cerebral cortex

57. Select the term that best describes the spinal cord tissue shown in the following figure.

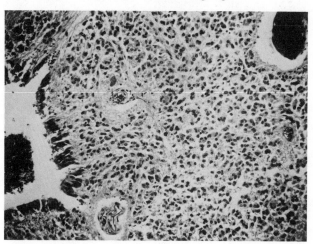

(A) Normal
(B) Ependymoma
(C) Astrocytoma
(D) Myelitis
(E) Acute trauma

58. The patient whose brain is shown in the following figure would most likely show which of the following sets of clinical features?

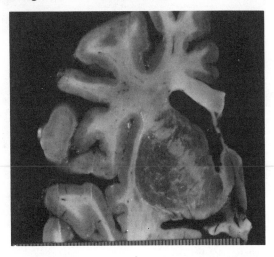

Used with permission of Lea & Febiger, from *Scientific Approaches to Clinical Neurology* (p 1238), by Goldensohn ES and Appel SH, © 1977. Courtesy of Dr. Jans Muller.

(A) Birth hypoxia, mental retardation, and athetoid cerebral palsy
(B) Onset of dementia and choreiform movements in the third decade
(C) Onset of dementia and wing-beating tremor in the second decade
(D) Parkinsonism appearing 20 years after encephalitis
(E) Carbon monoxide poisoning at 21 years of age

59. The condition shown in the figure below is best described as

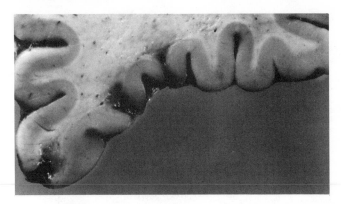

(A) normal brain
(B) demyelinating disease
(C) birth hypoxia
(D) head trauma
(E) pseudolaminar necrosis

60. The history of the patient whose brain is shown in the figure below would be most likely to contain which of the following information?

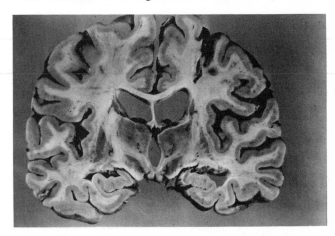

(A) Head trauma
(B) Treated chronic lymphatic leukemia
(C) Cardiac arrest with a period of survival
(D) Implantation of shunt for relief of hydrocephalus
(E) Chorea and dementia

61. The brain shown in the following figure is best described as illustrating

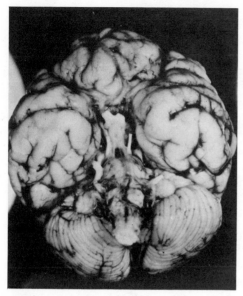

Used with permission of DeMyer W: The face predicts the brain. *Pediatrics* 34:259, 1964. Copyright American Academy of Pediatrics 1964.

(A) normal brain
(B) atrophy of the cerebellum
(C) pontine hypertrophy
(D) uncal herniation
(E) arhinencephalia

62. The tissue shown in the figure below is best described as

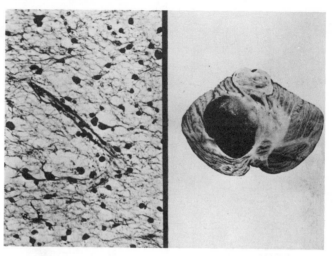

(A) normal brain
(B) edema
(C) scar formation
(D) astrocytoma
(E) ischemic infarction

63. The tissue illustrated in the figure below is best described as

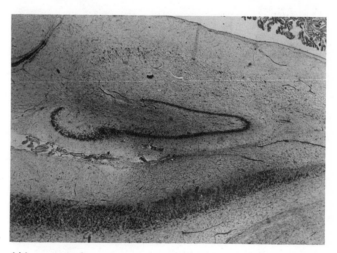

(A) normal
(B) hippocampal sclerosis
(C) rabic encephalitis
(D) granulovacuolar degeneration
(E) atrophy of the dentate gyrus

DIRECTIONS: Each question below contains four suggested answers of which **one** or **more** is correct. Choose the answer

A	if	1, 2, and 3	are correct
B	if	1 and 3	are correct
C	if	2 and 4	are correct
D	if	4	is correct
E	if	1, 2, 3, and 4	are correct

64. The electron photomicrograph of peripheral nerve appearing below exhibits

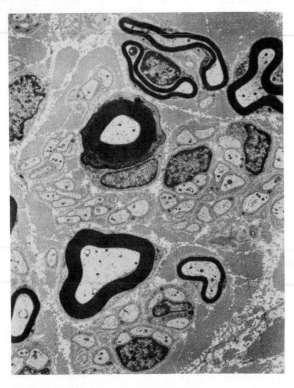

(1) an absence of myelinated fibers
(2) numerous inflammatory cells
(3) active Wallerian degeneration
(4) endoneurial proliferation

65. A patient with cardiac arrest resulting in brain death is maintained on a respirator for 72 hours. At autopsy, the brain would typically show which of the following?

(1) Collapse of the ventricles with extreme swelling
(2) Extreme firmness of the white matter to palpation
(3) Universal necrosis of neurons
(4) Thrombosis of most or all large cerebral arteries

66. Sudden neurologic deterioration of a patient with a brain abscess would suggest which of the following possibilities?

(1) Dissemination of the intracranial abscess to a heart valve
(2) Internal herniation of the brain
(3) Diffuse cerebritis
(4) Rupture of the abscess into the ventricle

67. Focal slowing of nerve conduction velocity at sites of chronic nerve entrapment, with normal conduction velocities distally, is related histologically to which of the following pathological changes?

(1) Lymphocytic infiltration
(2) Nerve trunk edema
(3) Atrophy of the endoneurium
(4) Segmental demyelination

68. Cerebral vessels, as compared to extracranial vessels, appear to have which of the following characteristics?

(1) Much thicker arterial walls in relation to the size of the lumen
(2) Tighter and more extensive junction zones between the endothelial cells
(3) More numerous pinocytotic vesicles in the endothelial cells
(4) Well developed internal elastic membranes

69. Lipochrome (lipofuscin) may be characterized as

(1) an intracellular pigment that resists degradation
(2) accumulating in many types of aging neurons
(3) accumulating in the neurons of infants with Batten-Mayou disease
(4) having an association with brain enlargement (megalencephaly)

70. Typical findings in the biopsy of aged muscle include

(1) lipofuscin accumulation
(2) grouped atrophy (motor unit type)
(3) random atrophy
(4) occasional enlarged muscle fibers

71. Genetically determined anatomic megalencephaly may occur in association with which of the following?

(1) Neurofibromatosis
(2) Tuberous sclerosis
(3) Achondroplastic dwarfism
(4) A simple dominant hereditary condition

72. Neuropathies with predominantly Schwann cell degeneration (segmental degeneration of Goumbault and Stransky) rather than primary axonal degeneration include

(1) acute idiopathic polyneuritis (Landry-Guillain-Barré syndrome)
(2) most cases of Charcot-Marie-Tooth peroneal muscular atrophy
(3) diphtheria
(4) diabetic neuropathy

DIRECTIONS: The groups of questions below consist of lettered choices followed by several numbered items. For each numbered item select the **one** lettered choice with which it is **most** closely associated. Each lettered choice may be used once, more than once, or not at all.

Questions 73-76

For each clinical history that follows, select the figure to which it is most closely related.

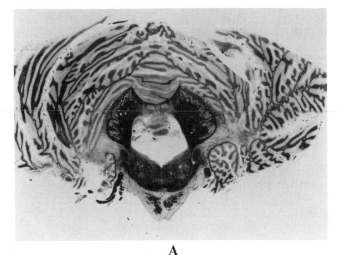

A

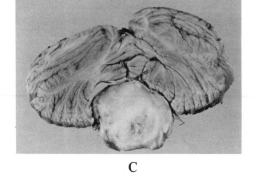

C

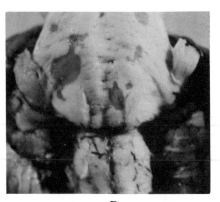

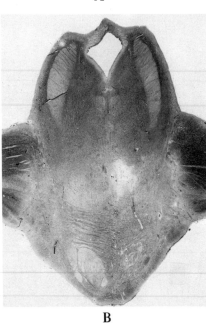

B

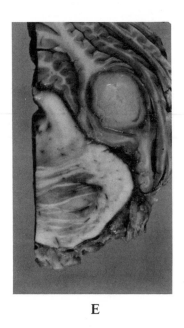

D

73. A 34-year-old woman with a history of 8 years of intermittent unsteadiness of gait, some slurring of speech, mild weakness, and several days of blurred vision. Other findings include minimal dysarthria, weakness of adduction of one eye and nystagmus in the abducting eye, mild bilateral dystaxia, and brisk muscle stretch reflexes with bilateral extensor toe signs

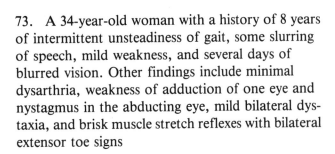

E

74. A 12-year-old boy with a 2-year history of gradually increasing spastic quadriparesis leading to anarthria and aphagia, who finally becomes totally paralyzed except for vertical eye movements

75. A 51-year-old man who for several years noticed the insidious, gradually progressive onset of unsteadiness in walking. He began to have dysarthria and dysphagia. Physical examination disclosed bilateral nystagmus in all fields of gaze, severe dystaxia with terminal tremor, brisk muscle stretch reflexes, but only questionable extensor toe signs. His sensory system and intellect remained intact. The patient died from aspiration pneumonia

76. An elderly patient with emphysema and a chronic cough who had increasing difficulty walking and mild mental confusion for several weeks. A few days prior to death, he became febrile and refused food and drink. He lapsed into coma over a 36-hour period and was pronounced dead on arrival at the hospital

Questions 77-79

For each diagnosis listed below, select the figure to which it is most closely related.

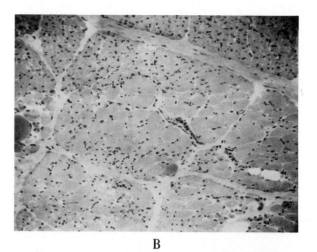

B

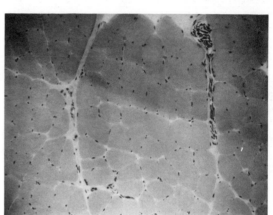

C

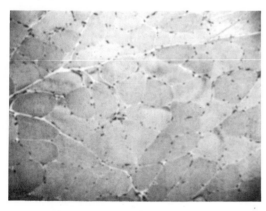

A

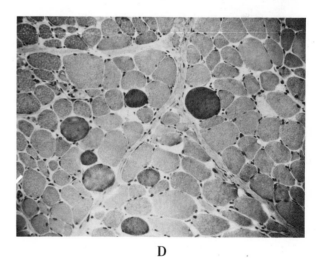

D

E None of the above

77. Normal muscle

78. Neurogenic atrophy in an adult

79. Muscular dystrophy

Questions 80-84

For each pattern of demyelination or dys-myelination described below, select the disease to which it is most closely related.

   (A) Pelizaeus-Merzbacher disease (aplasia axialis congenita)
   (B) Sudanophilic leukodystrophy
   (C) Metachromatic leukodystrophy
   (D) Krabbe's globoid cell leukodystrophy
   (E) Adrenoleukodystrophy

80. The absence of myelin affects the parieto-occipital region most prominently, but does extend into the frontal regions, often somewhat asymmetrically. The lesion shows three zones, visible on cut section and by CAT scan

81. Typically, the brain shows more or less symmetrical tigroid patches of myelinated fibers, against an unmyelinated background of white matter. No enzymatic deficiencies are known

82. The centrum ovale shows diffuse demyelination tending to affect the periventricular region maximally and sparing the arcuate fibers. No enzymatic abnormalities are recognized

83. The brain and peripheral nerves contain an excess of material that stains brown with basic dyes

84. The brain shows a diffuse demyelination, and the peripheral nerves show a segmental demyelination. Microscopic sections of cerebral white matter show accumulations of large spherical cells, many of which contain more than one nucleus

Neuropathology
Answers

46. The answer is A. *(Bell, vol 12. p 93.)* The organisms most commonly found in brain abscesses are streptococci, staphylococci, and pneumococci. Each of the other choices in the question contains at least one organism that may occur, but is uncommon—*Nocardia asteroides, Pseudomonas, Clostridium, and Amoeba*. Knowledge of the probable organism that causes an infection is important, because the clinician often has to start antibiotic medication before the suspected organism is actually identified. In many clinics, conservative treatment of abscesses with antibiotics has replaced more aggressive surgical drainage of brain abscesses. Surgical treatment is still indicated in certain instances if conservative treatment is unsuccessful or if the mass effect of the lesion threatens to cause herniation of the brain.

47. The answer is A. *(Bell, vol 12. p 93.)* Brain abscesses associated with congenital heart disease usually are solitary. The number and distribution of brain abscesses provide some clue as to the cause. Therefore, knowledge of distributional patterns becomes important. Abscesses from mastoiditis or sinusitis tend to be adjacent to the site of infection. Thus, a frontal lobe abscess would be unlikely to have originated in the mastoid. Such an abscess would most likely be blood-borne and the clinician should suspect the lungs or heart as the organs of origin. Many chronic lung conditions serve as a source of brain abscesses. Lung abscesses themselves and bronchiectasis, for example, may provide the primary source of an infected embolus that could travel to the brain.

48. The answer is E. *(Blackwood, ed 3. p 413.)* The periventricular nodules of tuberous sclerosis characteristically occur along the thalamocaudate seam (sulcus terminalis). This characteristic distribution helps to distinguish these nodules from other periventricular lesions. Their profusion along the sulcus terminalis leads to a "dripped wax" effect resembling congealed wax drippings. The lesions also regularly occur in the cortex, and may even be located in the white matter. The nodules of tuberous sclerosis consist of peculiar neural cells that are difficult to classify as either neuronal or glial. Some nodules may undergo malignant transformation, but most are hamartomatous with a potentiality for growth that is similar to the surrounding normal tissue.

49. The answer is C. *(Adams, ed 2. pp 719-720. DeMyer, ed 3. pp 258-259.)* A particular syndrome characterized by unsteadiness of gait, little or no dystaxia on formal testing of the legs, and sparing of the arms is related to degeneration of the anterior vermis and adjacent parts of the anterior lobe. All neurons of this region are affected, the Purkinje neurons perhaps more so than others. This syndrome is the closest approximation to an anterior lobe syndrome in humans. In animals, destruction of the anterior lobe leads to disturbances of posture, but also results in greatly increased extensor muscle tone. Electrical stimulation of the anterior lobe inhibits extensor tone in the decerebrate animal. How these animal experiments are to be reconciled with the role of the anterior lobe in humans is unclear.

50. The answer is E. *(Adams, ed 2. pp 952-953.)*   Some denervation atrophy occurs fairly often in muscles of patients who have polymyositis. Thus, this finding neither invalidates the diagnosis nor suggests a second disease process. Presumably, it indicates inflammatory involvement of the vasa nervorum of the peripheral nerves, with infarction and subsequent denervation atrophy of parts of the muscle. A muscle biopsy in and of itself is insufficient for the diagnosis of a neuromuscular disease. Some dystrophic muscle shows a considerable inflammatory component but absence of denervation atrophy. The biopsy should be integrated with the full range of clinical data to achieve a final diagnosis.

51. The answer is E. *(Adams, ed 2. pp 952, 968-969.)*   Differentiation between muscular dystrophy and polymyositis by muscle biopsy is often difficult. The biopsy in both disorders can show inflammatory cells and necrosis, and a mixture of atrophic and large fibers. The presence of numerous regenerating fibers favors polymyositis, but regenerating fibers also occur in Duchenne's dystrophy. Hence, this feature is not pathognomonic. The clinician cannot relegate the diagnosis to the histopathologist. Because of the difficulties in interpreting a single biopsy, some clinicians more or less routinely sample two muscles during the initial investigation, believing that a more accurate diagnosis can be achieved by combining the observations from the two samples.

52. The answer is E. *(Adams, ed 2. p 979.)*   Arthrogryposis multiplex congenita refers to the condition of an infant born with more than one joint in a fixed position. Thus, it is a descriptive clinical term instead of a true diagnosis. Arthrogryposis is a symptom complex of varied causes rather than a disease entity with a specific, universally acknowledged pathogenesis. Any mechanism that interferes with mobility during intrauterine development may produce the clinical picture of multiple fixed joints. Oligohydramnios, which hampers intrauterine motility, or prolonged paralysis of the fetus by curare-like drugs may cause the syndrome in experimental animals. The pathogenetic mechanisms may involve hypoplasia or destruction of ventral horn neurons, destruction of nerves, and disease of muscle or connective tissue. Children born with their legs fixed in flexion and adduction are likely to have the myopathic variety of the arthrogrypotic syndrome.

53. The answer is D. *(Adams, ed 2. pp 979-981.)*   The muscle biopsy of a patient affected by the Kearns-Sayre syndrome of ophthalmoplegia and retinitis pigmentosa shows ragged red Type I fibers in the Gomori stain. The other biopsy findings mentioned in the question occur in one of the various congenital myopathies, several of which may also affect the ocular or cranial nerve muscles. In central core disease, the central parts of the fibers stain positively with the periodic acid-Schiff reaction for carbohydrates. In nemaline myopathy, bacillus-like rods occur in the muscle fibers. The muscle biopsy shows central nuclei in centronuclear myopathy. These various biopsy findings are virtually diagnostic of the disease in question.

54. The answer is C. *(Cooper, ed 3. p 94.)*   The best current theory of the pathogenesis of myasthenia gravis is that it is an autoimmune disease with circulating antibodies against cholinergic receptor sites in skeletal muscle. Various parts of the cell membrane may have structural differences. The differences in the surface of the cell may elicit antibodies against only a particular site on the cell, such as its receptor. As a refinement of this concept, it is now possible to detect genetically determined differences in the surface membrane of cells, and to make antibodies that will seek out only the genetic mutants in a population of cells. Earlier hints of the exquisite specificity of receptor sites came from the observation of a difference in the action of nicotine and muscarine on what are now considered to be cholinergic endings. The recognition of alpha and beta receptors and their subclassification indicates a similar specificity of catecholaminergic receptors.

55. The answer is B. *(Bell, vol 12. p 97.)* Although the cerebrospinal fluid (CSF) cell count varies from normal to several hundred in patients with brain abscess, the usual range is 10-100 cells per mm³. Counts above 100 suggest the presence of bacterial meningitis. The CSF cell count alone thus lacks reliability as evidence either for or against a brain abscess. The diagnosis must rest on demonstration of the lesion by computerized axial tomography (CAT) scan or angiography. The diagnosis of a brain abscess should be made early, prior to the advent of coma, because of the improved prognosis if the abscess is discovered and treated at that stage. The onset of coma generally indicates that the cerebrum has begun to herniate and compress the brain stem.

56. The answer is D. *(Blackwood, ed 3. pp 383-385.)* The figure that accompanies the question shows a 5-week-old infant's brain, cut coronally at the level of the red nuclei and mid-thalamus. The caudate nuclei occupy only the lateral angle of the lateral ventricles and are of normal size. The cingulate sulci clearly demarcate the cingulate gyri. The cortex appears normal in disposition and lacks evidence of gross abnormalities such as reduction in width or pseudolaminar necrosis. Although this is an infant's brain and is yet to become fully myelinated, the proportion of white to gray matter is reduced. The very thin internal capsule and smallness of the centrum semiovale establish this fact, which is well reflected in the hypoplasia of the corpus callosum. In addition, the fornices, which adhere to the undersurface of the corpus callosum, are tiny. The infant has a type of craniosynostosis called craniotelencephalic dysplasia, characterized by orbital hypotelorism and extreme upward and anterior bulging of the frontal region of the skull. The few infants described with this type of craniosynostosis have been mentally retarded. A concomitant deficiency in brain white matter may be the cause for the mental retardation.

57. The answer is B. *(Russell, ed 4. pp 204-219.)* The figure accompanying the question shows a cellular neoplasm, an ependymoma. The tissue illustrated features spaces lined by ependymal cells and a fairly uniform-appearing cellular background, but with rosette formation. The tumor has incited little stromal or blood vessel proliferation. The presence of cilia and blepharoplasts is characteristic of ependymomas, but requires phosphotungstic acid-hematoxylin for demonstration. Ependymomas occur most frequently in the region of the fourth ventricle, but they may occur in the hemispheric white matter and in the spinal cord, where, in company with astrocytomas, they rank as the two most common intrinsic neoplasms. Ependymomas occur predominantly in childhood and adolescence, but also may affect adults. These tumors tend to grow slowly, but constitute difficult neoplasms to manage because of their location in the fourth ventricle or spinal cord and their resistance to nonsurgical modalities of treatment.

58. The answer is A. *(Goldensohn, pp 1237-1243.)* The brain section accompanying the question shows a marbled appearance of the caudate nucleus, a condition called status marmoratus. The white mottling results from abnormal patches of myelinated fibers. Although the exact nature of the patches is controversial, the patches probably represent a state of hypermyelination from investment of glial fibers with myelin sheaths. The condition usually affects the caudate-putamen and may also involve the thalamus and cerebral cortex. In the cerebral cortex, the lesion forms the so-called plaques fibromyeliniques. Status marmoratus most frequently follows a perinatal hypoxic episode. The affected patient shows a clinical picture of athetoid cerebral palsy. No other disorder that affects the basal ganglia after the age of infancy can cause the typical appearance of status marmoratus. Therefore, its presence in the brain fixes at least the age of onset and usually the mechanism as well, which is hypoxia or related birth difficulties.

59.   The answer is D. *(Blackwood, ed 3. pp 329-332.)*   In the figure accompanying the question, the brain shows localized defects in the continuity of the cortical ribbon. These defects affect the cortex at the surface or crest of the gyri and spare the deeper-lying cortex in the depths of the sulci. The defects extend slightly into the underlying white matter. The part of the brain shown is a coronal section through the orbital surface of the frontal lobe. The orbital plate of the skull fits into the concavity of the frontal lobe at the bottom of the section. The destruction of the crest of the sulci with little extension into the white matter, and its occurrence on the orbital surface of the frontal lobes, is virtually pathognomonic of cerebral contusion of either the coup or contrecoup type. Although initially hemorrhagic, the gross blood is removed and the chronic stage of the lesion persists for the life of the individual, in the form shown. In addition to the orbital surface, other sites of predilection for these lesions are the tips of the temporal lobes and the lips of the sylvian fissure.

60.   The answer is C. *(Blackwood, ed 3. pp 62-68.)*   The figure accompanying the question shows a wedge-shaped defect extending down from the cerebral surface into the deep white matter of the superior frontal gyrus, near its junction with the middle frontal gyrus. This lesion, an infarct, occupies the junction zone between tissue irrigated by the anterior cerebral artery and the middle cerebral artery. Such a lesion, a junction zone or watershed infarct, most typically follows an episode of sudden systemic hypotension with oligemic hypoxia of the brain. Cardiac arrest is the usual cause of the sudden systemic hypotension. The junction between the major arteries therefore represents the zone vulnerable to the oxygen deficiency. Autoregulation of the cerebral blood vessels permits them to dilate to keep the cerebral blood flow constant, even though the systemic pressure drops to between one-third and one-half of its normal level. As autoregulation fails, the vulnerable zones undergo infarction first. If circulation is restored, the remainder of the brain may survive, as in this case. The characteristic location and shape of the lesion would argue against many of the other possible etiologic agents, such as trauma. Although the brain does show mild ventricular dilation, the lesion is unlikely to have been caused by a shunt implanted to treat hydrocephalus—such shunts are placed more posteriorly than the site of the lesion and away from the posterior frontal region, which is depicted in the figure.

61.   The answer is E. *(Vinken, pp 431-478.)*   The brain shown in the figure accompanying the question lacks an interhemispheric fissure separating the frontal lobes, which remain undivided across the midline. It also lacks olfactory bulbs and tracts, and correspondingly lacks the sulcus rectus on the orbital surface of the frontal lobe that normally overlies each olfactory bulb and tract. The absence of olfactory bulbs and tracts, together with failure of the frontal lobes to divide, classify this anomaly as a malformation in the arhinencephalia (holoprosencephaly) category. In this type of malformation, the normal division of the brain into mirror image halves is curtailed. Patients with arhinencephalia usually have midline defects of the face—orbital hypotelorism, flat nasal bridge, and a median or bilateral lateral cleft of the upper lip—which, when present in pathognomonic patterns, permit identification of the type of associated brain malformation.

62.   The answer is D. *(Russell, ed 4. pp 152-191.)*   The tissue shown in the figure accompanying the question features a branched, rather uniform-appearing cell with numerous microcysts—an astrocytoma. Mitoses are absent. The tissue shown came from a hemispheric mass in an adult. The microcystic nature of the deeper portions of astrocytomas may reflect the tendency of the tumor to outstrip its blood supply. Occasionally a single large cyst constitutes the bulk of an astrocytoma and allows surgical decompression to relieve the mass effect of the lesion. Astrocytomas infiltrate and merge gradually with the surrounding tissue. Astrocytomas occur in all parts of the central nervous system. Although benign in a histologic sense, the neoplasms often cannot be extirpated because they are situated in the brain stem or spinal cord. More easily treatable are the cystic astrocytomas of the cerebellum and the astrocytomas of the optic nerve. Astrocytomas in these latter locations can often be cured, in contrast to those situated elsewhere.

63. The answer is B. *(Blackwood, ed 3. pp 775-778.)* The figure accompanying the question shows hippocampal sclerosis. The vulnerable parts of the pyramidal layer of the hippocampus, sections H1 and H3-5 of Somer, have disappeared. The dentate gyrus is preserved. This type of hippocampal sclerosis may result from hypoxia and is characteristic of the neuropathologic findings in a significant percentage of epileptic persons who come to autopsy. Granulovacuolar degeneration may affect the pyramidal neurons of the hippocampus in aging and senile dementia, but in these conditions the lesion is not limited to a Somer's sector. In rabic encephalitis, Negri bodies occur in the pyramidal neurons of the hippocampus, but these bodies, as in the case of vacuolar degeneration, require much higher magnification than shown in this figure in order to be visualized.

64. The answer is D (4). *(Blackwood, ed 3. pp 688-694.)* The electron photomicrograph accompanying the question shows some myelinated axons as well as numerous unmyelinated ones. Each myelinated axon is associated with only one Schwann cell, whereas many unmyelinated axons receive their investment from the enfolded surface membrane of a single Schwann cell. The section shows an absence of both inflammatory cells and of active Wallerian degeneration. It does exhibit a conspicuous proliferation of the endoneurium, as evidenced by the numerous transversely cut collagen fibers, appearing as dots outside the cell membranes. This section thus represents a quiescent neuropathy. The specimen came from the distal part of a nerve injured some years previously.

65. The answer is B (1, 3). *(Blackwood, ed 3. pp 78-79.)* The so-called "respirator brain" typically shows extreme swelling of the gray and white matter accompanied by collapse of the cerebral ventricles. Although in some instances the tissue feels fairly firm, typically it is very soft. Usually, the brain shows transforaminal and transtentorial herniation. Microscopically, the brain shows universal death of all neurons. The endothelial cells swell tremendously, occluding the smaller vessels. While the veins and venous sinuses typically contain thrombi, the larger arteries usually remain patent. The necrosis of tissue and absence of blood flow may or may not involve the spinal cord. Thus, in patients with a dead brain, some spinal reflexes may remain—although of course these patients will lack evidence of reflexes mediated through the brain stem.

66. The answer is C (2, 4). *(Bell, vol 12. p 97.)* Sudden deterioration of a patient known to have a brain abscess most probably indicates brain herniation or rupture of the abscess into the ventricles. An understanding of these mechanisms is important because prompt heroic treatment to relieve intracranial pressure or to irrigate the ventricles may save the patient. Diffuse cerebritis **precedes** the development of an abscess. Although an infection can metastasize from heart valve to brain, the reverse is virtually unknown. Another cause of sudden deterioration of a patient with a brain abscess is intracranial hemorrhage, either intraparenchymal or subarachnoid. The bleeding may come about in some patients by rupture of a mycotic aneurysm (with or without a concomitant brain abscess). In these patients, angiography may disclose one or many aneurysms. Most mycotic aneurysms arise from bacterial endocarditis, which is also a common cause of brain abscesses.

67. The answer is D (4). *(Adams, ed 2. p 882.)* Focal slowing of conduction velocity at entrapment sites, with preserved distal conduction, is related to segmental or local demyelination of the nerve. The preservation of the distal axons and their myelin sheaths accounts for the preserved conduction velocity. The nerve trunk edema and lymphocytic infiltration that may be seen in various peripheral neuropathies are not the usual lesions at entrapment sites. The endoneurium undergoes proliferation and thickening rather than atrophy. Surgical treatment by decompression or transposition of the nerve trunk may allow restoration of function, regeneration of the myelin sheaths, and an increase in conduction velocity across the lesion site.

68. The answer is C (2, 4). *(Cooper, ed 3. p 19.)* Cerebral vessels have thinner walls in relation to lumen size than do extracranial vessels, with the thinness coming at the expense of the adventitia and media. On the other hand, the internal elastic membrane is well developed. Electron microscopy shows that the endothelial cells of cerebral vessels have tighter-appearing and more extensive junction zones and lack pinocytotic vesicles. Pinocytotic vesicles are regarded as agents in the transportation of macro- and micromolecular substances. The scarcity of pinocytotic vesicles in cerebral endothelial cells may reflect the fact that the blood-brain barrier plays a prominent role in excluding substances, particularly certain macromolecular substances, that pass through extracerebral capillaries.

69. The answer is A (1, 2, 3). *(Blackwood, ed 3. p 7.)* Lipochrome is a pigment that accumulates in aging neurons. In light microscopy, it appears as a yellowish brown amorphous mass. It accumulates near the axon hillock of many neurons, and has a predilection for pyramidal cells of the cortex, ventral motor neurons, and the olivary and dentate nuclei. In some dementias, lipochrome may fill much of the cytoplasm of neurons. Although lipochrome is rarely evident in the neurons of infants and young children, it is the most conspicuous intracellular lesion in Batten-Mayou disease (ceroid lipofuscinosis). In spite of this lipochrome accumulation in the neurons in Batten-Mayou disease, brains affected by this disorder are atrophic and lower in weight than normal. This finding stands in contrast to certain other degenerative diseases, such as the mucopolysaccharidoses, in which the intracellular product causes brain enlargement, therefore a metabolic megalencephaly.

70. The answer is E (all). *(Adams, ed 2. p 977.)* Aged muscle shows lipofuscin accumulation, both grouped and random atrophy, and an occasional enlarged fiber. Lipofuscin, the pigment of aging, accumulates in muscle fibers. It is the predominant abnormality seen in light microscopy in brain and muscle in Batten-Mayou disease, to which an analogy with aging has been drawn. The grouped fiber atrophy reflects the loss of ventral horn cells due to aging, and is the usual histological pattern of muscle in any disease that destroys ventral horn neurons. Random muscle fiber atrophy may represent the primary death of an occasional muscle fiber per se in aging, as contrasted to the grouped atrophy secondary to neuron loss. The occasional enlarged fiber may represent use hypertrophy in a fiber still capable of responding. The interpretation of a muscle biopsy is thus strongly dependent on the age of the patient. Lipofuscin in a muscle biopsy from an infant would suggest Batten-Mayou disease, but in muscle from an aged individual it would be regarded as normal.

71. The answer is E (all). *(Blackwood, ed 3. pp 390-391. DeMyer, Neurology 22:634-643, 1972.)* **Anatomic** megalencephaly may occur in a number of genetic conditions — neurofibromatosis, tuberous sclerosis, achondroplastic dwarfism, and as a simple dominant hereditary condition. The oversized and overweight brain in affected patients results from an excessive number or size of neurons rather than from distention by an abnormal metabolic product. In the **metabolic** megalencephalies, however, the oversized and overweight brain results from the accumulation of an abnormal metabolite, such as a ganglioside, which distends neurons. The genetic pattern of the anatomic megalencephalies tends to be autosomal dominant, while the genetic pattern of the metabolic megalencepalies tends to be autosomal recessive.

72. The answer is A (1, 2, 3). *(Adams, ed 2. pp 882, 888-889.)* Acute idiopathic polyneuritis, most cases of peroneal muscular atrophy, diphtheria, infantile metachromatic leukodystrophy, and Krabbe's disease produce segmental demyelination, as does lead poisoning in which segmental demyelination was described by Goumbault and Stransky. The loss of myelin accounts for the extremely low nerve conduction velocities that characterize these conditions. The advent of nerve biopsy, usually performed on the sural nerve (a purely sensory nerve), has served to clarify the pathogenesis of a variety of neuropathies predominantly affecting either myelin sheaths or axons. Some neuropathies predominantly affect axons, with the demyelination secondary to Wallerian degeneration of the axon. Thus, depletion of the peripheral nerves in disorders such as amyotrophic lateral sclerosis and some hereditary neurogenic atrophies results from primary disease of the ventral motoneurons with secondary axonal degeneration and peripheral nerve demyelination.

73-76. The answers are: 73-D, 74-C, 75-A, 76-E. *(Bell, vol 12. pp 93-97. Blackwood, ed 3. pp 470-477, 623-624. Russell, ed 4. pp 181-183.)* Figure D shows the ventral aspect of the pons and medulla with the Vth nerve roots still attached to the lateral aspect of the basis pontis. On its surface, the basis pontis shows numerous dark, depressed areas, which stand out because of the whiteness of the normal tissue. The whiteness is the result of the myelinated fiber systems that form much of the bulk of the basis pontis. These fiber systems comprise part of the cortico-ponto-cerebellar circuit involved in the coordination of voluntary movement. The dark, depressed areas are the typical surface lesions of multiple sclerosis. These lesions, scattered throughout the white matter of the cerebrum, brain stem, and spinal cord, give rise to the neurologic signs indicating multiple system involvement that characterize the typical clinical course of multiple sclerosis.

Figure C shows an enlarged medulla, still in situ in relation to the cerebellum. The lesion, a brain stem glioma, has obliterated the normal markings of the medulla and distorted its outline. The central region of the tissue, just ventral to the center of the medullary section, shows some cystic degeneration that indicates regional differences in the neoplasm. Brain stem gliomas most frequently affect children and grow slowly, usually originating from the basis of the brain stem. They produce a gradually evolving quadriparesis, although some intermittence of signs early in the course may hint at another diagnosis. Terminally, the patient described in question 74 retained only vertical eye movements, all other movements having been abolished by the interruption of the other corticofugal motor pathways. The pathways for vertical eye movements run directly to the oculomotor nuclei of the midbrain without descending through the basis, and may be spared when the pathologic process involves the rest of the stem. The clinical state is the so-called "locked-in" syndrome. Histologically, the tumor was composed of astrocytes with glioblastomatous transformation in selected areas.

Figure A consists of a myelin stained section through the pons and cerebellum. The section shows a complete loss of the myelinated fiber pathways, which run from the basis pontis into the cerebellum. Correspondingly, the basis pontis has lost most of its bulk. The cerebellar white matter per se has become completely demyelinated. In striking contrast, the corticospinal tracts in the basis pontis stand out with well-preserved myelin, as does the amiculum around the dentate nuclei and the superior cerebellar peduncle just medial to the dentate nuclei. Just dorsal to the basis pontis, the fiber systems of the tegmentum (particularly the medial lemnisci), retain their myelination. This specimen shows the typical findings of olivo-ponto-cerebellar degeneration, which generally manifests in adults with a gradually progressive course of cerebellar signs. The disease may appear sporadically or with a familial pattern. A clear biochemical lesion has yet to be identified in this degenerative disease.

Figure E, a hemisection of the pons with the cerebellum in situ, shows extreme thickening of the basilar meninges around the basis pontis, and an abscess in the overlying cerebellar hemisphere. The abscess shows a well-developed capsule indicating that it has been present for some weeks. The pons appears to be free of compression or distortion. The clinical features and postmortem findings suggest that the patient described in question 76 had a lung infection that produced a cerebellar abscess. The abscess smouldered for several weeks and then seeded the subarachnoid space, to produce the terminal meningitis.

77-79. The answers are: 77-C, 78-A, 79-D. *(Blackwood, ed 3. pp 848-871.)* Figure C shows normal muscle. All muscle fibers have a uniform coloration and show faint stippling, indicating minimal ice crystal artifact. The fibers have a fairly uniform size. The outline of each fiber has a gently polyhedral or polygonal shape in the trichrome-stained frozen section. The nuclei are all subsarcolemmic in location. Very little endomysial connective tissue is present, but the perimysium is evident and contains blood vessels. Inflammatory cells are absent. A segment of normal peripheral nerve appears at the left of the section.

Figure A shows neurogenic atrophy in an adult. The muscle fibers stain fairly uniformly. The large fibers have the usual polyhedral outline, and their nuclei maintain a subsarcolemmic location. Inflammatory cells are absent. The abormal feature consists of groups of collapsed profiles of atrophic muscle fibers. These appear in clusters and may show some rounding of their nuclei, which do not appear flattened against the sarcolemma as in the normal fibers. This pattern indicates a neurogenic atrophy in mature muscle. It contrasts with figure B, which shows the typical pattern of neurogenic atrophy in a child. In this case, the child exhibits Werdnig-Hoffmann disease, and the customary feature of neurogenic atrophy in infants is the rounding of the atrophic fibers rather than the polyhedral flattening as seen in figure A.

Figure D shows muscular dystrophy. The diagnostic features consist of some variation in fiber size with enlargement of some fibers and rounding of the contour. The increased space between the individual muscle fibers indicates an accompanying fibrosis. Later, much more necrosis and inflammation may occur with fatty replacement. The serum creatine phosphokinase (CPK) will be highest during the early stages of dystrophy. Histochemical stains in dystrophy will show a poor differentiation of fiber types. Although the microscopist can suspect Duchenne's muscular dystrophy from the section, the same features may occur in other dystrophies. Thus, the final diagnosis of the type of dystrophy depends on a blending of the total clinical information and genetic history with the physical findings and the muscle biopsy.

80-84. The answers are: 80-E, 81-A, 82-B, 83-C, 84-D. *(Blackwood, ed 3. pp 541-557.)* The demyelinating diseases are a heterogeneous group of disorders, often genetic in origin, in which the pattern of myelin deficiency differs from one disease to another—often differing so much as to constitute a decisive diagnostic feature. However, the pathologic distribution of the demyelination is only one feature in the nosology of the disease.

In adrenoleukodystrophy, a sex-linked recessive disorder and the commonest form of leukodystrophy in males, the loss of myelin predominantly affects the parieto-occipital regions of the brain but does extend frontally. The demyelination shows three zones. The central zone exhibits little or no myelin and appears quiescent histologically, showing only glial scarring. The second zone contains some surviving myelin and preserved axons, and displays a prominent perivascular inflammatory reaction. The most peripheral of the three zones shows scattered demyelination with axonal preservation and the presence of numerous para-aminosalicylic acid (PAS)-positive and sudanophilic macrophages. In adrenoleukodystrophy, the localization of the most intense inflammation in the second zone differs from multiple sclerosis, which exhibits the most intense inflammation at the periphery of the lesion. Clinically, the male child with adrenoleukodystrophy usually appears normal at birth and in early infancy, beginning to show neurologic retrogression between 3-12 years of age. The bronze skin, reflecting the adrenal insufficiency, provides a clinical clue to the type of neurologic disorder pressent.

In Pelizaeus-Merzbacher disease, a sex-linked recessive disorder, the brain classically shows patches of myelinated fibers scattered through otherwise amyelinated white matter; but some brains that are genetically and clinically associated with this disorder lack myelin entirely. Thus, the classical pathologic finding of tigroid patches of myelin constitutes only one link in the chain of diagnostic evidence for identifying a disease. The absence of myelin probably represents a failure of myelin formation rather than demyelination as such. Pelizaeus-Merzbacher disease is manifested in the neonatal period by oscillating eye movements. Cases of so-called adult-onset Pelizaeus-Merzbacher disease, which at autopsy show tigroid patches of preserved myelinated fibers, probably have little relation to the classical entity; nor does Cockayne's syndrome, which also shows similar preserved myelin patches.

In sudanophilic leukodystrophy, the demyelination affects the centrum ovale diffusely but tends to concentrate in the periventricular zone and to spare the arcuate fibers. The arcuate fibers consist of the short association fibers of a hemisphere that connect one area of cortex with the neighboring areas. These short association fibers curve around the depth of the gyri, from which they receive the name "arcuate." The arcuate fibers are preserved in some other types of leukodystrophy, such as globoid cell leukodystrophy. In sudanophilic leukodystrophy, the myelin degeneration products stain orthochromatically with dyes and, as implied in the name "sudanophilic," the degeneration products have an affinity for sudan black. The sudanophilia by itself fails to constitute a pathognomonic feature. The sudanophilic material has a high content of esterified cholesterol. Similar sudanophilic degradation products of myelin occur in a variety of disorders ranging from phenylketonuria to head injuries.

In metachromatic leukodystrophy, a metabolic product accumulates in the central and peripheral nervous systems. This substance appears brownish in cresyl violet or thionin stains, which ordinarily produce a blue color. The term meta- indicates this alteration in tinctorial reaction. The basic defect usually is a deficiency in the lysosomal enzyme, *aryl* sulfatase A. In other cases, multiple sulfatases are deficient. The metabolic substance that accumulates in the tissues consists of sulfatides, which are sulfuric acid esters of cerebrosides. The discovery of the fact that the metachromatic substance consisted of a lipid led to the renaming of metachromatic leukodystrophy as sulfatide lipidosis, placing it with the disorders of lipid metabolism rather than with the demyelinating diseases. The disease typically manifests in infants or children and has a sex-linked recessive inheritance pattern.

In Krabbe's globoid cell leukodystrophy, demyelination affects the central and peripheral nervous systems. Affected patients have a defect in galactocerebroside β-galactosidase. The outstanding pathologic feature is the presence of globoid cell macrophages that appear as clumps in the white matter and often have multiple nuclei. The macrophages and Schwann cells contain abnormal tubules on electron microscope sections. Globoid leukodystrophy follows a recessive inheritance pattern. It usually manifests by neurologic retrogression in the young infant, and the patient is usually dead by 4 years of age.

Neurophysiology

DIRECTIONS: Each question below contains five suggested answers. Choose the **one best** response to each question.

85. Stimulation of the supplementary motor area produces movements that are

(A) more discrete and isolated than those produced in area 4
(B) more consistently contralateral than those produced in area 4
(C) complex and bilateral, involving trunk and legs
(D) restricted to the face and hand
(E) restricted to release of sphincters

86. Cerebellar dysfunction is most severe when the lesion involves the

(A) spinocerebellar tracts
(B) frontopontine tract
(C) temporopontine tract
(D) pontocerebellar tract
(E) superior cerebellar peduncle

87. The troponin-tropomyosin system has which of the following actions?

(A) Excites the myosin to contract
(B) Inhibits the contractile protein actin
(C) Unites with excess magnesium ions
(D) Splits adenosine triphosphate (ATP)
(E) None of the above

88. In most individuals, interruption of the corpus callosum is likely to cause apraxia of the

(A) right and left extremities
(B) right extremities only
(C) left extremities only
(D) arms only
(E) legs only (gait apraxia)

89. In the neuropathies that primarily affect axons, as contrasted to those that primarily cause Schwann cell degeneration, the nerve conduction velocity is usually

(A) 10-15 m/sec
(B) 35-40 m/sec
(C) 50-80 m/sec
(D) more than 80 m/sec
(E) too variable to have diagnostic significance

90. In electroencephalography, the contingent negative variation consists of a

(A) negative wave in schizophrenic patients
(B) rapid oscillation during depth recording from the septal region
(C) downward deflection of the oscilloscope tracing that is recording hippocampal potentials during memorization
(D) slow wave seen over the parietal cortex after electrical stimulation of a peripheral nerve
(E) slow wave that appears prior to a response to a stimulus about which the subject has been forewarned

91. A patient with a T10 level spinal cord lesion who attempts to sit up from a supine position will exhibit an umbilicus that

(A) migrates downward (caudad)
(B) migrates upward (rostrad)
(C) migrates laterally
(D) is protrusive
(E) does not move

92. The duration of posthyperventilation apnea in patients with diffuse bilateral cerebral disease is

(A) prolonged because of release of the brain stem inhibitory center from cerebral suppression
(B) prolonged because of loss of the drive to breathe that comes from an intact cerebrum
(C) reduced because of oversensitivity of the carotid bodies to oxygen saturation
(D) reduced because of hippocampal lesions
(E) the same as in normal subjects

93. A hypertensive patient with the acute onset of Broca's aphasia (predominantly expressive with poverty of speech) and a right central facial palsy also shows a tendency for deviation of the eyes to the left. The most probable cause of the eye deviation is

(A) a separate destructive lesion in the right frontal eye field
(B) an extension of the lesion into the left frontal eye field
(C) an interruption of corticobulbar fibers at the brain stem level
(D) a lesion of the left occipital lobe
(E) a lesion of the right occipital lobe

94. The sternocleidomastoid muscle acts to turn the head

(A) contralaterally, tilt it contralaterally, and flex it
(B) contralaterally, tilt it ipsilaterally, and protrude it
(C) contralaterally, tilt it contralaterally, and retract it
(D) ipsilaterally, tilt it ipsilaterally, and extend it
(E) ipsilaterally, tilt it ipsilaterally, and protrude it

95. After interruption of the right Vth nerve, a patient's mandible responds in which of the following ways?

(A) Deviates to the left when opened
(B) Deviates to the right when opened
(C) Opens in the midline
(D) Cannot be opened
(E) Shows an overbite when closed

96. If the head of an infant is turned to one side to elicit the tonic neck reflex, the normal infant responds by

(A) extending the ipsilateral arm and leg and flexing the contralateral arm and leg
(B) extending the contralateral arm and leg and flexing the ipsilateral arm and leg
(C) extending the ipsilateral arm and contralateral leg
(D) extending the contralateral arm and ipsilateral leg
(E) displaying none of the above reflexes

97. After caloric-induced nystagmus, volitional visual fixation has which of the following effects on nystagmus?

(A) Augments the nystagmus
(B) Inhibits the nystagmus
(C) Increases the slow component
(D) Increases the fast component
(E) None of the above

98. The accommodation or "near reflex" of the eyes consists of

(A) pupillodilation, convergence, and lens thickening
(B) pupillodilation, intorsion, and lens thickening
(C) pupilloconstriction, divergence, and lens thickening
(D) pupilloconstriction, convergence, and lens thickening
(E) pupilloconstriction, extorsion, and ptosis

Questions 99-103

Two experimental animals are subjected to the following surgical procedures. The first animal has a complete transection of the nervous system at the medullocervical junction (encéphale isolé); the second animal has a complete transection at the midcollicular level of the midbrain (cerveaux isolé). Both animals are stabilized and past the immediate shock of the operation.

99.   After stabilizing from the operation, which animal(s) would require permanent artificial respiration?

(A) Neither animal
(B) The animal with the medullocervical transection only
(C) The animal with the midbrain transection only
(D) Both animals
(E) Available data make prediction impossible

100. A stimulating electrode is applied to a sensory peripheral nerve in the leg of each animal, and the potentials are recorded over the parietal cortex. An evoked response would occur in

(A) neither animal
(B) the animal with the medullocervical transection only
(C) the animal with the midbrain transection only
(D) the animal with the midbrain transection only, if it receives concomitant stimulation of its auditory system
(E) both animals

101. A brain stem auditory evoked response (BAER) test would show some recordable response in

(A) neither animal
(B) the animal with the midbrain transection only
(C) the animal with the medullocervical transection only
(D) the animal with the medullocervical transection only, if it receives concomitant visual stimulation
(E) both animals

102. The two animals are subjected to photic stimulation while recording electrodes are in place over the occipital regions of their brains. A visual evoked response would occur in the occipital cortex in

(A) neither animal
(B) the animal with the medullocervical transection only
(C) the animal with the midbrain transection only
(D) the animal with the midbrain transection only, if it receives concomitant auditory stimulation
(E) both animals

103. A psychoactive drug is given to the two animals while an EEG is being run. The drug causes the EEG of the animal with medullocervical transection to show generalized low-amplitude fast activity, but has little effect on the EEG of the second animal. The best interpretation of the effect of the drug on the EEG is that the drug

(A) acts on the cerebral cortex through some system that ascends through the midbrain
(B) acts through the cerebellum
(C) acts through the hypothalamus
(D) directly affects the cerebral cortex
(E) bypasses the reticular activating system and stimulates ascending sensory pathways

DIRECTIONS: Each question below contains four suggested answers of which **one** or **more** is correct. Choose the answer

A	if	1, 2, and 3	are correct
B	if	1 and 3	are correct
C	if	2 and 4	are correct
D	if	4	is correct
E	if	1, 2, 3, and 4	are correct

104. Contraction myoedema (slow waves of contraction that ripple over the muscle during a postural change) is very likely to be associated with

(1) complaints of stiffness and tightness in the muscles
(2) percussion myoedema
(3) slow relaxation after voluntary contraction of muscles
(4) delayed relaxation of muscles involved in stretch reflexes

105. Relaxation of muscle depends on

(1) union of troponin-tropomyosin with calcium
(2) enzymatic hydrolysis of the actin-myosin complex
(3) union of magnesium with the myosin
(4) calcium uptake by the sarcoplasmic reticulum

106. Characteristics of conduction aphasia include which of the following?

(1) Fluent paraphasia with retention of prosody
(2) Retention of comprehension and awareness of word errors
(3) Striking inability to repeat words or nonsense syllables
(4) Interruption of the arcuate fasciculus and overlying cortex

107. The electrically excitable somatomotor area of the cerebrum extends

(1) somewhat rostral to area 4
(2) over the medial crest of the hemisphere
(3) somewhat behind the central sulcus
(4) onto the insular cortex

108. Methods for diagnosis of latent tetany consist of

(1) hyperventilation
(2) muscle or nerve percussion
(3) tourniquet test (Trousseau's sign)
(4) induction of hypermagnesemia

109. A temporary increase in muscle strength on repetitive contractions may be seen with some frequency in

(1) myotonic dystrophy
(2) McArdle's phosphorylase deficiency
(3) myasthenia gravis
(4) small cell carcinoma of the lung

110. In a patient with hemiballismus, a second lesion is likely to abolish the movements associated with the disease if it is situated in the

(1) motor cortex
(2) ventrolateral nucleus of the thalamus
(3) pyramidal tract
(4) dentate nucleus

111. Myoedema is seen with some regularity in which of the following disorders?

(1) Myotonic dystrophy
(2) Cachexia
(3) Polymyositis
(4) Hypothyroidism

112. In the absence of a histological lesion of the peripheral neuromuscular system, persistent muscle spasm at rest that intensifies with muscle use is characteristic of

(1) tetanus
(2) myotonic dystrophy
(3) black widow spider bite
(4) McArdle's disease

```
SUMMARY OF DIRECTIONS

   A        B        C       D        E

 1, 2, 3   1, 3     2, 4     4      All are
  only     only     only    only    correct
```

113. Carotid sinus stimulation may result in syncope as a consequence of

(1) reflex bradycardia
(2) reflex hypotension, a depressor response
(3) a central mechanism without bradycardia or hypotension
(4) reflex sympathetic vasoconstriction of cerebral vessels

114. Conditions that may produce or enhance fasciculations include

(1) severe dehydration
(2) organophosphate poisoning
(3) exercise in untrained individuals
(4) hypocalcemia

115. Percussion irritability of muscle is decreased by

(1) hypocalcemia
(2) hyperkalemia
(3) hypomagnesemia
(4) vitamin D intoxication

116. Patients with Broca's aphasia frequently exhibit

(1) a contralateral central type of facial palsy
(2) dysgraphia with either the right or left hand
(3) some degree of loss of speech comprehension
(4) jargon speech and neologisms

117. The myasthenic syndrome of Eaton-Lambert differs from myasthenia gravis by showing

(1) a predilection for proximal muscles of the limbs and girdles
(2) a decremental response in the EMG after repetitive nerve stimulation
(3) an association with carcinoma
(4) uniformly better response to anticholinesterase medication

118. Electrical stimulation of the nucleus locus ceruleus would result in

(1) an increase of methoxyhydroxyphenylethyleneglycol (MHPG) in the brain tissue and CSF
(2) activation of tyrosine hydroxylase in the norepinephrinergic neurons of the nucleus
(3) increased uptake of norepinephrine at the axonal endings of the neurons of the nucleus locus ceruleus
(4) widespread activation of the CNS with decreased threshold to stimulation of the majority of neurons of the reticular formation

119. Diagnostic features of pseudonystagmus include which of the following?

(1) It occurs at one or another extreme of gaze
(2) It disappears or dampens upon moving the eyes slightly back toward the primary position
(3) It is a jerk nystagmus with the fast phase in the direction of gaze
(4) Affected individuals usually complain of oscillopsia and vertigo

120. Central nervous system disorders associated with hypotonia include

(1) profound mental retardation
(2) congenital blindness
(3) Down's syndrome
(4) cerebellar destruction

DIRECTIONS: The group of questions below consists of lettered choices followed by several numbered items. For each numbered item select the **one** lettered choice with which it is **most** closely associated. Each lettered choice may be used once, more than once, or not at all.

Questions 121-124

For each ocular movement listed below, choose the ocular rotatory muscle that is most closely involved.

(A) Superior oblique muscle
(B) Superior rectus muscle
(C) Inferior rectus muscle
(D) Inferior oblique muscle
(E) Medial rectus muscle

121. Elevation of the eye (with the eye abducted)

122. Intorsion of the eye (with the eye abducted)

123. Depression of the eye (with the eye adducted)

124. Elevation of the eye (with the eye adducted)

Neurophysiology
Answers

85. The answer is C. *(Adams, ed 2. p 38.)* The supplementary motor area produces complex, frequently bilateral movements of the axial muscles and legs, although a full somatotopic representation does exist. The most discrete contralateral movements come from area 4. Isolated sphincter movements cannot be obtained from the supplementary area. The role of the supplementary area in brain function remains to be determined. It may be responsible for some return of voluntary function after pyramidal tract destruction, because it has bilateral projections. Blood flow studies show an increased activity of the supplementary motor area during complex volitional movements, and aphasia has been reported after infarction of the region.

86. The answer is E. *(Adams, ed 2. p 65.)* Lesions of the afferent systems to the cerebellum cause relatively little clinical dysfunction. For example, a high cervical cordotomy performed to relieve pain, involving sectioning of the entire ventral spinocerebellar tract on one side, results in little, or merely transient, dysfunction. Some damage may occur to the cerebellar cortex or white matter, with little clinical defect. The most severe signs of cerebellar dysfunction are due to lesions of the efferent system (such as destruction of the superior cerebellar peduncle), or with large, severely destructive lesions of the cerebellar cortex and deep white matter. As with lesions elsewhere, the clinical expression of the lesion will vary with the age of the individual when the lesion occurs, the size of the lesion, and the rate of tissue destruction.

87. The answer is B. *(Adams, ed 2. p 872.)* The troponin-tropomyosin system inhibits the contractile protein actin, preventing its union with myosin. The latter event leads to muscular contraction. After depolarization (induced by the action potential) spreads to the interior of the muscle fiber, calcium is released from the sarcoplasmic reticulum, where it is stored. Calcium binds to the troponin-tropomyosin protein that inhibits the combination of actin and myosin. The interaction of actin and myosin leads to the rapid release of energy by splitting of ATP, a reaction that provides the energy for contraction. Muscle relaxation, which is an active process, occurs when calcium reunites with the sarcoplasmic reticulum.

88. The answer is C. *(Adams, ed 2. p 42.)* Interruption of the corpus callosum is likely to cause apraxia of only the left extremities. The theory is that the locus for motor schema (or the ideation for movement) is located in the left hemisphere of right-handed individuals, presumably in the left posterior parasylvian area. Interruption of the corpus callosum would disrupt the transfer of information from this locus in the left hemisphere to the right. Since the right hemisphere directs movement of the left extremities, the defect would be expressed in the left extremities. Since the connections through the deep white matter between the left posterior parasylvian region and the left motor cortex remain intact, apraxia of the right extremities, which are controlled by the left motor cortex, would be absent.

89.   The answer is B.   *(Adams, ed 2. p 882.)*   In the primary neuropathies with "dying-back" (retrograde) or Wallerian (orthograde) degeneration, the conduction velocity is usually in the 35-40 meter per second range, thus only slightly reduced from normal. Those nerve fibers that remain conduct at approximately their normal rate. In the neuropathies that cause primarily Schwann cell degeneration, the conduction velocity is profoundly reduced, often to the range of 10-15 meters per second. This fact is in keeping with the supposition that one role of the myelin sheath is to increase conduction velocity. Both toxic-metabolic neuropathies and heredofamilial neuropathies may be associated with primarily axonal or myelin sheath degeneration.

90.   The answer is E.   *(Barchas, pp 60, 82.)*   The contingent negative variation is a slow negative wave that appears in the EEG while the subject awaits a stimulus that follows a warning stimulus. If the subject is asked to press a telegraph key after a warning signal and a tone, the contingent negative variation in the EEG appears in the time interval between the warning signal and the tone. The amplitude of the contingent negative variation can be used to measure the effects of drugs on the responsiveness of the subject.

91.   The answer is B.   *(DeMyer, ed 3. p 186.)*   When a patient with a T10 level spinal cord lesion attempts to sit up, the umbilicus migrates upward (rostrally). The T8 and T9 spinal cord segments innervate the abdominal muscles rostral to the umbilicus and the T11 and T12 segments innervate the muscles caudal to the umbilicus. The intact upper abdominal muscles, acting unopposed by the paralyzed lower muscles, pull the umbilicus rostrally—the classical Beevor's sign, which appears after a T10 level spinal cord lesion. In other words, the umbilicus migrates in the direction of pull of the intact muscles. Normally, the pull exerted by the upper and lower abdominal muscles is equal and opposite, leaving the umbilicus centered.

92.   The answer is B.   *(Plum, ed 3. p 33.)*   The duration of posthyperventilation apnea after a patient completes five rapid voluntary deep inhalations and exhalations is less than 10 seconds in normal subjects, and is prolonged in subjects with diffuse cerebral disease. The reduction in CO_2 results in the apnea. The prolongation of posthyperventilation apnea in patients with bilateral cerebral disease illustrates the fact that part of the drive to breathe comes from an intact, functioning cerebrum. Loss of cerebral function from bilateral cerebral disease reduces the drive to breathe, not only after hyperventilation but also in obtundation or even in sleep, contributing to sleep apnea.

93.   The answer is B.   *(DeMyer, ed 3. pp 136-137.)*   Deviation of the eyes to the left due to a cortical lesion and in association with Broca's aphasia and a central facial palsy suggests extension of the lesion into the adjacent frontal eye fields. Destruction of this region eliminates the vector acting to turn the eyes (and head) to the right. The right frontal center, intact and acting unopposed by its destroyed mate, turns the eyes to the left. Lesions in the other locations listed in the question could affect eye turning, but parsimony favors a single lesion rather than multiple ones.

94.   The answer is B.   *(DeMyer, ed 3. pp 166-167.)*   The sternocleidomastoid muscle acts to turn the head contralaterally, tilt it ipsilaterally, and protrude it. One can readily confirm the role of the muscle by palpating it during these actions. The usual clinical test for the action of the muscle is to test contralateral head rotation, but the muscle's strength in the other maneuvers is also easily tested and its action easily observed. Knowledge of its other actions sometimes helps in the analysis of hysterical paralysis. In involuntary movement disorders with spasmodic torticollis, the overaction of the sternocleidomastoid muscle frequently causes head tilt as well as rotation. However, the other neck muscles also frequently are involved in head turning and head tilting. Hence, surgical section of the sternocleidomastoid alone fails in the treatment of spasmodic torticollis. The head may continue to tilt and turn in the absence of this muscle.

95. The answer is B. *(DeMyer, ed 3. pp 146-148.)* After interruption of the right Vth nerve, the affected patient's mandible deviates to the right. A patient with unilateral paralysis of the lateral pterygoid muscle will show ipsilateral deviation of the mandibular tip on opening the jaw and weakness of jaw movement contralaterally. The action of the lateral pterygoid is to protrude the mandible, depress its tip, and move it to the opposite side. These actions depend on the origin and insertion of the pterygoid muscles and the manner of suspension of the mandible. When a patient with a unilateral Vth nerve lesion and lateral pterygoid paralysis opens the jaw, the opposite, intact pterygoid protrudes the mandible to the weak side.

96. The answer is A. *(DeMyer, ed 3. pp 138-139.)* An infant whose head is turned to one side extends the ipsilateral arm and leg and flexes the contralateral arm and leg. While normal infants in the age range of 2-4 months will spend considerable amounts of time in the tonic neck reflex (TNR) posture and will, to some degree, exhibit the TNR when the examiner turns the infant's head, the normal infant readily struggles out of it and the response fatigues. Abnormality is evidenced by a machine-like response that persists. Such an infant has some disturbance in cerebral control of movement and generally will have some form of cerebral palsy. The TNR also may appear in infants with degenerative diseases of the cerebrum.

97. The answer is B. *(DeMyer, ed 3. p 285.)* Deliberate visual fixation inhibits caloric or vestibular nystagmus. The cortical influence thus overrides the vestibular mechanism. A dancer uses this phenomenon to inhibit vestibular symptoms induced by a series of spins or pivots. The dancer deliberately fixates the eyes on some stationary point, then retains fixation as long as possible while the body turns. Then the dancer snaps the head around to resume fixation as long as possible, while the body turns independently of the head. Thus, during most of the turn, the eyes and head remain fixed while the body turns. Both the inhibitory effect of visual fixation and the brief time occupied by turning the head reduce the vestibular stimulation.

98. The answer is D. *(DeMyer, ed 3. p 63.)* To accommodate for near vision requires the eyes to converge, the lens to thicken, and the pupils to constrict. Convergence aims the visual axis of each eye at the near target. Thickening of the lens increases its ability to focus the more divergent rays from the near object on the retina, and pupilloconstriction narrows the aperture that admits light rays to the retina, producing a pinhole camera effect. The nervous system coordinates these three actions into a single reflex. However, as a person reaches the fifth decade, loss of lens elasticity prevents the normal thickening that should occur to accommodate for near vision. The affected person then complains of blurred vision for near objects, a condition called presbyopia.

99. The answer is B. *(Carpenter, p 156. DeMyer, ed 3. p 379.)* After the stage of shock immediately following the operation described in the question, only the animal with the medullocervical transection should require permanent artificial respiration. Although the entire brain plays some role in breathing, the critical region extends through the reticular formation of the pontomedullary tegmentum. If this area is intact and in continuity with the spinal cord, the animal will show sufficient automatic breathing to maintain life. In the animal with transection at the medullocervical junction, all descending pathways from the respiratory centers that drive the respiratory muscles are interrupted. The spinal cord, when isolated from the brain stem, lacks the ability to maintain breathing; but an intact pontomedullary tegmentum and spinal cord retain that ability.

100. The answer is A. *(DeMyer, ed 3. p 434.)* In the experimental animals described in the question, the parietal electrodes would record no response (in either animal) to peripheral nerve stimulation in the leg. The afferent pathways—the medial lemniscus or spinothalamic tracts—are transected in both animals. The animal with the medullocervical junction transection would show a parietal response in the face area to trigeminal nerve stimulation, since its pathway through the pons and midbrain would remain intact. The animal with midbrain transection would lack such a response.

101. The answer is E. *(DeMyer, ed 3. p 434.)* A brain stem auditory evoked responses (BAER) test would show a recordable response in both of the experimental animals described in the question. It would be more complete and better show the waves attributed to the rostral brain stem in the animal with the medullocervical transection than in the animal with the midbrain transection; but even in the latter animal, the earlier waves, attributable to the pathway from the auditory nerve through the pons, would appear.

102. The answer is E. *(DeMyer, ed 3. p 434.)* A visually evoked driving response should occur in response to photic stimulation in both of the experimental animals described in the question. In each case, the retino-geniculo-calcarine tract remains intact and can drive the occipital cortex. To interrupt this tract, the transection would have to be at the diencephalic level to section the optic tract or the lateral geniculate bodies.

103. The answer is A. *(Barchas, pp 53-62.)* The conclusion drawn from the experiment described in the question is that the psychoactive drug activated the cerebral cortex in the animal by acting through some system ascending rostrally through the midbrain. Since the basis of the midbrain contains only corticofugal fibers, and the collicular plate lacks ascending systems to the cortex in general, the ascending system driving the low-amplitude fast EEG activity must run through the midbrain tegmentum. Furthermore, it must have widespread connections with the cortex. If the drug acted directly on the hypothalamus, thalamus, or cortex, it should have caused the same effect in the two animals. Thus, the midbrain transection removed some ascending influence that was present in the animal with the medullocervical transection.

104. The answer is E (all). *(Adams, ed 2. p 943.)* Contraction myoedema and percussion myoedema, stiffness of muscles, and slow relaxation of muscle all occur together in hypothyroidism, in association with complaints of weakness. These findings, in association with the classical symptoms of dry skin and husky voice, establish a diagnosis of hypothyroid myopathy. The physical findings in hypothyroidism separate hypothyroid myopathy from conditions involved in the differential diagnosis of muscular disease such as dystrophy, polymyositis, and the myotonias.

105. The answer is D (4). *(Adams, ed 2. pp 872-873.)* Muscle relaxation is an active metabolic process that requires the union of calcium with the sarcoplasmic reticulum. Deficiency of calcium or of the energy mechanisms that bind it to the sarcoplasmic reticulum interferes with muscular relaxation. Contraction of muscle—as seen in certain disorders with exercise intolerance—may reflect a disturbance in the metabolism of the ionic binding required for muscle relaxation. This process, like contraction itself, is ATP-dependent.

106. The answer is E (all). *(Adams, ed 2. pp 330-331.)* The characteristics of conduction aphasia include fluent paraphasia with retention of prosody, retention of comprehension, awareness of word errors, striking inability to repeat words or nonsense syllables, and a lesion that usually interrupts the arcuate fasciculus. Wernicke proposed a major center for the reception of language in the posterior superior temporal region, and a center for expression in the posterior inferior frontal region. Separation of these two regions by interruption of the intervening cortex of the supramarginal gyrus and inferior parietal lobule and of the interconnecting white matter, predominantly the arcuate fasciculus, produces conduction aphasia. The arcuate fasciculus is a large bundle of fibers, which, as the name implies, arc around the sylvian fissure from the temporal lobe to the frontal lobe. A major distinction between conduction aphasia and Wernicke's aphasia is that the ability to comprehend speech and to recognize word errors is lost in Wernicke's aphasia and retained in conduction aphasia.

107. The answer is A (1, 2, 3). *(Adams, ed 2. p 37.)* The somatomotor area as defined by electrical stimulation extends anterior to area 4, over the medial crest of the hemisphere, and behind the central sulcus into the parietal lobe. The somatomotor area does not extend into the insular cortex, which belongs to the limbic-visceral systems. The somatomotor area as electrically defined corresponds to no single cytoarchitectural, lobar, or sulcal boundary. Discovery of the area depended solely on physiological criteria, i.e., the somatomotor responses to electrical stimulation and the paralysis that followed ablation of this area.

108. The answer is A (1, 2, 3). *(Adams, ed 2. pp 943, 1000.)* Several tests bring out latent tetany: hyperventilation (which blows off CO_2), muscle or nerve percussion, and the placing of a tourniquet around the upper arm. Ischemia caused by the tourniquet results in muscle spasm and produces a peculiar hand position. Increasing blood levels of calcium or magnesium would tend to further depress, rather than elicit, latent tetany. Ischemia and reduction in CO_2 elicit latent tetany by chemical changes. Direct percussion with a percussion hammer or fingertip is a mechanical method of demonstrating the excessive irritability of axonal or muscle membranes produced by tetany (Chvostek's sign).

109. The answer is D (4). *(Adams, ed 2. p 992.)* A paradoxical increase in the strength of muscular contraction may occur in patients with small cell carcinoma of the lung. Affected patients complain of weakness that increases with use; but they may show a temporary increase in strength, measurable both clinically and by electromyography. This feature helps to distinguish the myasthenic state of affected patients from true myasthenia gravis, in which continuous use of a muscle reduces its strength.

110. The answer is A (1, 2, 3). *Adams, ed 2. pp 58-59. DeMyer, ed 3. p 230.)* Hyperkinesias such as hemiballismus require an intact circuitry to drive, originate, or mediate the movements associated with the disease. Most instances of ballistic hyperkinesias or tremors may be abolished by lesions of either the ventrolateral nucleus of the thalamus, the motor cortex on which it plays, or the pyramidal tract that issues from the motor cortex. This circuitry must be intact for the movement disorder to appear. It is a striking paradox that pyramidal tract interruption not only reduces or paralyzes voluntary movement, but also reduces or abolishes involuntary movements. Some decades ago, attempts were made to alleviate involuntary movement by pyramidal tract interruption through surgery. The operation did alleviate involuntary movement, but too often left the patient with some paralysis. However, induction of thalamic lesions, if effective, reduces the involuntary movements without causing paralysis.

111. The answer is C (2, 4). *(Adams, ed 2. p 943.)* Myoedema is a bump-like mound of muscle that follows percussion of the muscle with the point of a percussion hammer. While it can occur in otherwise normal individuals, it is seen with some regularity in cachexia and hypothyroid myopathy. Unlike myotonia, it is electrically silent in electromyography (EMG). Neither myotonia nor myoedema occurs as a feature of Duchenne's dystrophy. Myoedema, a purely local phenomenon limited to the point of percussion, does not result in a movement of the part activated by the muscle. By its duration, percussion myoedema is easily differentiated clinically from percussion irritability, which is a quick contraction and relaxation of the muscle. Moreover, percussion irritability may be sufficiently strong to move the part served by the muscle, such as slight dorsiflexion of the foot after percussion of the tibialis anterior muscle. Percussion myoedema never causes movement of this type, but is confined to the point of percussion.

112. The answer is B (1, 3). *(Adams, ed 2. p 1002.)* Tetanus and black widow spider bite both produce persistent muscle spasm of resting muscle. The spasm is intensified by use, but histologic lesions in the muscle are absent. In myotonic dystrophy, the myotonia appears only after use of the muscle, without causing spasm of a resting muscle. Similarly, in McArdle's disease, exercise induces muscle cramps that are relieved by rest. In both disorders, the lesion apparently is primary in the muscle and can be demonstrated by histologic or histochemical study of a muscle biopsy. The muscle spasm of tetanus or black widow spider bite is thought to reflect a pathophysiologic alteration induced by a toxin affecting the central nervous system, although peripheral mechanisms may also contribute. In any event, histologic lesions are absent in the peripheral neuromuscular complex of patients with tetanus and black widow spider bites.

113. The answer is A (1, 2, 3). *(Adams, ed 2. p 252. DeMyer, ed 3. pp 401-404.)* Carotid sinus stimulation may cause reflex bradycardia, arterial hypotension without bradycardia, and a central type of response possibly due to cerebral ischemia or to some unrecognized mechanism. Carotid sinus stimulation does not produce syncope as a result of sympathetic vasoconstriction of cerebral vessels. In a patient suspected of carotid sinus syncope, all three mechanisms or combinations of mechanisms should be considered, and the patient properly monitored for each by ECG, EEG, and blood pressure recordings. Carotid sinus stimulation should be performed only under conditions in which possible cardio-respiratory arrest can be properly managed. It should be avoided in patients who are elderly, have heart disease, or are at risk for cerebrovascular accidents.

114. The answer is E (all). *(Adams, ed 2. pp 878-879.)* Conditions that produce fasciculations range from exercise to organophosphate poisoning. Exercise in untrained individuals and severe dehydration are intrinsic causes for the membrane instability that results in the motor unit discharges constituting the fasciculations. Organophosphates are extrinsic anticholinesterase agents that increase the amount of acetylcholine. Low calcium blood levels likewise increase membrane instability. These non-neurologic causes of fasciculations need to be distinguished from the primarily neurologic disorders associated with fasciculations. Benign fasciculations, which are fasciculations appearing in otherwise healthy individuals, also must be differentiated from fasciculations due to neuronal disease. In patients with benign fasciculations, there is no known evidence of toxic-metabolic disorder, atrophy or weakness, or EMG indications of denervation.

115. The answer is C (2, 4). *(Adams, ed 2. p 874.)* Percussion irritability reflects the state of excitability of the sarcolemmal membrane of the muscle fibers. Alterations in ionic concentrations affect membrane excitability. Both hyperkalemia and vitamin D intoxication (by raising calcium blood levels) cause a depression in the excitability of the muscle and cause it to lose its direct response to percussion. On the other hand, denervation of muscle (as in the peripheral neuropathies), results in a preserved or exaggerated response of the muscle to percussion, but it reduces or abolishes muscle stretch reflexes. Thus, muscle percussion has direct bedside value in clinical practice.

116. The answer is A (1, 2, 3). *(Adams, ed 2. pp 327-329. DeMyer, ed 3. pp 352-353.)* While the cardinal feature of Broca's aphasia is sparse, telegraphic speech consisting of nouns and verbs with few prepositions, articles, or conjugations, patients with this disorder also frequently show a contralateral facial palsy of central type, dysgraphia, and some degree of loss of speech comprehension. Jargon speech or neologisms, which characterize Wernicke's aphasia, are absent. The lesion of Broca's aphasia typically involves the posterior inferior part of the frontal lobe. Since the motor area for the face is adjacent, it is frequently affected by the lesion, resulting in a contralateral central type of facial palsy.

117. The answer is B (1, 3). *(Adams, ed 2. p 992.)* The Eaton-Lambert syndrome differs from myasthenia gravis by showing a predilection for proximal limb muscles and girdles and an association with carcinoma. It shows an incremental response in the EMG after repetitive nerve stimulation, whereas myasthenia shows a decremental response. The muscle weakness of the Eaton-Lambert syndrome responds poorly to anticholinesterase medication. The Eaton-Lambert syndrome may appear in advance of any overt signs of the primary neoplasm. Its presence should initiate a screening examination for an occult neoplasm.

118. The answer is A (1, 2, 3). *(Cooper, ed 3. pp 163, 173.)* The nucleus locus ceruleus contains norepinephrinergic neurons. Stimulation of the nucleus would demonstrate the following general principles: An increase in the activity of a pathway is reflected by an increase in the end product of its neurotransmitter, the end product in this case being methoxyhydroxyphenyl-ethyleneglycol (MHPG); the enzymes that are rate-limiting in the production of the transmitter will be increased, in this case tyrosine hydroxylase; and the increased release of the transmitter at the endings will cause an increased uptake, presumably for recycling. The evidence for the functional effect of stimulation of the nucleus locus ceruleus is that it tends to hyperpolarize the trans-synaptic neuron, which increases its threshold for firing.

119. The answer is A (1, 2, 3). *(DeMyer, ed 3. p 142.)* Pseudonystagmus characteristically occurs when an individual gazes fully in one direction or another, disappears with a slight shift of the eyes back to the midline, and has a jerk component in the direction of gaze. This is a benign type of nystagmus, evident in many otherwise normal individuals, and is not associated with either oscillopsia or vertigo. Oscillopsia and vertigo **are** associated with an acquired type of pathologic nystagmus, but are absent with pseudonystagmus or congenital nystagmus.

120. The answer is E (all). *(DeMyer, ed 3. p 212.)* Many disorders of the central nervous system are associated with hypotonia rather than with the customary spasticity or rigidity. These include many syndromes with profound mental retardation (such as the Prader-Willi syndrome and even some of the diffuse hypoxic encephalopathies), congenital blindness, Down's syndrome, and cerebellar destruction. In some instances of cerebral palsy, the affected child goes through an early period of months of hypotonia before spasticity or spasticity and athetosis supervene. Thus, hypotonia in an infant does not necessarily indicate a neuromuscular disease. In newborn infants with spinal cord trauma, the stage of spinal shock may produce hypotonia. Thus, the diagnosis of hypotonia in infants requires a very thorough history, physical examination, and a systematic consideration of the many possible causes.

121-124. The answers are: 121-B, 122-A, 123-A, 124-D. *(DeMyer, ed 3. p 55.)* With the eye abducted, the most effective elevator is the superior rectus muscle, and the most effective intorter is the superior oblique muscle. With the eye adducted, the most effective depressor is the superior oblique muscle, and the most effective elevator is the inferior oblique muscle. All of these muscles change their actions depending on the position of the eye.

A distinction has to be made between the strongest and most effective action of an ocular rotatory muscle and all of its possible actions. In testing the main, or most effective, action of muscle, this action should be isolated from the secondary or tertiary actions of the muscle. The muscle has some help in its secondary and tertiary actions, allowing for some compensation by other muscles; but the eyeball can be rotated into a position that calls for the sole or principal action of the muscle. This position provides the best and most exclusive test of the integrity of the muscle.

To test the integrity of the left inferior rectus muscle, for example, a physician asks a patient to look down and to the left. The outward rotation of the eye by the lateral rectus muscle places the eyeball in such a position that the only muscle that will turn the eye down is the inferior rectus muscle. With the eye in the primary position or medially rotated, some of the depressant action of the inferior rectus muscle is dissipated, either in adduction or intorsion—actions that it shares with other muscles. To understand these secondary and tertiary actions, the origin and insertion of the muscles must be known. In addition, the line of pull of each muscle must be analyzed in terms of vectors, whereupon the relationship of the vectors to the axes of the eyes can be understood.

Neurochemistry

DIRECTIONS: Each question below contains five suggested answers. Choose the **one best** response to each question.

125. The biochemical abnormality that is shared by the inborn errors of the urea cycle and that has neurologic manifestations is which of the following?

(A) A great increase in urea excretion
(B) Large amounts of prehepatic bilirubin in the blood
(C) High blood ammonia levels
(D) High serum uric acid levels
(E) Deficiency of brain carbamyl phosphate synthetase

126. Within hours after ligation of a sympathetic nerve, an accumulation of excessive catecholamine would be found in the

(A) dendrites
(B) perikaryon
(C) axon proximal to the ligature
(D) axon distal to the ligature
(E) synaptic terminals

127. A victim of chronic alcoholism who drinks steadily and vomits frequently presents with progressive muscle weakness of several weeks duration. Examination discloses minimal signs of peripheral neuropathy, but the weakness of the muscles seems greatly out of proportion. As a guide to immediate treatment of the weakness, the most important laboratory test for this patient would be

(A) an EMG
(B) a serum CPK level
(C) a serum cortisol level
(D) a serum calcium level
(E) a serum potassium level

128. In Duchenne's pseudohypertrophic muscular dystrophy, the serum CPK value is

(A) roughly constant throughout the course of the disease
(B) greatly elevated prior to overt, clinically apparent weakness
(C) greatly elevated only in later stages of the disease
(D) increased as the weakness becomes severe
(E) unrelated to the stage of the disease

129. An 8-year-old child experiences several episodes of extreme irritability, unsteadiness of gait, and a skin rash in response to sunlight. His parents are second cousins. The single most important diagnostic test would be

(A) an EEG with photic stimulation
(B) a CAT scan
(C) a urinary amino acid screen
(D) a serum lipid profile
(E) a liver biopsy

130. The rate of transport of metabolic substances from the perikaryon to the periphery in peripheral nerves is estimated to be in the range of

(A) 1 mm-1 m/day
(B) 1-10 m/day
(C) 1 m/min
(D) 10 m-100 m/min
(E) 45-60 m/sec

131. The most important mechanism for inactivating or terminating the action of catecholamine neurotransmitter released at the synaptic cleft is thought to be

(A) irreversible binding of the catecholamine with the postsynaptic membrane
(B) energy-dependent reuptake of the transmitter by the presynaptic neuron
(C) inherent instability of the neurotransmitter
(D) addition of sulphate radical by sulphatases
(E) isomerization from the D to the L form

132. The "second messenger" theory of the mechanism of action of neurotransmitters (and other signaling substances such as hormones) suggests that the primary messenger substance

(A) releases a second substance into the synaptic cleft
(B) releases a second substance that inactivates the degradative enzymes for the neurotransmitter
(C) activates the enzyme-controlled metabolism of cyclic nucleotides
(D) blocks the energy-dependent expulsion of sodium
(E) acts on the DNA to alter the encoded genetic constitution of the cell

133. After release into the synaptic cleft, acetylcholine is removed mainly by

(A) passive diffusion into the interstitial fluid and CSF
(B) engulfment into the postsynaptic membrane by pinocytosis
(C) return to the presynaptic ending by passive diffusion
(D) enzymatic hydrolysis with presynaptic uptake of choline
(E) long-term binding to the presynaptic surface

134. Approximately half the patients with the clinical syndrome of Friedreich's ataxia have a biochemical abnormality involving

(A) lipoamide dehydrogenase deficiency
(B) an absence of hypoxanthine-guanine phosphoribosyltransferase
(C) low serum B_{12} levels
(D) agammaglobulinemia
(E) high blood ammonia levels

135. The problem in identifying glutamic acid as a neurotransmitter is that

(A) none of the enzymes that could act on it can be isolated from the nervous system
(B) it fails to pass the blood-brain barrier
(C) it may also have a significant role in intermediary metabolism
(D) it cannot be demonstrated in the CNS
(E) it cannot be shown, by iontophoresis, to have any effect on neuronal polarization

136. Striatal dopamine is located in highest concentration in the

(A) perikarya of striatal neurons
(B) glia
(C) dendrites
(D) synapses
(E) perivascular space

DIRECTIONS: Each question below contains four suggested answers of which **one** or **more** is correct. Choose the answer

A	if	1, 2, and 3	are correct
B	if	1 and 3	are correct
C	if	2 and 4	are correct
D	if	4	is correct
E	if	1, 2, 3, and 4	are correct

137. In the normal metabolism of pyruvate, the pathways consist of which of the following?

(1) Transamination to form alanine
(2) Oxidative decarboxylation to form CO_2
(3) Reduction to lactate
(4) Carboxylation to oxaloacetate

138. Correct statements about the metabolism of acetylcholine include which of the following?

(1) An active uptake system returns acetylcholine to the interior of the presynaptic neuron
(2) The cholinergic neurons manufacture both the acetyl group and the choline group
(3) The rate-limiting factor is the availability of acetyl groups
(4) Acetylcholinesterase hydrolyzes acetylcholine to acetic acid and choline

139. The amount of neurotransmitter in presynaptic endings may be increased by which of the following probable mechanisms?

(1) Active reuptake of previously released transmitter
(2) Transport from the perikaryon
(3) In situ synthesis of the transmitter by activation of enzymes in the synapse
(4) In situ synthesis of more of the enzymes that produce neurotransmitters

140. Glutamate functions in the brain as

(1) a putative excitatory neurotransmitter
(2) a precursor of γ-aminobutyric acid
(3) an ammonia scavenger in detoxification
(4) an energy source in coupled phosphorylation

141. In systemic diseases (excluding familial periodic paralysis), correct statements about weakness associated with low or high levels of potassium include which of the following?

(1) It affects all muscles equally
(2) It is usually severe if the serum level drops below 3.8 mEq/L or exceeds 5.1 mEq/L
(3) It is corrected by edrophonium
(4) It is associated with absent or reduced muscle stretch reflexes

142. Major differences between serotonin and catecholamine metabolism include no apparent

(1) feedback inhibition of serotonin synthesis
(2) active uptake mechanism for serotonin
(3) activation of a secondary messenger by serotonin as contrasted to catecholamines
(4) depletion of serotonin by reserpine

143. Neurologic diseases that may be associated with red or brown urine include

(1) McArdle's disease
(2) porphyria
(3) alcoholic myopathy
(4) polymyositis

144. The neurosecretory granules isolated from catecholaminergic neurons of the peripheral and central nervous system are characterized by

(1) having a high concentration of dopamine or norepinephrine
(2) having the complete system of enzymes for synthesis of catecholamines
(3) containing high concentrations of ATP and ATPase
(4) lacking a distinct membrane under electron microscopy

145. Correct statements concerning serotonin, norepinephrine, and histamine include which of the following?

(1) The metabolic pathway to each begins with an essential amino acid
(2) The precursor undergoes decarboxylation
(3) Monoamine oxidase is involved in their inactivation or degradation
(4) Each of the substances has a potent vasoactive effect

146. Acetylcholine fulfills criteria for a neurotransmitter at

(1) neuromuscular junctions on skeletal muscle
(2) motor neuron collaterals to Renshaw cells
(3) preganglionic endings in the paravertebral ganglia of the autonomic system
(4) Purkinje cell synapses on the midline cerebellar nuclei

147. Characteristics of monoamine oxidase (MAO) include which of the following?

(1) It converts catecholamines to their corresponding aldehydes by oxidative deamination
(2) It exists only in a single unique form specific for catecholamines
(3) It is located in high concentration in mitochondria
(4) It is the rate-limiting enzyme in the catecholamine metabolic pathway

148. In its metabolic pathway, γ-aminobutyric acid (GABA) may be described as

(1) being derived from glucose and glutamic acid
(2) undergoing transamination and subsequently entering the Krebs cycle
(3) undergoing a rapid increase in concentration in postmortem tissues
(4) producing many derivatives that could act as neuromodulators or neurotransmitters

149. In regard to its distribution, γ-aminobutyric acid may correctly be described as

(1) being confined to the CNS
(2) being present in much higher concentrations in the ventral rather than dorsal horns
(3) having a very low concentration in white matter
(4) having a very low concentration in the basal ganglia and substantia nigra

150. Central cholinergic pathways are thought to include which of the following?

(1) Collaterals from the ventral horn motor neurons to the Renshaw cells
(2) Afferents to the hippocampus from the septum and diagonal band
(3) Primary afferent fibers of the auditory and visual systems
(4) Projections from the majority of the raphe nuclei

151. Neurotransmitters found in very high concentrations in the striatum include

(1) dopamine
(2) norepinephrine
(3) serotonin
(4) glycine

152. Evidence that glycine may be a neurotransmitter is reflected in which of the following statements?

(1) The inhibitory striatonigral tract is glycinergic
(2) The inhibitory action of the Purkinje cell is glycinergic
(3) Glycine is well established as an excitatory neurotransmitter in several central tracts
(4) Glycine is an inhibitory substance on spinal neurons

153. The theory that neurotransmitter is released by exocytotic dumping of the contents of neuro-secretory granules is consistent with which of the following statements?

(1) It explains the quantal release of neuro-transmitter
(2) It requires a high rate of protein synthesis to replace the soluble protein contained within the neurosecretory granules
(3) It may be too slow to account for the rapid rate of release of transmitter in response to tetanic stimulation
(4) It appears to contradict the evidence that the most recently formed norepinephrine is preferentially released

154. Characteristics of prostaglandins include which of the following?

(1) They are constructed from long chain fatty acids
(2) They are well established as primary neuro-transmitters
(3) They are diffusely distributed in neural and extraneural tissues
(4) They act universally to excite nerve and muscle cells

DIRECTIONS: The groups of questions below consist of lettered choices followed by several numbered items. For each numbered item select the **one** lettered choice with which it is **most** closely associated. Each lettered choice may be used once, more than once, or not at all.

Questions 155-158

For each procedure or operation described below, choose the neurotransmitter that it would deplete.

  (A) Glycine in the spinal cord
  (B) Dopamine and norepinephrine in the central and peripheral nervous system
  (C) Taurine
  (D) Glutamic acid
  (E) Catecholamines and serotonin from the cerebral cortex

155. Destruction of the granule cells in the cerebellum or section of dorsal roots

156. Destruction of interneurons (by controlled hypoxia)

157. Administration of 6-hydroxydopamine

158. Transection of the medial forebrain bundle

Questions 159-162

For each of the neurotransmitters listed below, choose the precursor with which it is most closely associated.

  (A) Tyrosine
  (B) Tryptophan
  (C) Glutamic acid
  (D) Glucose or citrate
  (E) Alanine

159. Acetyl group of acetylcholine

160. Serotonin

161. Dopamine

162. Gamma-aminobutyric acid

Questions 163-166

Match the following.

  (A) Endorphins
  (B) Enkephalins
  (C) Substance P
  (D) Angiotensin
  (E) Vasopressin

163. Putative pain transmitter found in high concentration in the dorsal horn neurons of the substantia gelatinosa

164. Peptides discovered by the Aberdeen group of Hughes and Kosterlitz that imitate the action of the opiates and have a widespread distribution in interneurons with short axons

165. A peptide mainly found in the periventricular regions like the pineal body and pituitary glands, which causes profound thirst when injected into the third ventricle

166. Generic term for a large class of neuropeptides with morphine-like activity

Questions 167-170

For each action listed below, select the putative neurotransmitter(s) to which it is most closely related.

  (A) γ-Aminobutyric acid and glycine in CNS
  (B) Glutamate and aspartate in CNS
  (C) Dopamine, norepinephrine, serotonin in CNS
  (D) Norepinephrine in the peripheral nervous system
  (E) Tryptophan

167. Essentially always excitatory

168. Essentially always inhibitory

169. Predominantly inhibitory but may have some excitatory actions

170. Known to have definite mixture of excitatory and inhibitory actions

Neurochemistry Answers

125. The answer is C. *(Stanbury, ed 4. p 381.)* A biochemical abnormality that is shared by the inborn errors of the urea cycle is an increase in the blood ammonia level. The formation of urea via the urea cycle is both the only known metabolic pathway for urea synthesis in humans and the major pathway for ammonia detoxification. Patients with an inborn error of the urea cycle have a deficiency of one of the five enzymes that lead to the biosynthesis of urea. When urea fails to be produced because of a block along the pathway of urea production, ammonia will accumulate in the body tissues and fluids. Ammonia accumulation leads to vomiting, lethargy, convulsions, hypotonia, coma, and mental retardation. Exacerbations may be related to the ingestion of large amounts of dietary protein. Although hepatomegaly may occur, there is no evidence of jaundice. The best single screening test for a urea cycle disorder is a blood ammonia level determination. The specific defect is subsequently identified by the abnormal pattern of amino acid excretion in the urine, and direct demonstration of the particular enzyme defect by biochemical assay of the patient's cells.

126. The answer is C. *(Cooper, ed 3. pp 150-151.)* After a ligature is placed around a sympathetic nerve, catecholamine accumulates just proximal to the ligature. The accumulation begins shortly after the ligature is placed. This observation supports the supposition that the neurotransmitter substance is manufactured in the perikaryon and transported down the axon to the terminals for storage and release. The idea that a substance originates in the central nervous system and undergoes transportation distally is an ancient theory in the history of medicine. We no longer speak of this substance as "animal spirits" but as neurohumors. Ramón y Cajal was one of the first scientists to demonstrate the distention of nerves proximal to a ligature, but he of course lacked the biochemical tools to demonstrate the nature of the accumulated substance.

127. The answer is E. *(Adams, ed 2. p 959.)* Muscle weakness in alcoholic persons may represent a true myopathy, although these individuals may also have severe neuropathy. Associated with the myopathy may be an increased or decreased level of serum potassium. The hypokalemic myopathy may be associated with loss of potassium from vomiting and diarrhea. **High** potassium levels may be associated with accompanying renal damage. Immediate treatment of the muscle weakness is to correct the potassium balance. The other determinations—CPK, cortisol, calcium, and EMG studies—may be helpful in the overall evaluation of the patient, but fail to provide useful guides to restoration of muscle strength.

128. The answer is B. *(Adams, ed 2. pp 962-963.)* In pseudohypertrophic muscular dystrophy, the serum CPK value is greatly elevated prior to overt clinical manifestations. It remains high during the early clinical course and drops later as the muscle mass is reduced. Thus, the CPK determinations help in early diagnosis of the disease in infants, prior to clinical signs of the weakness. High CPK values also are present in the fetus, and CPK measurement of fetal blood levels can lead to a prenatal diagnosis. CPK exists in at least three isoenzymes—from muscle, heart, and brain. Muscle CPK blood levels are elevated in Duchenne's dystrophy, as is the cardiac isoenzyme. Normally the serum contains no brain CPK.

129. The answer is C. *(Stanbury, ed 4. pp 1575-1576.)* The combination of intermittent episodes of unsteady gait (ataxia), emotionality, and a photosensitive skin rash in a patient coming from a consanguineous mating suggests Hartnup disease. This disease is a recessively inherited error of metabolism characterized by a deficiency in the gastrointestinal and renal transport of tryptophan and certain other monoaminomonocarboxylic amino acids. The critical diagnostic test for Hartnup disease is the demonstration of the pattern of excessive excretion of monoaminomonocarboxylic acids in the urine. The direct selection of this single, simple urine screening test eliminates the need for further laboratory testing.

130. The answer is A. *(Cooper, ed 3. pp 112-113.)* The rate of axoplasmic transport of substances is variously estimated as 1 mm-1 m/day. Interestingly, the rate of regeneration of axons is in the range of 1-5 mm/day, which approximates the rate of slow axoplasmic flow. Whether axoplasmic flow increases or decreases during regeneration remains in dispute. The rate of transport of metabolic substances down the axon (1 mm-1 m/day) contrasts with the rate of propagation of the nerve impulse, which is in the range of 45-60 m/sec. This vastly greater rate of impulse propagation underscores its electrical nature in contrast with axoplasmic flow, which involves the movement of ions, molecules, or even macromolecules.

131. The answer is B. *(Cooper, ed 3. pp 148-149.)* Probably the most important mode of inactivation of catecholamine neurotransmitter at the synaptic cleft is an energy-dependent reuptake of the substance into the presynaptic neuron. Whatever the mechanism, apparently it is efficient because little of a catecholamine such as norepinephrine overflows into the circulation, in spite of strong stimulation of sympathetic nerves. While degradation by monoamine oxidase (MAO) or catechol-*O*-methyltransferase (COMT) accounts for much of the inactivation of released catecholamine neurotransmitter, the inhibition of these enzymes fails to potentiate the effect of nerve stimulation. In favor of the importance of active reuptake is the fact that a sympathetic neuron can concentrate catecholamines from surrounding media by a ratio as great as 10,000 to 1.

132. The answer is C. *(Cooper, ed 3. pp 282-287.)* Just how the primary chemical messenger—whether neurotransmitter or hormone—activates the target cell to do its job of secreting, contracting, or firing an impulse, is one of the fundamental questions of cell biology. Current theory suggests that the combination of the neurotransmitter with its receptor activates nucleotide cyclase and sets into play a series of enzymatically dependent events that provide the energy for the subsequent actions of the target cell. A whole series of "Koch's postulates" has been developed to justify the recognition of a second messenger mechanism, just as they have been developed to justify recognition of a particular substance as a primary neurotransmitter.

133. The answer is D. *(Cooper, ed 3. p 76.)* The removal and inactivation of acetylcholine after its release appears to be mainly dependent on enzymatic hydrolysis. The choline part of the molecule is then actively transported back into the presynaptic cell by an energy-dependent mechanism. The availability of choline appears to be the limiting factor in acetylcholine synthesis, and this mechanism of active return of choline may be a mechanism for conservation of a rate-limiting metabolite. In some instances, the entire neurotransmitter molecule is taken up by the presynaptic ending and presumably can be recycled many times without undergoing degradation or resynthesis.

134. The answer is A. *(Blass, Neurology 8:280-286, 1979.)* In assaying patients with the clinical syndrome of Friedreich's ataxia, about one half of them have a deficiency in the pyruvate dehydrogenase complex of enzymes. The third member of the pyruvate dehydrogenase complex, lipoamide dehydrogenase, appears to be the deficient enzyme. Oxygen transport deficits, deficits of purine metabolism (absence of phosphoribosyltransferase), and low B_{12} levels have been eliminated as defects in Friedreich's ataxia. Whether the deficiency of pyruvate metabolism accounts for the clinical and pathological findings of Friedreich's ataxia remains uncertain. There also may be a deficiency in the high-density lipoproteins (α-lipoproteins) that could lead to a defect in cell membranes. Such a deficiency would better explain the phenotypic similarity between Friedreich's syndrome and some other syndromes with Friedreich-like features, such as the abetalipoproteinemia of Bassen-Kornzweig.

135. The answer is C. *(Cooper, ed 3. pp 252-254.)* Glutamic acid can be demonstrated to have excitatory effects on crustacean muscle and mammalian neurons. It and the enzymes that metabolize it can be isolated from nervous tissue. The main problem in identifying glutamic acid as a neurotransmitter is that it has a role in intermediary metabolism, which gives it a much more ubiquitous distribution in comparison to other putative neurotransmitters like dopamine, which can be localized to specific neurons and specific tracts.

136. The answer is D. *(Adams, ed 2. p 52.)* Fractionation of the striatum with subsequent chemical analysis shows the highest concentrations of dopamine in the synaptosomal fraction. This observation indicates that the striatum, rather than producing its own dopamine, receives it from elsewhere via axonal transport. Its accumulation in the synaptosomes suggests that it plays a neurotransmitter role. The nigrostriatal pathway apparently provides the majority of dopaminergic synapses for the striatum. Interruption of this pathway or degeneration of the substantia nigra is associated with a severe decrease in the dopamine content of the striatum.

137. The answer is E (all). *(Blass, Neurology 8:280, 1979.)* The glycolytic cycle through pyruvate is almost the only energy-producing pathway available to the central nervous system. Pyruvate is a crucial product of glycolysis via the Embden-Meyerhof pathway. In its normal metabolism, pyruvate is transaminated to form alanine, undergoes oxidative decarboxylation to form CO_2, is reduced to lactate, or may undergo carboxylation to oxaloacetate. The transamination of pyruvate to alanine is reversible, allowing alanine to be a precursor for gluconeogenesis through pyruvate. After passing through the pyruvate dehydrogenase complex of enzymes, pyruvate enters the Krebs cycle as acetyl coenzyme A. The formation of pyruvate is stimulated by conditions that interfere with oxidative metabolism, causing the accumulation of pyruvate in conditions such as hypoxia or shock. Conversely, pyruvate may increase because of a block in its pathway through the pyruvate dehydrogenase complex of enzymes.

138. The answer is D (4). *(Barchas, pp 42-43.)* In the metabolism of acetylcholine, the rate-limiting factor is the availability of choline, which apparently is manufactured mostly in the liver and transported to the neurons. Acetylcholinesterase hydrolyzes acetylcholine to acetic acid and choline. An active transport mechanism returns choline, but not the entire acetylcholine molecule, to the neuron. One stumbling block in acetylcholine research has been the lack of a drug that specifically blocks the uptake of choline.

139. The answer is A (1, 2, 3). *(Cooper, ed 3. p 16.)* Probable mechanisms for increasing the amount of neurotransmitter in synaptic endings include active reuptake, in situ synthesis of the transmitter, and transport of the transmitter from the perikaryon. It seems improbable that the synapse could increase the amount of contained neurotransmitter by in situ synthesis of the enzymes that produce the transmitter. The enzymes are protein substances that presumably can be produced only by the metabolic machinery located in the perikaryon. The enzymes in the synapse are thought to travel from the perikaryon by axoplasmic transport.

140. The answer is E (all). *(Cooper, ed 3. pp 52-53.)* Glutamate has numerous roles in the CNS. It is a putative excitatory neurotransmitter, a precursor of γ-aminobutyric acid, an ammonia scavenger, and is involved in energy metabolism. It also is a structural amino acid for protein synthesis. Glutamine and other putative amino acid neurotransmitters can be derived from glucose, and glutamate is involved in many other metabolic reactions including proline, glutathione, and N-acetylaspartate production.

141. The answer is D (4). *(Adams, ed 2. p 874.)* The weakness from increased or decreased levels of potassium in systemic electrolyte disturbances tends to spare the cranial nerves (ocular and bulbar) and respiratory muscles, affecting the trunk and extremity muscles most severely. It usually fails to become severe until the serum potassium level falls below 2.5 mEq/L or rises above 7 mEq/L (depending on the other electrolyte abnormalities). Extreme flaccid paralysis requires serum potassium levels below 2.5 mEq/L. The muscle stretch reflexes are reduced with either high or low potassium levels. In contrast, abnormally high serum calcium levels result in decreased reflexes, whereas abnormally low serum calcium levels result in increased reflexes.

142. The answer is B (1, 3). *(Cooper, ed 3. pp 210-212.)* Although serotonin and catecholamine metabolism share many features, serotonin synthesis differs in its apparent freedom from feedback inhibition. There is strong evidence for activation of a secondary messenger by catecholamines, as has been demonstrated in the effect of stimulation of the nucleus locus ceruleus on the Purkinje cells. Reserpine depletes both catecholamines and serotonin, which has confounded the correlation between neurohumoral levels and behavior.

143. The answer is E (all). *(Adams, ed 2. p 875.)* A number of neurologic diseases may produce reddish brown discoloration of the urine. The color results from hemoglobin or myoglobin pigments. The pigmented urine in most instances of neuromuscular disease results from necrotic or injured muscle, which liberates myoglobin, or from the biosynthesis of heme. The liberated pigment damages the kidney, leading to renal failure. Renal failure poses a threat to survival in many neuromuscular diseases that might not, in themselves, be fatal, including McArdle's disease, porphyria, alcoholic myopathy, and polymyositis.

144. The answer is B (1, 3). *(Cooper, ed 3. p 140.)* Subcellular particles called neurosecretory granules isolated from catecholaminergic neurons have high concentrations of dopamine or norepinephrine, and of ATP and ATPase. The ATP may bind the norepinephrine within the granules by means of a salt linkage. The granules lack the complete enzyme systems for the synthesis of the catecholamines. Electron microscopy shows that the granules have a dense core and a well-developed outer membrane. The very structure of these so-called neurosecretory granules raises questions as to whether they could fuse with the presynaptic membrane and release their neurotransmitter contents rapidly enough to account for synaptic transmission. An alternate theory is that they form a long-term storage system rather than the immediately mobile neurotransmitter that responds so quickly to the arrival of the nerve impulse.

145. The answer is E (all). *(Cooper, ed 3. pp 55, 301.)* The metabolic pathway to serotonin begins with tryptophan, to norepinephrine with phenylalanine or tyrosine, and to histamine with histidine. Tryptophan, phenylalanine, and histidine all are essential amino acids. Each of the amino acids undergoes decarboxylation. Monoamine oxidase may be involved in the activation or degradation of serotonin, norepinephrine, and histamine. All three substances produce vasoactive agents. Tryptophan produces tryptamine and tyramine, and phenylalanine produces norepinephrine and epinephrine, all of which are vasopressors (as is serotonin), whereas histamine is a vasodilator.

146. The answer is A (1, 2, 3). *(Cooper, ed 3. p 91.)* Acetylcholine fulfills criteria for a neurotransmitter at neuromuscular junctions on skeletal muscles, motor neuron collaterals to Renshaw cells, and preganglionic endings in the paravertebral ganglia. It also is the presumptive neurotransmitter in the postganglionic parasympathetic terminals. Cholinergic transmission also may occur in the hippocampus from the diagonal band and septum, thus from rhinencephalic structures at the base of the forebrain. The habenulointerpeduncular tract also may be cholinergic. Other suggested cholinergic systems include the ascending reticular activating system, the primary afferents in auditory and visual systems, and some dorsal root fibers. The subject of cholinergic transmission in the cerebral cortex remains unsettled. In almost all known instances, acetylcholine acts as an excitatory transmitter, although evidence for inhibitory transmission exists for some sites. The Purkinje cells strongly inhibit the midline nuclei, and the transmitter is thought to be γ-aminobutyric acid (GABA).

147. The answer is B (1, 3). *(Cooper, ed 3. pp 145-148.)* Monoamine oxidase (MAO) converts catecholamines to their corresponding aldehydes by oxidative deamination. It exists in more than one form and lacks specificity for catecholamines, acting on a number of other substances including serotonin, tryptamine, and tyramine. It is generally regarded as existing in highest concentration in the mitochondria. It is not a rate-limiting enzyme in the catecholamine pathways. In spite of the presumed role of MAO in inactivating various biogenic amines that could serve as neurotransmitters, the action of these transmitters appears to be unaffected by the inactivation of MAO.

148. The answer is E (all). *(Cooper, ed 3. pp 234-238.)* γ-Aminobutyric acid (GABA) has an amino acid precursor, glutamic acid, but also can be derived from glucose. GABA undergoes transamination and then may enter the Krebs cycle. A striking fact about GABA is that it can produce a large number of compounds that may have neuromodulator or neurotransmitter actions. It can produce compounds that have anesthetic action or that may depress or excite some neurons. Thus, the metabolic derivatives of GABA are under intensive study at this time. One problem in assessing GABA levels or the effects of chemical manipulations on the GABA content of the CNS is that GABA undergoes a very rapid rise in concentration in postmortem tissues, which may result from activation of glutamic acid decarboxylase at death.

149. The answer is A (1, 2, 3). *(Cooper, ed 3. pp 224-226.)* γ-Aminobutyric acid (GABA) and its synthesizing enzyme glutamic acid decarboxylase are confined to the CNS, including the retina, which is embryologically derived from the CNS. GABA is found in much higher concentrations in the gray matter than in the white matter, in keeping with its presumed role as a neurotransmitter. It is found in high concentrations in the ventral horns, where inhibitory effects do occur, rather than in the dorsal horns, where excitatory neurotransmitters predominate. A GABA pathway is believed to run from the striatum to the pallidum and substantia nigra; the synthesizing enzyme for GABA (glutamic acid decarboxylase) and its degradative enzyme (GABA-transaminase) are in high concentration in these regions.

150. The answer is A (1, 2, 3). *(Cooper, ed 3. pp 90-91.)* Although technical difficulties prevent the establishment of acetylcholine as a neurotransmitter in central pathways as firmly as in the peripheral nervous system, some central pathways are thought to be cholinergic. The most likely pathways include Renshaw collaterals from the ventral horn motor neurons, hippocampal afferents from the diagonal band and septum, the habenulointerpeduncular tract, the ascending reticular activating system, and primary afferents from the auditory and visual systems. Several other central cholinergic pathways are suggested. On the other hand, many central pathways lack evidence of being cholinergic; many, such as the raphe nuclei, which appear to be serotonergic, have other putative neurotransmitters.

151. The answer is B (1, 3). *(Adams, ed 2. p 51.)* The striatum contains several putative neurotransmitters in high concentration, including dopamine, serotonin, acetylcholine, γ-aminobutyric acid (GABA), and polypeptides. It contains low amounts of norepinephrine and glycine. The high concentrations of dopamine and serotonin and low amounts of norepinephrine are thought to reflect the density of innervation of the striatum by the various tegmental nuclei. In particular, the low concentration of norepinephrine reflects only a slight innervation of the striatum by the norepinephrinergic pathways arising in such tegmental nuclei as the locus ceruleus.

152. The answer is D (4). *(Cooper, ed 3. pp 247-252.)* The weight of evidence for glycine as a neurotransmitter suggests that it may be an inhibitory transmitter in spinal interneurons, but its presence in these neurons and its release at their terminals has yet to be proved. The striatonigral tract, which is considered to be inhibitory, apparently utilizes γ-aminobutyric acid (GABA) as its transmitter rather than glycine. The Purkinje cell also is thought to exert inhibition by release of GABA rather than glycine. Satisfactory evidence to establish glycine as an excitatory transmitter in the mammalian nervous system is lacking.

153. The answer is E (all). *(Cooper, ed 3. pp 142-144.)* The exact mechanism of storage and release of neurotransmitter remains uncertain, particularly in the CNS. Exocytotic fusion of the neurosecretory granule with the presynaptic membrane, dumping the contents of the granule into the synaptic cleft, is one favored explanation. This theory would explain the quantal release of neurotransmitter in specific increments. The loss of the soluble protein in a secretory granule would require a local mechanism for rapid replacement, a process yet to be established. *A priori*, a process requiring exocytosis would seem to be too slow to account for the rapid release that follows tetanic stimulation. Again, if the most recently formed norepinephrine is the first to be released, the likelihood of its undergoing a process of incorporation into a vesicle that then would have to fuse with the presynaptic membrane seems remote.

154. The answer is B (1, 3). *(Cooper, ed 3. pp 294-299.)* The prostaglandins are constructed from long chain fatty acids that fold upon themselves to form a five-carbon atom ring structure in their midportion. The ring has oxygen linkages forming either ketones or hydroxyl groups. The prostaglandins are widespread in both the body and brain. Their widespread distribution in the brain argues against their having a specific role as a neurotransmitter, which would require that they be concentrated in particular neuronal groups or tracts. Instead, prostaglandins are conjectured as being local modulators that work through cyclic adenosine monophosphate (AMP) to produce excitatory or inhibitory effects. The effect observed may vary with the state of the neuronal systems being acted upon. Prostaglandins are released from active neural tissue and can be found in the cerebrospinal fluid. The prostaglandins apparently act in very small concentrations. Although it is difficult to state their physiologic role, some prostaglandins do appear to inhibit the effects of stimulation of the sympathetic nervous system.

155-158. The answers are: 155-D, 156-A, 157-B, 158-E. *(Cooper, ed 3. pp 113-116, 251, 253, 303.)* By certain manipulations, the experimenter can deplete the nervous system of specific substances presumed to be neurotransmitters. Controlled hypoxia causes a selective necrosis of interneurons in the spinal cord. The glycine content of the spinal gray matter is reduced, offering one line of evidence that glycine may be the transmitter that mediates the inhibitory effect of these neurons.

The intravenous administration of 6-hydroxydopamine causes a chemical sympathectomy in the peripheral nervous system, or in the central nervous system when given by intraventricular injection. The drug causes a fairly specific destruction of catecholamine-containing neurons.

Transection of the medial forebrain bundle interrupts the ascending pathways that convey axons from the catecholaminergic neurons of the pontomesencephalic tegmentum and the serotonergic neurons of the raphe. These axons synapse in the cerebral cortex, where they release their transmitter.

These and similar techniques are beginning to clarify the biochemical specification of neural pathways. The older methods of analyzing pathways depended on the ability of silver to precipitate on axons, or on the development or loss of myelin. The biochemical reactions of pathways may help to identify pathways of similar function that had not previously been recognized as related. It may also be possible to trace and classify short pathways that cannot be studied by classical methods. Finally, it may become possible by administration of a drug to interrupt the action of specific pathways and thus to bring about some desired clinical goal.

159-162. The answers are: 159-D, 160-B, 161-A, 162-C. *(Cooper, ed 3. pp 120-121, 197, 227.)* The precursor of the acetyl group of acetylcholine is glucose or citrate; of serotonin, tryptophan; of dopamine, tyrosine; and of γ-aminobutyric acid (GABA), glutamic acid. These precursor substances, occurring in the diet, undergo several metabolic transformations to gain activity as neurotransmitters. With some further slight metabolic transformation, the neurotransmitter loses its capacity to excite or inhibit the postsynaptic neuron. The elaborate metabolic pathway involved insures that only the exact substance rather than a substance that happens to enter the blood, will affect the function of the neurons.

The precursors of acetylcholine differ from the other precursors in this group. The precursors of serotonin, dopamine, and GABA are all amino acids. The acetyl group of acetylcholine is readily available from the catabolism of glucose. The choline that comes from the diet is the rate-limiting moiety of acetylcholine synthesis. Choline is taken up for recycling by the presynaptic ending, after the splitting of acetylcholine by cholinesterase at the synapse.

The recycling of one moiety of a transmitter, choline, appears to be unusual. The biogenic amines are transformed by undergoing methylations or hydroxylations. In the case of amino acid related transmitters, inactivation may ultimately involve deamination. Serotonin is inactivated by both oxidation and deamination. The end product of this process is 5-hydroxyindoleacetic acid. The carboxyl group of the acetic acid replaces the amino grouping on the terminal carbon of the aliphatic portion of the molecule.

163-166. The answers are: 163-C, 164-B, 165-D, 166-A. *(Cooper, ed 3. pp 264-273.)* Nervous tissue and the gastrointestinal tract contain a large number of peptides that have neurotransmitter-like effects on neurons and smooth muscle. These peptides consist of chains or, perhaps in some instances, rings of amino acids. When injected into the ventricular region, they may have profound effects on consciousness, motor reactivity, and autonomic responses such as thirst. Such peptides also combine with opiate receptors; opiate antagonists block their action.

The term "endorphins" has become a generic term for a large group of neuroactive peptides of the kind mentioned above, whereas the term "enkephalins" is usually reserved for the two specific peptides discovered by Hughes and Kosterlitz of the Aberdeen group of investigators.

Substance P is found in high concentration in the substantia gelatinosa, where it has been linked to transmission of pain impulses, but it also ocurs in small neuronal systems throughout the CNS. In Huntington's chorea, the amount of substance P in the substantia nigra is considerably reduced.

Angiotensin is highly concentrated in periventricular organelles such as the pineal body and pituitary gland. Like other neuropeptides, it may profoundly alter fluid intake and fluid balance.

167-170. The answers are: 167-B, 168-A, 169-C, 170-D. *(Cooper, ed 3. pp 144, 210, 250.)* From the evidence now available, γ-aminobutyric acid and glycine are regarded as essentially inhibitory transmitters, glutamate and aspartate as essentially excitatory, and the biogenic amines as inhibitory in the CNS. Tryptophan is not a putative transmitter, but serves as the precursor for serotonin. In the peripheral nervous system, norepinephrine has both excitatory and inhibitory effects. The fact that adrenergic substances cause constriction of some smooth muscles and inhibition of others led to the proposal by Ahlquist of alpha and beta receptors. For example, adrenergic drugs constrict vessels in the skin, mucosa, and kidney but dilate vessels to skeletal muscle.

The molecular mechanism that causes one smooth muscle cell to contract and another to relax in response to the same chemical messenger remains unknown. The difference in response might be mediated at the receptor site or in the release of a second messenger in the receptor cell.

The inhibitory or excitatory effects of the neurotransmitter on smooth muscle and neurons can be differentially affected by drugs. Strychnine, for example, will block the inhibitory effects of glycine on the spinal cord, causing the experimental animal to exhibit reflex excitability, convulsions, and spasms of all voluntary muscles. Sensory stimuli produce violent muscle spasms because the excitatory effects are unopposed by corresponding inhibition.

Neuropharmacology

DIRECTIONS: Each question below contains five suggested answers. Choose the **one best** response to each question.

171. Which of the following sequences lists agents in the correct ascending order of the time required for them to reduce intracranial pressure?

(A) Hyperventilation, mannitol, dexamethasone (Decadron)
(B) Mannitol, hyperventilation, dexamethasone
(C) Mannitol, dexamethasone, hyperventilation
(D) Dexamethasone, mannitol, hyperventilation
(E) Dexamethasone, hyperventilation, mannitol

172. A patient lacking available history is brought in off of the street with delirium, pupillodilatation, dry, flushed skin and mucous membranes, peculiar myoclonus-like twitchings, tachycardia, and fever. The clinical condition appears to be deteriorating during a period of 45 minutes of observation. The drug of choice for treatment would be which of the following?

(A) Edrophonium
(B) Thiamine
(C) Phenobarbital
(D) Physostigmine
(E) Metocurine iodide (Metubine)

173. To dilate the pupil without paralyzing accommodation, the examiner would use a drug that

(A) blocks parasympathetic endings
(B) blocks sympathetic endings
(C) stimulates parasympathetic endings
(D) stimulates sympathetic endings
(E) does none of the above

174. A patient with a history of drug abuse is brought to an emergency room with obtundation, a respiratory rate of 7/min, and pinpoint pupils, but no other frank neurologic signs. A glucose test-tape shows a normal blood glucose level. The patient is intubated. The most appropriate management of this patient would involve which of the following measures?

(A) Immediate CAT scan
(B) Administration of pure oxygen
(C) Intravenous bolus of 50% glucose
(D) Administration of intravenous naloxone
(E) Immediate lumbar puncture

175. Local anesthetic agents like procaine are thought to act by

(A) inhibiting cyclic AMP
(B) inhibiting the oxidative enzymes of the mitochondria in the perikaryon and synaptic endings
(C) blocking pyridoxal-dependent enzymes of the catecholamine metabolic pathway
(D) blocking the voltage-dependent transient rise in membrane permeability to sodium
(E) completing depolarization

176. Of the several drugs that have value in the relief of spasticity, the one that acts directly on skeletal muscle is which of the following?

(A) Diazepam (Valium)
(B) Dantrolene
(C) Mephenesin
(D) Cyclobenzaprine
(E) Methocarbamol

177. A 6-year-old hyperactive child with generalized motor seizures is hospitalized and started on treatment with phenytoin (Dilantin) capsules. She weighs 30 kg (66 lb). The dosage has been gradually increased to 500 mg/day during a period of several weeks. Phenytoin blood levels are in the range of 1-3 μg/ml and have not changed much with the increasing dose. The best treatment plan would be which of the following?

(A) Switch to phenytoin suspension
(B) Switch to valproic acid
(C) Add carbamazepine (Tegretol)
(D) Add trimethadione (Tridione)
(E) Add phenobarbital

178. The most widely accepted theory to explain tachyphylaxis by sympathomimetic drugs is which of the following?

(A) Irreversible binding of the neurotransmitter at the receptor site
(B) Stimulation of degradative enzymes
(C) Increased flushing of intercellular fluid through the synapse
(D) Displacement of neurotransmitter from the presynaptic terminals
(E) Release of dopamine-beta-hydroxylase

179. In a patient suspected of having ocular myasthenia, no improvement in the ptosis or ocular palsy and no subjective complaints or objective signs of cholinergic stimulation appeared after initial injection of 2 mg of edrophonium followed by 1 mg every 30 seconds for a total dose of 10 mg. The most appropriate management of this patient is to

(A) conclude that the patient does not have myasthenia gravis and discontinue testing
(B) perform the same test using neostigmine
(C) perform a curare test
(D) perform a Jolly test (look for decremental response after repetitive nerve stimulation)
(E) administer additional edrophonium until improvement occurs or signs or symptoms of cholinergic overactivity appear

180. Administration of morphine to a patient with paraplegia due to a complete cord transection would have which of the following effects?

(A) Increase in the response to pain inflicted rostral to the spinal transection
(B) Increase in the spasticity of the paralyzed limbs
(C) Increase in the reflex withdrawal of the paralyzed limbs to noxious stimulation
(D) Decrease in the nerve conduction velocity caudal to the transection
(E) None of the above

181. The primary mechanism of the anticonvulsant action of phenytoin (Dilantin) is currently thought to be which of the following?

(A) Increasing the amount of γ-aminobutyric acid in the cortex
(B) Binding with glutamic acid receptor sites at synapses
(C) Depolarization of all neuronal membranes
(D) Blockage of sodium channels in resting membranes
(E) Stimulation of acetylcholinesterase

182. A minimally retarded 14-year-old boy has required blood levels of 18-22 μg/ml of phenytoin (Dilantin) for control of seizures. His parents observe that for several months the patient has exhibited increasing lassitude, declining school performance, fatigability, and irritability; however, he has not had seizures. His blood levels of phenytoin and his neurologic examination have remained the same for several years. Which of the following combinations of tests would be most likely to lead to the diagnosis?

(A) EEG and CAT scan of the head
(B) EMG and serum CPK level
(C) Prothrombin time and SGOT level
(D) Neuropsychologic testing and psychiatric consultation
(E) Blood cell count and serum folate level

183. The psychotrophic drug most likely to cause a pigmentary retinopathy is

(A) chlorpromazine (Thorazine)
(B) haloperidol (Haldol)
(C) thioridazine (Mellaril)
(D) amphetamine
(E) imipramine (Tofranil)

184. A 5-year-old epileptic boy has received pheno-barbital for 4 years. His parents report that in recent months he often complains of pain in his back and extremities and that he seems less active and weaker than previously. The neurologic examination fails to disclose definite abnormalities, but the child coop-erates poorly for strength testing. The test battery most likely to establish the diagnosis in this patient is

(A) nerve conduction velocity and an EMG
(B) serum calcium and alkaline phosphatase levels, and bone radiographs
(C) serum folate and B$_{12}$ levels, blood cell count and bone marrow examination
(D) C-reactive protein, erythrocyte sedimentation rate, and antistreptolysin titer
(E) SGOT, serum bilirubin, and prothrombin time

185. A manic-depressive patient recently started on lithium treatment begins to show diarrhea, ataxia, fasciculations, tremor, overactive muscle stretch reflexes, and seizures. The blood lithium level is 1.5 mEq/L. The best interpretation of these find-ings is that the

(A) correct diagnosis of delirium tremens was overlooked
(B) symptoms and lithium blood level are com-patible with lithium intoxication
(C) patient has acute hyperthyroidism
(D) lithium has precipitated a catecholaminergic crisis
(E) patient must have received a stimulant medication and should have a toxicology screening

186. The disorder of involuntary movement most likely to respond to anticonvulsant medication is

(A) chorea
(B) essential tremor
(C) familial paroxysmal choreoathetosis
(D) athetoid cerebral palsy
(E) Gilles de la Tourette's syndrome

187. A striking difference in the response of the nigrostriatal system to mechanical or pharmaco-logic interruption of impulse flow, as contrasted to the other catecholaminergic systems, is that the interruption results in

(A) increased storage of dopamine in the axonal terminals, and increased production
(B) great increase in acetylcholine in the striatum
(C) immediate switch to serotonin neurotrans-mission
(D) no change in the production or storage of dopamine because of steady-state kinetics of the system
(E) extreme depletion of dopamine in the striatum

188. Which of the following statements concerning routine use of anticonvulsants after the diagnosis of brain abscess is most nearly true?

(A) It is the usual practice in many centers
(B) It is not indicated unless seizures occur
(C) It should be strongly avoided because of possible obtundation
(D) It interferes with the effectiveness of antibiotics
(E) It may increase the intracranial pressure

DIRECTIONS: Each question below contains four suggested answers of which **one** or **more** is correct. Choose the answer

A	if	1, 2, and 3	are correct
B	if	1 and 3	are correct
C	if	2 and 4	are correct
D	if	4	is correct
E	if	1, 2, 3, and 4	are correct

189. Relatively common, well-established toxic effects of chronic administration of therapeutic amounts of phenytoin (Dilantin) in humans include which of the following?

(1) Degeneration of Purkinje cells
(2) Liver necrosis
(3) Aplastic anemia
(4) Peripheral neuropathy

190. A patient inadvertently receives an excessive dose of intramuscular chlorpromazine (Thorazine) and develops hypotension that requires treatment. The patient is placed in a recumbent position and should receive

(1) plasma expanders
(2) isoproterenol
(3) norepinephrine
(4) epinephrine

191. Correct statements concerning opiate receptors include which of the following?

(1) They are relatively numerous in the limbic system, diencephalon, and spinal cord
(2) They combine with endogenous polypeptides as well as morphine
(3) They have an affinity for naloxone
(4) They produce an identical response to the various opiates

192. A drug that disarranges microtubules would also be expected to

(1) uncouple oxidative phosphorylation
(2) arrest cell division in metaphase
(3) impair entry of glucose into the neuron
(4) impair axoplasmic transport

193. Which of the following features distinguish a myasthenic crisis from a cholinergic crisis?

(1) Predominance of weakness in the ocular and bulbar muscles
(2) Incontinence of bowel and bladder
(3) Tongue fasciculations, pupillodilatation, and bradycardia
(4) Increased strength after injection of 8 mg of edrophonium

194. In preparing to treat a patient who has parkinsonism with L-dopa, a physician should do which of the following?

(1) Discontinue ordinary over-the-counter vitamin preparations
(2) Discontinue anticholinergic parkinsonian drugs
(3) Begin with 0.5 to 1.0 g of L-dopa in divided doses
(4) Administer a monoamine oxidase inhibitor

195. A patient suffering from an overdose of an anticholinesterase drug would display which of the following autonomic effects?

(1) Tachycardia
(2) Abdominal cramping
(3) Dry skin
(4) Salivation

196. Administration of morphine is contraindicated in the presence of

(1) acute head injury with mild obtundation
(2) hypovolemic shock
(3) asthma
(4) cor pulmonale

197. Pharmacologic agents that paralyze by depolarization of the end-plates in skeletal muscle include

(1) pyrophosphates
(2) succinylcholine
(3) edrophonium
(4) quarternary ammonium compounds

198. Manipulations that increase the action of tyrosine hydroxylase in catecholaminergic neurons include which of the following?

(1) Administration of monoamine oxidase inhibitors
(2) Administration of tyramine
(3) Administration of 6-hydroxydopamine or α-methyl-p-tyrosine (AMPT)
(4) Increased activity of the catecholaminergic neurons

199. An epileptic woman in satisfactory mental condition who requires continuous anticonvulsant medication informs her physician that she wants to have a baby. The physician should adhere to which of the following principles or procedures?

(1) The woman should be urged not to have a child, because anticonvulsant drugs are teratogenic
(2) The anticonvulsant medication should be stopped
(3) The woman should receive megadoses of folic acid
(4) The woman should receive vitamin K near term

200. Which of the following statements apply to the pharmacology of tardive dyskinesia?

(1) It is thought to result from hypersensitivity of cholinergic receptors
(2) It occurs most commonly in patients receiving benzodiazepines
(3) It disappears when the offending neuroleptic drug is stopped
(4) It may be prevented by intermittently stopping neuroleptic medication

201. Which of the following statements apply to benztropine?

(1) It is synthesized from a combination of active groups of atropine and diphenhydramine (Benadryl)
(2) In ordinary doses, it may be dangerous in the very young, the elderly, or in chronically ill persons
(3) It is very often effective in both drug-induced and naturally-occurring parkinsonism
(4) It is ineffective when given intravenously

202. Most major antipsychotic drugs produce which of the following pharmacologic actions?

(1) Production of involuntary movement syndromes
(2) Antiemesis
(3) Sedation and decreased response to stimuli
(4) Alpha-adrenergic blockade

203. Difficulties in using valproic acid concurrently with other anticonvulsants include which of the following?

(1) Alterations in the blood levels of other anticonvulsants
(2) Reduction in efficacy of major anticonvulsants
(3) Precipitation of absence status epilepticus when used with benzodiazepines
(4) Very slow development of valproic acid blood levels

DIRECTIONS: The group of questions below consists of lettered choices followed by several numbered items. For each numbered item select the **one** lettered choice with which it is **most** closely associated. Each lettered choice may be used once, more than once, or not at all.

Questions 204-207

For each of the drugs listed below, select the graphic formula which is the parent compound.

204. Clonazepam

205. Phenobarbital

206. Ethosuximide

207. Phenytoin (Dilantin)

Neuropharmacology Answers

171. The answer is A. *(Gilman, ed 6. pp 184-186.)* Control of cerebral edema requires intimate knowledge of the varying times required for different antiedema agents to act. This knowledge is necessary in order to judge whether any improvement observed in a patient may be attributed to the treatment. The effect of hyperventilation becomes apparent within minutes. Hyperventilation "blows off" CO_2, the most potent cerebral vasodilator known, and permits constriction of cerebral blood vessels. The reduction in the volume of intracranial blood leads to an almost immediate reduction in pressure. The patient's neurologic signs (such as obtundation, eye signs, or immobility) resulting from the edema should promptly improve. Mannitol infusion requires up to half an hour to produce clinical improvement, which should last several hours. Then, 12 to 18 hours later, dexamethasone (Decadron)—if administered at the outset—will show its effects. In the interim, additional doses of mannitol can be given.

172. The answer is D. *(Gilman, ed 6. p 426.)* The combination of delirium, pupillodilatation, dryness of skin and mucous membranes, tachycardia, and fever exhibited by the patient presented in the question suggests cholinergic (muscarinic) blockade, which most commonly would be due to ingestion of atropinelike drugs, including the tricyclic antidepressants. The drug of choice both for therapy and as a diagnostic aid is physostigmine, a potent peripheral and central anticholinesterase. Physostigmine, like many other anticholinesterases, penetrates the blood-brain barrier to counteract the central effects of the cholinergic blocking agents. It must be administered cautiously and the patient monitored in an intensive care unit (ICU) because of the tendency of this drug to cause cardiac arrhythmias and hypotension. Phenothiazines, which have cholinergic blocking action, would only worsen the patient's condition. Phenobarbital would further impair the patient's sensorium. A preferable anticonvulsant would be diazepam. Edrophonium would have muscarine and cholinergic effects peripherally, but not centrally, and would act for too short a period of time. Metrocurine iodide (Metubine) would block the nicotinic action of acetylcholine on skeletal muscle (which would not prove beneficial) and thiamine would be ineffective, although not harmful.

173. The answer is D. *(DeMyer, ed 3. p 98.)* To dilate the pupil without paralyzing accommodation requires a drug that stimulates sympathetic endings on the pupillodilator muscle, the only muscle of the eyeball innervated by the sympathetic nervous system. The parasympathetic nervous system innervates two muscles—the ciliary muscle required to adjust the lens thickness in accommodation, and the pupilloconstrictor muscle. A parasympathetic blocking agent would result in pupillodilatation, but it would paralyze the ciliary muscle and prevent lens thickening during accommodation. A drug that paralyzes the ciliary muscle is called a cycloplegic. During the action of the cycloplegic, the patient will have blurred vision because of the lack of ability to control lens thickness, and because of the large pupil that permits the light rays to traverse the periphery of the lens.

174. The answer is D. *(Gilman, ed 6. p 510.)* The clinical picture of the patient described in the question suggests morphine intoxication. A dose of intravenous naloxone provides the critical immediate diagnostic test by reversing the respiratory depression and pupilloconstriction. The result becomes apparent within a few minutes, and the test may be repeated two or three times. If a response fails to occur, the diagnosis of morphine intoxication becomes doubtful. In a patient without morphine intoxication, naloxone would have no observable effect. In the event of a negative response to the test, one might then consider a CAT scan or lumbar puncture. Administration of glucose would not be helpful since the glucose test-tape shows normal blood glucose level (which also excludes diabetic coma). Although respiratory assistance is indicated, it would be unwise to administer pure oxygen. In the presence of morphine intoxication, the breathing response to CO_2 is relatively depressed; thus, the patient depends upon the hypoxia as a stimulus to breathe. Under this circumstance, pure oxygen, by removing the effective stimulus to breathe, may further impair ventilation.

175. The answer is D. *(Gilman, ed.6. p 301.)* Local anesthetics such as procaine appear to act by blocking the voltage-dependent transient rise in membrane permeability to sodium that accompanies the nerve impulse. As sodium exits from the cell during passage of the nerve impulse, the membrane shows an increasing conductance to sodium that is voltage-dependent. Apparently, the anesthetic agent binds with the cell membrane in such a way as to block the sodium ''pores'' that permit the inward flow of sodium with the passage of the impulse. The local anesthetics may bond with the mobile phosphate tails of the molecules in the external lipid layer of the membrane, and may occupy the sites normally occupied by calcium. The resting potential of the cell is maintained, and the metabolic processes per se appear to remain intact during local anesthesia.

176. The answer is B. *(Gilman, ed 6. pp 448-491.)* Most of the drugs that have value in the treatment of spasticity work mainly through the central nervous system. Mephenesin and methocarbamol depress spinal polysynaptic reflexes. However, not all agents that depress polysynaptic reflexes reduce spasticity. Other centrally acting drugs that are active against spasticity may have different actions. Baclofen, although chemically related to GABA, hyperpolarizes primary afferent terminals rather than depolarizing them as does GABA. Cyclobenzaprine, chemically related to the tricyclic antidepressants, also acts centrally but by an unknown mechanism. Only dantrolene appears to have its primary action on muscle, where it may reduce the amount of calcium released from the sarcoplasmic reticulum. Although dantrolene reduces reflex muscle contractions more than volitional muscle contractions, its tendency to cause weakness limits its value.

177. The answer is A. *(Gilman, ed 6. pp 453-454.)* Phenytoin (Dilantin) has always presented a problem of bioavailability. It crystallizes out of solution, and its solubility and absorption vary with a number of factors. In the event a patient (like the child presented in the question) has indeed ingested the medication as ordered, the best management if the blood phenytoin level fails to rise with ingestion of phenytoin capsules is to switch to the suspension form of the drug. This step would be in accord with one of the most fundamental principles in the treatment of seizures—selection of the one drug most appropriate for the type of seizure involved and increasing it to the point of either seizure control or evidence of toxicity, as monitored by clinical response and blood level. Adding a second drug or switching drugs would only complicate the therapy. Valproic acid and carbamazepine (Tegretol) are more dangerous. Trimethadione (Tridione) not only is ineffective against generalized seizures but may increase them; and phenobarbital, by inducing enzymes, might even decrease the already low level of phenytoin and aggravate the child's hyperactivity.

178. The answer is D. *(Gilman, ed 6. p 75.)* Tachyphylaxis refers to the decreasing effect of repeated doses or repeated infusions of a drug. The usual explanation is that those drugs displaying tachyphylaxis act indirectly by releasing some of the natural neurotransmitter stored at the presynaptic nerve endings. Because only a limited amount of neurotransmitter is available for release, the repeated administration of the drug fails to produce any further release. The amount available for release by the drug is judged to be quite small, because nerve stimulation will produce the expected response even though repeated drug administration becomes ineffective. The administration of the appropriate sympathomimetic drug also will elicit the response, showing that the receptors remain functional.

179. The answer is E. *(DeMyer, ed 3. pp 176-177.)* Edrophonium should be given to a suspected myasthenic person until either some improvement occurs in the muscle function being assessed, or some symptoms or signs of cholinergic overactivity become apparent. In a pharmacologic test of this type, the clinician titrates the drug rather than giving a predetermined mg/kg-amount of medication. The medication is given until an end point is reached. Signs of either an improvement in the disease or of overdose constitute the end point. A common mistake in testing for myasthenia is to give too little medication. Some myasthenic individuals have a tremendous tolerance for anticholinesterase medications. Unless the medication is pushed to tolerance, the pharmacologic test may fail to identify these patients. Under some conditions, it might be wise to try any of the other procedures mentioned—a neostigmine, curare, or Jolly test—but an adequate edrophonium test should be completed first.

180. The answer is E. *(Gilman, ed 6. p 500.)* In a paraplegic patient, morphine decreases the withdrawal response of the paralyzed limbs to noxious stimulation. This effect is thought to be due to the blocking effect of morphine on the excitatory pain impulses in lamina I and II of the spinal cord, in the substantia gelatinosa. Morphine affects the descending root of the Vth nerve similarly. Injection of opiates into the substantia gelatinosa abolishes the excitatory activity in lamina V produced by noxious stimulation. Naloxone blocks these spinal cord effects of morphine. On the contrary, convulsant-strength doses of morphine fail to affect the paralyzed extremities of a paraplegic animal, suggesting that the convulsive actions of the drug involve structures rostral to the spinal level. Morphine injection in ordinary doses fails to affect nerve conduction velocity or spasticity.

181. The answer is D. *(Gilman, ed 6. pp 310, 453.)* Although anticonvulsants may have several actions, phenytoin (Dilantin) is thought to restrict the flow of sodium ions across resting neuronal membranes as well as membranes undergoing electrically or chemically induced depolarization. Tetrodotoxin and saxitoxin appear to act in the same way. Phenytoin will even block the sodium channels held open by veratroidine. Electrically, phenytoin does tend to cause **hyper**polarization of neuronal membranes, rather than depolarization. There is no satisfactory evidence that phenytoin has any primary action either on the enzymes that produce or degrade neurotransmitters, or in blocking neurotransmitter function by binding with receptors.

182. The answer is E. *(Gilman, ed 6. p 454.)* The tests most likely to disclose the cause of gradual mental changes and fatigability in a previously stable epileptic patient receiving phenytoin (Dilantin) treatment are a blood cell count and serum folic acid level determination. Long-term therapy with phenytoin tends to depress folate levels, which may be associated with a change in mental state. In the patient presented in the question, an EEG and CAT scan would be unlikely to contribute to the diagnosis because the patient suffered no seizures and failed to show change in the formal neurologic examination. A serum CPK determination and an EMG likewise would be unavailing because phenytoin does not cause myopathy. Similarly, phenytoin rarely if ever causes liver damage to the extent that it would be reflected in an hepatic encephalopathy. Neuropsychologic testing and psychiatric consultation might document mental changes but would fail to reveal their cause.

183. The answer is C. *(Barchas, p 143.)* Thioridazine (Mellaril) may produce a pigmentary retinopathy that can permanently reduce visual acuity, but this is unlikely to occur with doses less than 800 mg/day. Chlorpromazine (Thorazine) may produce photosensitivity and pigmentation in the skin or cornea. Phenothiazines can cause star-shaped deposits in the cornea or in the ocular media, as well as inducing the formation of cataracts. Patients who receive high doses of phenothiazines, particularly thioridazine, should be monitored by periodic tests of visual acuity, ophthalmoscopic examination, and slit-lamp inspection of the cornea and lens. The ocular toxicity of drugs depends on various factors, including the preferential concentration of the drug in ocular tissues, concomitant ingestion of other drugs, and individual idiosyncracy. Finally, the ocular manifestations of the basic neurologic or psychiatric disease have to be separated from those attributable to the medication itself.

184. The answer is B. *(Gilman, ed 6. p 457.)* Patients receiving long-term anticonvulsant therapy tend to show a reduction in serum calcium and an increase in alkaline phosphatase levels. Some patients then develop frank osteomalacia and rickets, which manifest clinically by weakness and pains in the back and extremities. To establish the diagnosis requires a demonstration of low serum calcium and high alkaline phosphatase levels and radiographic changes of osteomalacia and rickets. While other disorders such as collagen-vascular disease and peripheral neuropathy might cause similar symptoms, the most likely diagnosis of pain and weakness would be anticonvulsant-induced rickets. Treatment with vitamin D may completely reverse the symptoms and signs. The activation of hepatic enzymes by anticonvulsants might lead to the increased hydroxylation of vitamin D to its less potent metabolite.

185. The answer is B. *(Barchas, pp 220-221.)* The appearance of diarrhea, ataxia, fasciculations, overactive muscle stretch reflexes, and seizures in a patient who has been started on lithium therapy is entirely compatible with lithium toxicity. Since the usual therapeutic range for lithium is between 0.8 to 1.2 mEq/L, the observed value of 1.5 mEq/L would support a diagnosis of lithium toxicity. Moreover, since the patient recently began treatment, this blood level probably represents a fairly rapid climb of the lithium level. Such sudden changes are more likely to cause symptoms than very gradual changes. To invoke a coexistent disorder in this patient would violate the principle of diagnostic parsimony. Many of the symptoms of lithium overdosage imitate other states like delirium tremens, barbiturate withdrawal, or a thyroid storm—all of which may be associated with signs of overactivity of the nervous system in the form of tremors, increased stretch reflexes, and seizures. A thyroid crisis would be unlikely in this patient, because the effect of lithium is to reduce the thyroid function.

186. The answer is C. *(Adams, ed 2. p 58.)* Familial dystonic choreoathetosis may respond to diazepam (Valium), although not to phenobarbital or phenytoin (Dilantin). In familial paroxysmal kinesigenic choreoathetosis, affected patients may respond to phenobarbital or phenytoin. These types of paroxysmal familial choreoathetoses differ from most other involuntary movement disorders, which are unresponsive to these anticonvulsant medications. Apparently, the neuronal instability that underlies these familiar conditions differs from that which causes the commoner types of chorea, or athetosis. Tremors in general respond to neither diazepam nor anticonvulsants. Patients with dystonia musculorum deformans may respond well to carbamazepine.

187. The answer is A. *(Cooper, ed 3. pp 173-176.)* Usually, when a neuronal pathway ceases to function or becomes less active, the synthesis and metabolism of the neurotransmitter are reduced accordingly. The nigrostriatal dopaminergic pathway seems to be anomalous in this regard. When impulse flow in this pathway is interrupted by mechanical or pharmacologic lesions, the amount of dopamine in the axonal terminals in the striatum increases, and the activity of the rate-limiting enzyme tyrosine hydroxylase also increases. Just how this increased enzyme activity occurs is unclear. Similar increases in the activity of tyrosine hydroxylase fail to occur in central norepinephrinergic pathways when they are quiescent. In fact, the norepinephrinergic pathways respond in the opposite way.

188. The answer is A. *(Bell, vol 12. p 98.)* Because of the frequency of seizures in the acute and chronic stage of brain abscesses, some authorities advocate routine use of prophylactic anticonvulsant medication. Obtundation can be avoided by monitoring anticonvulsant blood levels. Therapeutic levels of anticonvulsants neither interfere with antibiotic administration nor increase the intracranial pressure. Because other authorities object to routine anticonvulsant medication in brain abscess, the practice remains controversial.

189. The answer is D (4). *(Gilman, ed 6. p 454.)* All anticonvulsant drugs have adverse effects. A relatively common effect of chronic phenytoin (Dilantin) administration is peripheral neuropathy. Although it may fail to reach a symptomatic level, the neuropathy manifests by reduced conduction velocity of the peripheral nerves. The possible role of phenytoin in causing degeneration of Purkinje cells in humans remains controversial. The cerebellar atrophy caused by seizures may obscure the role of anticonvulsant drugs in this regard, but currently available evidence fails to establish phenytoin as a cause of Purkinje cell degeneration. Although aplastic anemia and liver necrosis occur with other anticonvulsants—such as valproic acid and carbamazepine—these effects, if they occur at all, are extremely rare with phenytoin.

190. The answer is B (1, 3). *(Barchas, pp 94, 144, 280.)* Phenothiazine-induced hypotension usually can be successfully managed by placing a patient in the recumbent position, fluid therapy, and administration of norepinephrine (4 mg in 500 ml by infusion), with titration of the dose by measurement of the patient's blood pressure. Norepinephrine, an alpha-adrenergic drug with little beta-adrenergic activity, is chosen in preference to isoproterenol and epinephrine, which are beta-adrenergic. The latter drugs may exacerbate the hypotension. Phenothiazines produce alpha blockade, and in the presence of such a blockade, the beta-adrenergic vasodilating activity of isoproterenol and epinephrine may worsen the hypotension. The alpha-adrenergic activity of norepinephrine does not have this adverse effect.

191. The answer is A (1, 2, 3). *(Gilman, ed 6. pp 521-522.)* The opiate receptors are relatively numerous in the limbic system, diencephalon, midbrain, and striatum. They combine with endogenous polypeptides, some of which may act as natural blockers of pain. Naloxone, a synthetic chemical relative of morphine, combines with the opiate receptors to reverse certain of the effects of morphine. The receptors do not produce an identical response to the various opiates. At least three classes of receptors have been identified—the mu, kappa, and sigmoid types. Of these, the mu type appears to be involved in the supraspinal type of analgesia, euphoria, physical dependence, and respiratory depression.

192. The answer is C (2, 4). *(Cooper, ed 3. p 11.)* Drugs like colchicine that cause a disarrangement in microtubules characteristically arrest cell division in metaphase and impair axoplasmic transport. Microtubules pull apart the chromosomes as the cell proceeds from metaphase to anaphase. The microtubules also appear to function in axoplasmic flow. Disarrangement of microtubules therefore impairs metaphase and axoplasmic flow.

193. The answer is D (4). *(DeMyer, ed 3. pp 175-177.)* Clinically, a myasthenic crisis and overmedication with anticholinergic medication may imitate each other closely. Weakness will usually predominate in the ocular and bulbar musculature, if that is the pattern of a patient's symptoms prior to treatment. However, in the myasthenic crisis, the amount of acetylcholine at the end-plate is too small, whereas after overdosage with anticholinesterase drugs, the amount may be excessive and lead to weakness from end-plate depolarization. The edrophonium test provides a quick way to differentiate a myasthenic crisis from overdosage. Edrophonium, a short-acting anticholinesterase, will improve a patient's strength in a myasthenic crisis and worsen it in a cholinergic crisis. In the former case, the patient needs more anticholinesterase medication, while in the latter, the patient needs less. A moderate dose of edrophonium may cause fasciculations and incontinence in nonmyasthenic patients, but not in myasthenic individuals who have a large tolerance to it.

194. The answer is B (1, 3). *(Gilman, ed 6. pp 477-482.)* In preparing to start a parkinsonian patient on L-dopa, a physician must take several precautionary steps. The patient should be ascertained to be free of serious systemic disease and should have a sound mentality. A baseline series of studies to include an ECG and tests of liver and kidney function should all show normal results. If the patient takes a proprietary vitamin preparation, it should be discontinued in favor of a special one without pyridoxine. Pyridoxine enhances the extracerebral metabolism of L-dopa by the pyridoxine-dependent enzyme L-amino acid decarboxylase. Exactly the opposite effect is desired. The peripheral decarboxylation of L-dopa can be reduced by the concurrent administration of carbidopa. Monoamine oxidase inhibitors are contraindicated because they increase the concentration of catecholamines or serotonin and may lead to cerebral excitation and hypertension. After completing all precautionary measures, the physician begins L-dopa with 0.5 to 1.0 gm per day in divided doses. Previous anticholinergic medications may be continued, at least during the early weeks before the dose of L-dopa reaches maximally effective levels.

195. The answer is C (2, 4). *(DeMyer, ed 3. p 177.)* A patient suffering from overdose of an anticholinesterase drug would experience abdominal cramping and salivation, but would show bradycardia rather than tachycardia, and sweating rather than dry skin. The anticholinesterase drugs increase the amount of acetylcholine at the end-plates of the autonomic and somatic nervous systems. The parasympathetic effects consist of pupilloconstriction and ciliary stimulation with blurred vision, salivary gland stimulation with salivation, vagal stimulation with bradycardia, and bowel and bladder stimulation with abdominal cramping, diarrhea, and micturition. The sympathetic effects consist of sweating, and the somatic muscle effects consist of fasciculations and cramps, particularly a feeling of tightness in myasthenic muscles. The reason that an anticholinesterase causes a sympathetic response (sweating) is that the postganglionic fibers to the sweat glands are cholinergic, even though the preganglionic fibers are adrenergic.

196. The answer is E (all). *(Gilman, ed 6. pp 507-508.)* Among the many contraindications to the administration of morphine are acute head injury with alteration of consciousness, hypovolemic shock, asthma, and cor pulmonale. When head injuries cause alteration of consciousness, the brain suffers concussion, contusion, or hemorrhage. The hemorrhage may be intraventricular, intraparenchymal, or in the meninges. In any event, the brain suffers from compression or edema; morphine, which increases intracranial pressure, worsens the condition. It also constricts the pupils, thereby masking pupillary changes that serve as a guide to the clinical state of the patient. In hypovolemic shock, morphine may worsen the hypotension. Morphine is generally contraindicated in any condition involving poor pulmonary function such as asthma or cor pulmonale, because its central effect may depress respiration and further impair breathing. Morphine also releases histamine, which constricts the respiratory passages.

197. The answer is A (1, 2, 3). *(Adams, ed 2. p 873.)* The pyrophosphates, succinylcholine, and edrophonium act as anticholinesterase agents. Acetylcholine accumulates at the end-plates because of inactivation of cholinesterase. The excess of acetylcholine at the end-plate keeps the end-plate in a depolarized state. The muscle is paralyzed because it is unable to respond to the arrival of new nerve impulses, which release more acetylcholine. Pyrophosphates are ingredients of some insecticides. The quarternary ammonium compounds also paralyze muscle but they act by blocking the receptor sites for acetylcholine.

198. The answer is D (4). *(Barchas, pp 24-30. Cooper, ed 3. pp 133-134.)* Tyrosine hydroxylase converts tyrosine to dihydroxyphenylalanine on its way to norepinephrine and epinephrine. The activity of tyrosine hydroxylase undergoes a homeostatic adjustment to the need for catecholaminergic neurotransmitter, but pharmacologic manipulation can also alter its activity. Increased neuronal activity requires more neurotransmitter and activates or increases the action of the synthetic enzymes like tyrosine hydroxylase that produce the transmitter. Administration of a MAO inhibitor will increase the amount of intraneuronal catecholamine, resulting in a feedback inhibition of tyrosine hydroxylase. Administration of tyramine increases the amount of intracellular catecholamine and also produces a feedback inhibition of catecholamine synthesis. Administration of 6-hydroxydopamine selectively kills catecholaminergic neurons and thus results in an absence of their contained enzymes, including tyrosine hydroxylase. Many drugs, like α-methyl-*p*-tyrosine and other amino acid analogs, will inhibit tyrosine hydroxylase, and some may find clinical application for that reason.

199. The answer is D (4). *(Gilman, ed 6. p 454.)* A physician should inform an epileptic woman that anticonvulsant drugs appear to be teratogenic, and thus they increase the risk of producing a malformed child. The physician does not advise her to avoid pregnancy. Having informed the patient of the reproductive risks involved, the physician leaves the ultimate decision to the patient who is mentally sound. Anticonvulsant medication should be continued throughout the pregnancy. Pregnancy has a variable effect on seizures and on the amount of medication required, and some pregnant women will require increased medication for seizure control. Even though anticonvulsants may depress folic acid metabolism, administration of large doses of folic acid (or any other chemical agent) may in itself be teratogenic. The woman should receive small doses of vitamin K near term because anticonvulsant drugs depress vitamin K-dependent coagulation factors in the baby and may lead to neonatal bleeding.

200. The answer is D (4). *(Gilman, ed 6. pp 407-413.)* Tardive dyskinesias occur most commonly in patients treated with phenothiazines or haloperidol. The most widely accepted current theory of pathogenesis is that the chronic pharmacologic blockade of dopamine receptors by the drugs leads to hypersensitivity. This theory might explain the observation that the tardive dyskinesia frequently fails to appear until discontinuation of the psychotrophic medication. The hypersensitive receptors, then unblocked, respond to the intrinsic dopamine released by dopaminergic synaptic terminals. Administration of dopa worsens the condition, as do anticholinergic (or more particularly antimuscarinic) drugs, by blocking the inhibitory effect of the cholinergic systems on the dopaminergic systems. Intermittent drug furloughs during long-term neuroleptic drug therapy are reputed to reduce the incidence of tardive dyskinesia.

201. The answer is A (1, 2, 3). *(Gilman, ed 6. p 486.)* Benztropine is synthesized from the active groupings of atropine and diphenhydramine (Benadryl). Thus, it has both anticholinergic and antihistaminic actions. It is effective when given orally for both naturally-occurring and drug-induced parkinsonism. It can be given intravenously to interrupt especially severe drug-induced parkinsonism, dystonia, or other involuntary movements. Because of its atropine-like activity, benztropine may be dangerous for very young, elderly, or chronically ill individuals. In the latter, it may block sweating and lead to hyperthermia in hot weather. It may augment a psychotic state in patients with organic dementia or in mentally ill patients taking neuroleptic medications. The symptoms of overdosage in any patient resemble those of atropine intoxication.

202. The answer is E (all). *(Barchas, pp 130-131.)* The major antipsychotic drugs, consisting of phenothiazines, thioxanthenes, and butyrophenones, share a number of pharmacologic properties. These include the production of involuntary movement syndromes, antiemetic properties, sedation and decreased response to stimuli, and alpha-adrenergic blockade. These common pharmacologic properties are thought to be related to the common sites of action in the nervous system. Centrally, the drugs affect the reticular formation, limbic, hypothalamic, and basal ganglia structures—all of which have short chain, polysynaptic pathways with numerous and varied chemical neurotransmitter systems. These pathways stand in contrast to the long sensory and motor tracts that operate through relatively few synapses and with a more restricted number of neurotransmitters. These long pathways and their functions are affected relatively less by the major antipsychotic drugs.

203. The answer is B (1, 3). *(Gilman, ed 6. p 463.)* Valproic (dipropylacetic) acid causes alterations, sometimes unpredictable, in the levels of other anticonvulsants. It elevates phenobarbital levels and may either increase or decrease phenytoin levels. It does not appear to reduce the therapeutic efficacy of these anticonvulsants, but when given with clonazepam (Clonopin) may precipitate absence status epilepticus. Concurrent administration of valproic acid and other anticonvulsant drugs does not materially impede the achievement of adequate blood levels of valproic acid. Valproic acid, like carbamazepine in being one of the fastest drugs to reach therapeutic blood levels, requires only 1-3 days to reach 95% of its steady state level.

204-207. The answers are: 204-D, 205-A, 206-C, 207-B. *(Gilman, ed 6. pp 448-474.)* Studies of the relationship of drug structure to pharmacologic effect show that many drugs with similar actions have a common structural grouping. Side chains or radicals attached to the common grouping change the potency and actions of the compounds.

In several anticonvulsant drugs, the common grouping is barbituric acid (figure A). Barbituric acid comes from the condensation of urea plus malonic acid to form a six-atom ring with four carbon atoms and two nitrogen atoms. The hydantoin ring (figure B) similarly may be regarded as the product of condensation of urea and glycolic acid. Urea thus forms a basic unit of both rings. The monoureides and diureides, as in barbituric acid and hydantoin, tend to appear in many centrally active compounds. For barbituric acid to have potent hypnotic and anticonvulsant properties, certain alkyl or aryl groups must replace the hydrogen atoms on position 5 of the barbituric acid ring. On the other hand, if the alkyl side chains on the 5th position are too long, the drug becomes a convulsant instead of an anticonvulsant. Phenobarbital has an ethyl and a phenyl grouping attached to the 5th position of its six-atom ring. Hydantoin has anticonvulsant action with two phenyl groups attached to the 5th position of its five-atom ring. Both phenobarbital and phenytoin have two carbonyl groups and two nitrogen atoms in their rings. While these correlations give us a satisfying sense of order, they do not permit us to understand how these drugs work.

Another group of ring structures with anticonvulsant properties derives from benzodiazepine (figure D). Again in a psychoactive drug, we find the familiar nitrogen-carbon ring, but this time with seven atoms. Benzodiazepines are thought to have greater effectiveness against anxiety than other anticonvulsants, but this action is difficult to prove, and the benzodiazepines are undoubtedly overprescribed for this purpose. By varying the groups attached to the positions on the benzodiazepine rings, biochemists have produced a family of compounds that vary greatly in their length of action and biotransformation. Thus, oxazepam has a half-life of about 5-15 hours and produces no active metabolites, while flurazepam has a half-life of around 100 hours and produces N-desalkylflurazepam.

In contrast to the foregoing families of drugs, dipropylacetate (valproic acid) (figure E) has no ring and consists of a relatively simple molecule; yet it, too, has strong anticonvulsant properties.

Neuroradiology

DIRECTIONS: Each question below contains five suggested answers. Choose the **one best** response to each question.

208. In the radiograph shown below, the most likely interpretation is

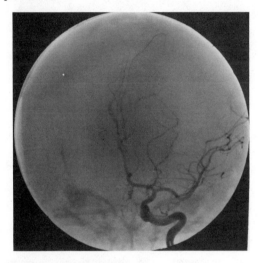

(A) normal angiogram
(B) subfalcial herniation
(C) aneurysm of the internal carotid artery
(D) upward displacement of the first segment (A1) of the anterior cerebral artery
(E) downward displacement of the first segment (M1) of the middle cerebral artery

209. The most reliable measure of orbital hypertelorism or hypotelorism in patients with malformation syndromes is the

(A) intercanthal distance
(B) external canthal distance
(C) interpupillary distance
(D) interorbital distance on skull radiographs
(E) lateral diameter of the skull

210. In the radiograph shown below, the most likely diagnosis is

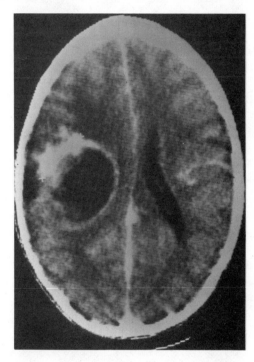

(A) cysticercosis
(B) astrocytoma
(C) intracerebral hematoma
(D) purulent abscess
(E) univentricular dilation

211. For a patient suspected of a chronic brain abscess, the single procedure that would provide the most information is

(A) lumbar puncture
(B) CAT with contrast
(C) angiography
(D) radioactive brain scan
(E) EEG

212. In the accompanying radiograph of a 5-year-old child, the most likely diagnosis is

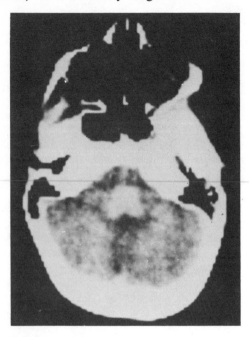

(A) cerebellar edema
(B) Arnold-Chiari malformation
(C) chordoma
(D) medulloblastoma
(E) brain stem glioma

213. In the accompanying radiograph of a 58-year-old man, the most likely diagnosis is

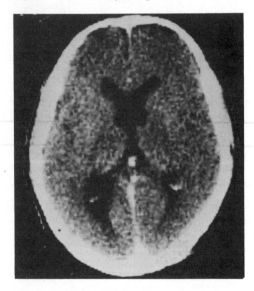

(A) pseudotumor cerebri
(B) late onset demyelinating disease
(C) presenile dementia of Alzheimer
(D) normal pressure hydrocephalus
(E) normal brain

214. The accompanying radiograph, in which the lesion showed faintly on the unenhanced scan, most probably indicates the presence of

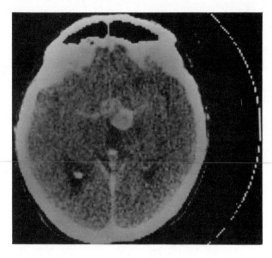

(A) an internal carotid aneurysm
(B) a colloid cyst of the third ventricle
(C) an astrocytoma of the anterior third ventricle
(D) a tuberculum sella meningioma
(E) a craniopharyngioma

215. In the accompanying radiograph of a retarded infant with microcephaly, the most likely diagnosis is

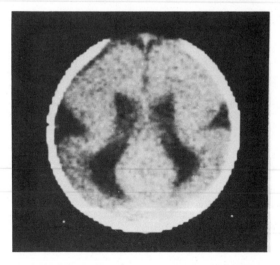

(A) microcephaly vera
(B) holoprosencephaly
(C) encephaloclastic porencephaly
(D) schizencephaly
(E) birth anoxia with infarction

216. In the radiograph shown below, the most likely diagnosis is

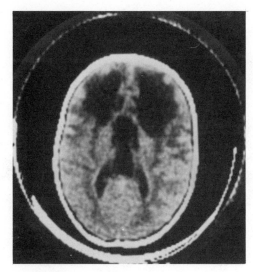

(A) bifrontal porencephaly
(B) obstructive internal hydrocephalus
(C) orbitofrontal contusion
(D) status postprefrontal lobotomy
(E) demyelinating encephalopathy

217. In the radiograph shown below, the most likely diagnosis is

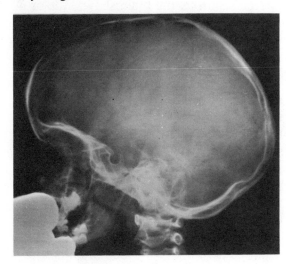

(A) normal child's skull
(B) sellar erosion
(C) pathologic frontal thinning
(D) obstruction of pharyngeal air space
(E) osteoporosis

218. The following angiogram is best described as displaying

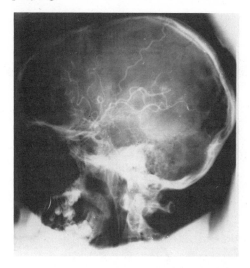

(A) normal vessels
(B) nonfilling of branches of middle cerebral artery
(C) a parasellar aneurysm
(D) arteriovenous shunting from the intracranial to extracranial vessels
(E) tumor blush in the posterior parietal region

219. The accompanying angiogram showed the same pattern in both cerebral hemispheres. The most likely diagnosis is

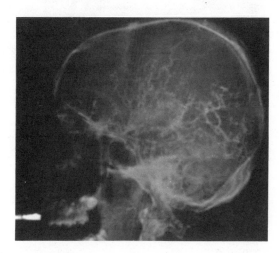

(A) normal tissue
(B) diffuse gliosis of the cerebral hemispheres (neurofibromatosis)
(C) multiple hamartomas
(D) multiple progressive arterial occlusions (moyamoya disease)
(E) congenital arteriovenous shunting

220. The calcified lesion in the accompanying radiographs is located in the

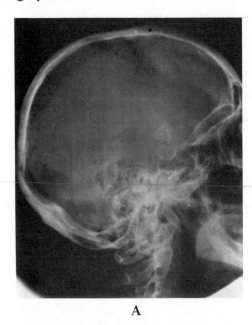

A

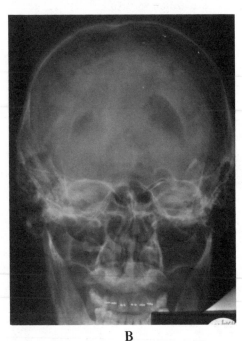

B

(A) suprasellar region
(B) frontal lobe
(C) temporal pole
(D) sylvian fissure
(E) skull

221. The large dark shadow shown in the posterior part of the following pneumoencephalogram represents

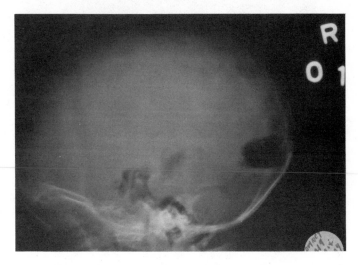

(A) normal cisterna magna cerebelli
(B) cerebellar atrophy
(C) a Dandy-Walker cyst
(D) a subarachnoid cyst of the posterior fossa
(E) occipital lobe porencephaly

222. After intravenous administration of radio-active norepinephrine, the brain shows little or no uptake, but it does show uptake after intraventricular injection. The best operational conclusion (as distinguished from an interpretation) to be drawn from this single experiment is that

(A) norepinephrine must pass from the blood into the CSF before entering the brain
(B) the blood-brain barrier excludes radioactive substances
(C) all substances pass more freely from the ventricular fluid into the brain than from the blood
(D) the ventricular fluid-brain barrier has a different permeability to radioactive norepinephrine than does the blood-brain barrier
(E) radioactive norepinephrine enters the brain from the intraventricular fluid at a different rate than from the blood

223. A 50-year-old female patient with the unenhanced CAT scan in the accompanying illustrations would most likely have which of the following?

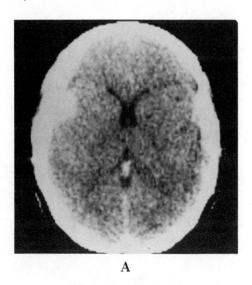

A

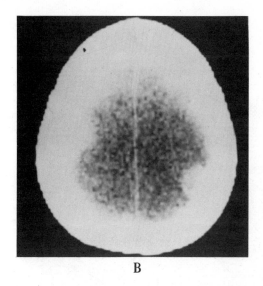

B

(A) Primary carcinoma of the breast
(B) Bronchiectasis with lung abscess
(C) Polycystic kidneys
(D) Paget's disease
(E) Multiple café au lait spots

DIRECTIONS: Each question below contains four suggested answers of which **one** or **more** is correct. Choose the answer

A	if	1, 2, and 3	are correct
B	if	1 and 3	are correct
C	if	2 and 4	are correct
D	if	4	is correct
E	if	1, 2, 3, and 4	are correct

224. The accompanying pneumoencephalogram shows which of the following?

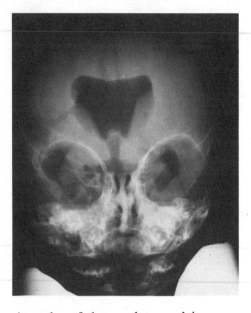

(1) Atrophy of the caudate nuclei
(2) Porencephaly
(3) Agenesis of the corpus callosum
(4) Absence of median plane structures

225. The accompanying angiogram shows which of the following features?

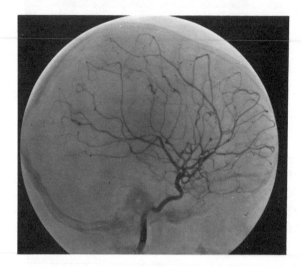

(1) Multiple berry aneurysms
(2) Upward displacement of the posterior cerebral arteries
(3) Peeling away of the vessels from the undersurface of the skull
(4) Internal hydrocephalus

226. A CAT scan of the head is characterized by which of the following statements?

(1) The usual angle of the CAT scan is 20-25 degrees to the cantho-meatal line
(2) The amount of radiation exposure from a CAT scan is about three times that of a routine skull series of five exposures
(3) The wider the window, the less the contrast on the reconstructed CAT image
(4) After passing through a patient's head, the photons that will produce the image impinge on an x-ray film

227. The accompanying radiograph is consistent with which of the following statements?

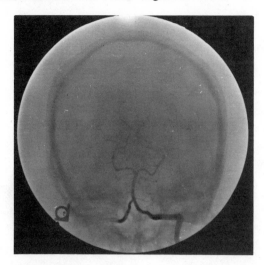

(1) One vertebral artery is pathologically small and stenotic
(2) The basilar artery appears to be normal
(3) The space between the bends of the posterior cerebral arteries is widened, indicating a midbrain mass
(4) The superior cerebellar arteries show a normal caliber

228. The lesion demonstrated in the accompanying radioactive brain scan would very likely be accompanied by clinical findings that include

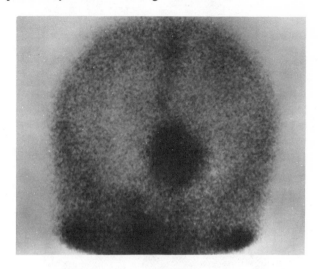

(1) mild personality changes
(2) ataxia
(3) unilateral anosmia
(4) visual hallucinations

DIRECTIONS: The groups of questions below consist of lettered choices followed by several numbered items. For each numbered item select the **one** lettered choice with which it is **most** closely associated. Each lettered choice may be used once, more than once, or not at all.

Questions 229-232

Match the vessels listed below with the letters on the radiograph.

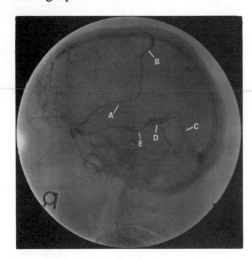

229. Basal vein of Rosenthal

230. Venous angle

231. Vein of Galen

232. Vein of Trolard

Questions 233-236

For each neuroanatomic structure listed below, choose the lettered structure on the radiograph to which it is most closely related.

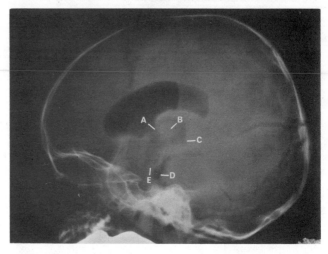

233. Interventricular foramen of Monro

234. Optic chiasm

235. Interpeduncular cistern

236. Massa intermedia

Questions 237-241

For each cranial nerve listed below, choose the skull aperture through which it passes.

    (A) Canal of Dorello
    (B) Superior orbital fissure
    (C) Jugular foramen
    (D) Stylomastoid foramen
    (E) Foramen lacerum

237. Xth cranial nerve

238. IIIrd cranial nerve

239. Ophthalmic division of the Vth cranial nerve

240. VIth cranial nerve

241. IXth cranial nerve

Neuroradiology
Answers

208. The answer is B. *(Taveras, ed 2. pp 656-657.)* The arteriogram accompanying the question shows a posterior or distal shift of the anterior cerebral vessels. The proximal part of the anterior cerebral artery begins to ascend in the midline, then shows a gentle arcing across the midline to the opposite side. The posterior cerebral artery fills on this angiogram, as does the middle cerebral artery. The carotid siphon shows its normal configuration. The distal type of shift of the anterior cerebral vessels indicates a posterior frontal or parietal mass. The more anterior the mass, the more the proximal parts of the anterior cerebral artery are involved in the shift. Then, the so-called rounded shift occurs in which the proximal part of the anterior cerebral artery forms a round curve across the midline and an abrupt return of the vessels under the falx to produce a notch effect on the frontal radiograph. The patient in question had a massive, high parietofrontal glioma. In addition to the arteriogram, the venogram also provides valuable evidence of a midline shift of the brain. The internal cerebral vein is nearly in the midline, and slight displacement can be read with accuracy. Moreover, since it is much nearer to the center of rotation of the head, it is less distorted than the anterior cerebral artery when the frontal film is not well-centered.

209. The answer is D. *(DeMyer, ed 3. p 5.)* The most reliable measure of ocular hypertelorism or hypotelorism is the interorbital distance as measured on posterior-anterior radiographs. Any measure of the spacing of the eyes based on the soft tissues, either the lids or eyeballs themselves, may produce a gross error. The intercanthal distance does not necessarily reflect the space between the eyes. Lateral displacement of the medial canthi relative to the orbital spacing regularly occurs in Down's and Waardenburg's syndromes and may lead to a spurious diagnosis of hypertelorism. In a patient with exotropia or esotropia, measurement of the interpupillary distance fails to reflect the anatomic spacing of the orbits. Measurement of the distance between the medial walls of the bony orbits on posterior-anterior radiographs is thus the most reliable way to determine the interorbital distance.

210. The answer is B. *(Taveras, ed 2. p 685.)* The radiograph accompanying the question shows a huge cystic lesion, with a peripheral ring of contrast medium enhancement. In the anterolateral aspect of the cyst, an enhancing nodule appears. These features would be most typical of a cystic astrocytoma of the cerebral hemisphere. Astrocytomas, wherever they appear—in the cerebrum, brain stem, or cerebellum—tend to form cysts. These may be small in size, but usually are large enough to compress adjacent tissue and add to the neurologic deficit, which improves after surgical drainage of the cyst. Cysticercosis cysts tend to be multiple and to show calcification. The cysts usually involve the choroid plexuses of the lateral ventricles, the fourth ventricle, and the basal meninges. A purulent abscess shows the enhancing ring, but lacks a discrete nodular mass. A hematoma would be uniformly radiodense rather than showing an enhancing ring.

211. The answer is B. *(Adams, ed 2. pp 489-490.)* For a patient suspected of a chronic brain abscess, the single procedure that provides the most information is the CAT scan. Although not pathognomonic, the characteristic ring around the lesion shown by contrast enhancement in the CAT scan, in connection with the clinical findings, provides sufficient evidence to treat the patient as having an abscess. Angiography, EEG, and the radioactive scan may be helpful, but they fail to provide the maximum amount of information. They can localize the lesion, but the EEG and radioactive scan fail to give information about internal herniation of the brain, nor do they discriminate between focal cerebritis and encapsulation. CAT scan thus provides a basis for surgical decisions and for the subsequent management of the patient. Definitive findings on the CAT scan obviate a need for EEG and radioactive scanning or angiography, thus greatly reducing the risk and expense to the patient.

212. The answer is E. *(Taveras, ed 2. pp 494-498.)* The radiograph accompanying the question shows an extreme increase in the radiodensity of the medulla oblongata. Autopsy examination confirmed the presence of a brain stem glioma. The radiograph shows that the cerebellar hemispheres and vermis have the normal radiodensity and configuration. The fourth ventricle is normal in size, shape, and position, thus excluding a medulloblastoma, a lesion that ordinarily occupies the fourth ventricle and distorts the cerebellar vermis. A chordoma would occupy the clivus, which forms the bony surface ventral to the medulla. Growing epidurally, chordomas compress the subarachnoid space ventral to the medulla. These tumors contain calcium and destroy the bone of the clivus, features absent in the radiograph. In the Arnold-Chiari malformation, the cerebellum and medulla occupy the rostral part of the cervical canal. The normal position of the cerebellum, medulla, and fourth ventricle rules out that malformation.

213. The answer is D. *(Adams, ed 2. pp 434-435.)* The radiograph accompanying the question shows a moderate increase in ventricular size without increase in the sulcal markings. The most likely diagnosis is normal pressure hydrocephalus. In presenile dementia, sulcal enlargement accompanies the ventricular enlargement. In pseudotumor cerebri, the ventricles are small-to-normal in size. In demyelinating diseases, the white matter becomes more radiolucent. Although the syndrome of normal pressure hydrocephalus remains controversial, Adams and Victor maintain that it is a valid entity if strict diagnostic criteria are applied. Assuming that a patient exhibits the triad of dementia, incontinence, and gait disorder, these authors advocate insertion of a shunt, which they state leads to reversal of the neurologic syndrome over a period of several weeks and even more rapid reduction in ventricular size.

214. The correct answer is A. *(Taveras, ed 2. pp 919-921.)* The radiograph accompanying the question shows a large, rounded, opacified aneurysm on the right side. It is filled with contrast material that also reveals the vessels of the anterior part of the circle of Willis. In the differential diagnosis of this lesion, several factors require consideration. The filling of the lesion by contrast material establishes it as highly vascular. Its location would be compatible with a variety of sellar and parasellar lesions. Hence, the diagnosis becomes one of a vascularized para- or suprasellar mass. Craniopharyngiomas and colloid cysts are not vascularized lesions but their surface vessels may become prominent. Gliomas of the third ventricle lack this pattern of rounded, regular opacification. Typically, a tuberculum sella meningioma (a highly vascular lesion) would present more anteriorly and more in the midline, as would an intrasellar lesion, although they can be asymmetrical. The location of the lesion is most typical for an aneurysm, as was conclusively shown by angiography.

215. The answer is D. *(Lemire, p 243.)* The radiograph accompanying the question shows symmetrical clefting along the line of the central sulcus, a condition called schizencephaly. The film shows that the cleft begins in incomplete operculatization of the insular region and extends up along the usual site of the central sulcus. Schizencephaly refers to bilaterally symmetrical clefts along the line of a major sulcus. These clefts are presumed to derive from a developmental error rather than from a destructive lesion. Therefore, although they represent defects in the cerebral wall, they differ from the encephaloclastic porencephalies due to a destructive process, most of which result from anoxia associated with cerebral infarction. The radiograph also shows only one sulcus in the frontal region, indicating pachygyria. In microcephaly vera the brain is miniaturized, but otherwise shows a fairly normal configuration. In holoprosencephaly, radiographs show incomplete separation of the hemispheres.

216. The answer is E. *(Cole, J Neurol Neurosurg Psychiatry 42:619-624, 1979.)* The radiograph accompanying the question shows maximal demyelination bifrontally. The third ventricle is greatly enlarged, but the type of demyelinating encephalopathy in this patient is Alexander's disease, as shown in this case by brain biopsy. The characteristic histopathological finding is Rosenthal fibers. These consist of club-shaped eosinophilic bodies strewn in the cerebral cortex and white matter. They presumably derive from degenerative changes in proliferated astrocytes. The CAT scan, showing intense demyelination of the frontal lobes, is almost pathognomonic for Alexander's disease, but the reason for the localization of the process is unknown. Another type of demyelinating encephalopathy, adrenoleukodystrophy, affects the occipital lobes maximally. Clinically, the patient with Alexander's disease, usually a young child or infant, shows a retrogressive syndrome with dementia, seizures, and increasing quadriparesis.

217. The answer is A. *(Taveras, ed 2. p 42.)* The radiograph accompanying the question shows a normal child's skull. The absence of the frontal sinus and the normal thinness of the frontal table indicate an immature individual. The frontal sinus develops and the diploic space thickens as the skull matures. The bone density, bone contours, and the adenoid tissue forming an indentation dorsally into the pharyngeal space all are normal.

218. The answer is B. *(Taveras, ed 2. pp 600-610.)* The radiograph accompanying the question demonstrates a lack of filling of the central and posterior parietal branches of the middle cerebral artery. The other two superior branches, the orbitofrontal and the operculofrontal arteries, do fill, as do the temporal branches of the middle cerebral artery. The vessel that appears to occupy the avascular region of the central and parietal branches and run diagonally to the vertex actually is an extracranial vessel, the superficial temporal artery. It is identified by its characteristic location and linear course with smaller undulations. The pericallosal branch of the anterior cerebral artery also fails to fill. In this patient, it filled from injection of the opposite carotid, a variation seen in normal individuals.

219. The answer is D. *(Taveras, ed 2. pp 902-909.)* The angiogram accompanying the question shows multiple neovascular channels that give a cloud-like appearance when filled with contrast material. The term moyamoya is the Japanese word for a cloud of smoke or haze. The disease was first described in Japanese, but affects other races. It typically presents as a progressive syndrome of multiple vascular accidents in an older child or young adult, with the patient having a series of strokelike clinical exacerbations such as alternating hemiparesis, hemianopia, dementia, and seizures. Although the exact pathogenesis of the condition remains in doubt, progressive occlusion of the carotid system apparently leads to rich anastomoses—a rete mirabile forming from vessels at the base of the brain and at its surface. Moyamoya disease tends to spare the vertebrobasilar system.

220. The answer is D. *(Taveras, ed 2. pp 205-218.)*   The radiographs accompanying the question show a calcified lesion that on the lateral view appears to be suprasellar in location, but on the frontal view is seen as being located in the stem of the sylvian fissure. Therefore, it is between the superomedial aspect of the temporal lobe and the inferior aspect of the frontal lobe. The angulation of the lesion on the frontal view exactly follows the angulation of the sylvian fissure. Here, the middle cerebral artery runs and follows the same angulation as the stem of the sylvian fissure. At autopsy, however, the lesion appeared to be unattached to the arteries and was easily shelled out. It thus constitutes a so-called brain rock, a calcareous mass of uncertain origin. These relatively benign lesions have to be distinguished from significant lesions, such as craniopharyngiomas.

221. The answer is A. *(Taveras, ed 2. pp 356-359.)*   The cisterna magna varies greatly in size. The one shown in the radiograph accompanying the question, while large, is within normal limits. Its size does not represent cerebellar atrophy. To read cerebellar atrophy in a pneumo-encephalogram requires demonstration of a reduction of folial size by the increased amount of air in the cerebellar sulci or by tomography. The cisterna magna may even extend upward above the tentorium through a defect in the posterior attachment of the tentorium to the occipital bone. The filling of the cisterna magna during this early phase pneumoencephalo-gram, before any air has entered the ventricular system, fails to indicate obstruction of the fourth ventricle inlets, which might be the case with a posterior fossa cyst. In addition, arach-noid cysts are seldom observed to fill from lumbar air injections.

222. The answer is E. *(Cooper, ed 3. pp 148-150. DeMyer, ed 3. p 40.)*   The results of the experiment described in the question show that radioactive norepinephrine enters the brain from the intraventricular fluid at a different rate than from the blood. This is an operational conclusion that asserts the experimental fact. The other conclusions either interpret the result by proposing some mechanism that was not actually operationally tested, or make unfounded generalizations. For example, it would be an interpretation to say that the intraventricular fluid-brain barrier differs from the blood-brain barrier, because no barrier was actually tested. What was actually measured was a difference in the uptake of one substance (radioactive norepinephrine) from two fluids—intraventricular fluid and blood. The reason the material failed to enter from the blood might be related to some chemical or physical property of the blood rather than some "barrier" per se. Conversely, a barrier between CSF and the brain may be nonexistent (and indeed none has been demonstrated), and many substances seem to pass freely from CSF to brain and brain to CSF. The errors caused by making unnecessary in-terpretations, and the failure to differentiate between observation and interpretation have led to much confusion in the field of psychopharmacology.

223. The answer is E. *(Adams, ed 2. pp 847-849.)*   The radiographs accompanying the question show three separate radiodense lesions adjacent to the inner surface of the skull. Their location and visibility on the unenhanced scan suggest meningiomas. The condition likely to be associated with multiple meningiomas is von Recklinghausen's disease (neurofibromatosis). Patients with neurofibromatosis have multiple café au lait spots, which consist of macular pig-mented spots scattered over the surface of the skin. These may appear at birth and become more conspicuous and deeply pigmented with maturation. Paget's disease causes a uniform thickening of the skull rather than local tumors. Polycystic disease of the kidneys is associated with multiple intracranial aneurysms that would not show as three discrete nodules on the in-ner surface of the skull. Brain abscesses also would not show on the unenhanced scan as areas of increased density. Breast cancer may involve skull and dura but produces irregular lytic lesions of the bone.

224. The answer is C (2, 4). *(Taveras, ed 2. p 344.)* The pneumoencephalogram accompanying the question shows porencephaly and absence of the septum pellucidum. Normally, the septum pellucidum forms a thin single or bi-leaved line on the frontal radiograph, which divides the two lateral ventricles and extends from the fornices to the corpus callosum. In the patient in question, the septum is congenitally absent. The third and lateral ventricles form a common chamber roofed by the corpus callosum. This patient also showed hypoplasia of the optic nerves, which classifies this malformation as opticoseptal dysplasia. Many patients with opticoseptal dysplasia also display porencephaly. In this case, a channel runs ventrolaterally through the cerebral wall from the dorsal aspect of one caudate nucleus to the expanded cavity of the porus itself, which reaches nearly to the surface of the cerebral wall. The caudate nuclei form their usual convexity in the lateral wall of the ventricles.

225. The answer is D (4). *(Taveras, ed 2. pp 724-731.)* The radiograph accompanying the question shows a broad curve of the anterior cerebral artery, because of straightening of its normal undulations. This finding occurs regularly as the ventricles enlarge from internal hydrocephalus, causing the corpus callosum to expand and thin out and stretch the anterior cerebral arteries. The posterior cerebral arteries have not filled from the carotid injection in this patient. They fill from the carotid circulation in only about 20 percent of affected individuals, filling from the vertebral injection in the remaining 80 percent. The arteries fail to indicate any aneurysms. The apparent nodules along the course of the cerebral arteries represent an end view of normal vessels. Mycotic aneurysms, however, do appear distally along the arteries, in contrast to the berry aneurysms of congenital origin that appear predominantly along the vessels at the base of the brain.

226. The answer is B (1, 3). *(Taveras, ed 2. pp 997-1000.)* CAT scan is based on the ability of a computer to enhance the differences in absorption of photons by tissues. The photons, after their generation by an x-ray tube, pass through a collimator, the patient's head, a second collimator and then are registered by a scintillation crystal. The computer processes the information from the scintillation crystal. No x-ray film is involved in this process. The usual angle of the photon beam through the head is about 20-25 degrees to the cantho-meatal (Frankfurt) line. This angle allows better visualization of the posterior fossa. The contrast achieved on the final readout depends on the width of the window chosen. The wider the window, the less the contrast; the images fade into one another. With a narrow window, only a small range of numbers is displayed as shades of gray or white, and all readings above or below the window width are represented as black or white.

227. The answer is C (2, 4). *(Taveras, ed 2. pp 778-796.)* The vertebral angiogram accompanying the question is normal. It shows filling of the terminal part of the opposite vertebral artery by regurgitation, which commonly happens. The vertebral arteries have the same caliber in only about 25 percent of individuals. Normal individuals may show severe hypoplasia or even absence of one vertebral artery. The posterior inferior cerebellar arteries, which usually derive from the vertebral arteries, likewise exhibit great variability from person to person. In the radiograph accompanying the question, the vertebral artery has its normal course and shows its normal terminal branching into the superior cerebellar arteries and posterior cerebral arteries. These arteries likewise have their normal caliber, course, and relationships. A midbrain mass that would separate the posterior cerebral arteries would also straighten out the undulations, which fails to occur in this case.

228. The answer is B (1, 3). *(Taveras, ed 2. p 989.)* The brain scan accompanying the question shows a dense unilateral frontal lesion, which by its location suggests a falx meningioma. Such lesions compress the nearby olfactory tract to produce unilateral anosmia, and compress the frontal lobe to cause mild personality changes. They may also cause seizures. However, the location of the lesion means that ataxia and visual hallucinations would be absent. Meningiomas are the easiest intracranial tumors to demonstrate by radiography. They may show on plain skull films because they contain calcium or cause hyperostosis. For similar reasons, they may show on the unenhanced CAT scan. Because of their vascularity, they visualize with any form of angiography and with radioactive scanning methods. Some meningiomas also may cause considerable cerebral edema. In such instances, the scan may show a much wider uptake of radioactive tracer.

229-232. The answers are: 229-E, 230-A, 231-D, 232-B. *(Taveras, ed 2. pp 620-634.)* Venography shows both the deep and superficial veins of the brain. The deep veins regularly demonstrated include the basal vein of Rosenthal (labeled "C" in the radiogram accompanying the question), the terminal or thalamostriate vein, the internal cerebral vein, and the vein of Galen (E).

The basal vein begins at the anterior perforated space that overlies the vallecula, in which the carotid artery bifurcates into the middle and anterior cerebral branches. The basal vein then runs backward across the base of the cerebrum to the midbrain, where it encircles the midbrain in the ambient cistern. It then joins the internal cerebral vein to form the vein of Galen. The vein of Galen in turn enters the straight sinus. The blood from the deep venous circulation mainly enters the left sigmoid sinus. The internal cerebral vein begins at the venous angle (A), where it has the terminal vein as one of its main tributaries and the septal vein as the other. The union of the terminal vein and septal vein to form the internal cerebral vein occurs at the interventricular foramen in most brains. In some brains it occurs behind the foramen, which then forms what is called the false venous angle.

In hydrocephalus, the true venous angle is widened as seen on frontal views because of lateral displacement of the ventricular wall to which the terminal vein is attached. Hemispheric tumors adjacent to the ventricular wall will shove the terminal vein medially, narrowing the venous angle.

The surface of the brain drains into the superficial venous system. Usually two large channels appear, one running up to the superior sagittal sinus as the vein of Trolard and the other running to the sigmoid sinus as the vein of Labbé.

The deep cerebral veins are often the sites of hemorrhage in birth trauma or hypoxia. The periventricular tissue or the ventricles themselves become distended with blood. The vein of Galen may form an aneurysmal dilation, which leads to obstructive hydrocephalus presumably because of mechanical compression of the midbrain aqueduct, and to heart failure because of the tremendous arteriovenous fistulation that evolves in these lesions. The superficial veins may be torn in birth injury or other forms of trauma to produce subdural bleeding, or they may undergo thrombosis from injury or as an idiopathic or even familial disorder. The patient in the latter case shows a strokelike syndrome with a hemorrhagic infarction. In infantile deyhydration, thrombosis of the superior longitudinal sinus was a frequent complication in the days before fluid therapy was understood.

233-236. The answers are: 233-A, 234-B, 235-E, 236-D. *(Taveras, ed 2. pp 310-314.)* Pneumoencephalography shows the details of the third ventricle much better than does CAT scan. The radiograph accompanying the question is a brow-up lateral view. Beginning at the aqueduct (labeled "C" in the radiograph), the air fills the third ventricle outlining a massa intermedia (D). This structure is rather large, indicating a young person since, in the senile brain, it decreases in size, according to Yakovlev. Tracing along the floor of the lateral ventricle, one finds an indentation (B) indicating the optic chiasm and forming the so-called fishmouth configuration. The anterior wall of the third ventricle, the lamina terminalis, can then be traced up to the connection between the lateral and third ventricles, the interventricular foramen of Monro (A). The superimposition of the two lateral ventricles, as well as their size, explains the darkness of their outline. Since the brow is up, the air has risen into the anterior horns.

Posteriorly, one sees a fluid level in each of the two ventricles. The fluid level differs because of asymmetrical emptying when air replaced the fluid, a normal finding. The air seen in the interpeduncular cistern (E) outlines the belly of the pons and runs up to a peak in the interpeduncular fossa at a site known as the posterior foramen cecum. Anteriorly, the air has been arrested by Lilequist's membrane, a normal veil that extends across from one IIIrd nerve to the other. This membrane limits the air during the early phase of pneumoencephalography until it slips by to fill the chiasmatic cistern, which, in the example pictured, is still unoccupied by air. Complete filling of these basal cisterns permits visualization of the bifurcation of the basilar artery into the posterior cerebral arteries and the IIIrd nerve trunk itself. The air will then extend around the midbrain to fill the cistern ambiens, which communicates with the pineal cistern. The communication of the basal vein of Rosenthal with the internal cerebral vein to form the vein of Galen follows the same course as does the cisterna ambiens.

237-241. The answers are: 237-C, 238-E, 239-E, 240-A, 241-C. *(Adams, ed 2. pp 469-470, 474.)* All of the cranial nerves pass through apertures in the base of the skull. Some apertures transmit more than one nerve. Characteristic syndromes occur when a lesion affects the conjunction of nerves at particular sites of exit from the skull.

Cranial nerves III, IV, VI, and the ophthalmic division of V run through the superior orbital fissure. The VIth cranial nerve runs through Dorello's canal at the medial tip of the petrous part of the temporal bone, in company with the inferior petrosal sinus. Both nerve and vessel then enter the cavernous sinus. Inflammation of the petrous bone involves the VIth nerve at the canal of Dorello and the nearby Vth nerve, producing Gradenigo's syndrome.

The IXth, Xth, and XIth cranial nerves all run through the jugular foramen in the posterior fossa. A lesion at this site, such as a tumor of the glomus jugulare, involves all three nerves (syndrome of Vernet).

In contrast to these apertures that transmit multiple cranial nerves, other apertures such as the optic canal and the hypoglossal canal transmit only one cranial nerve. The arteries traverse the apertures as follows: carotid arteries through the foramen lacerum, ophthalmic arteries through the optic canal, vertebral arteries through the foramen magnum, and middle meningeal arteries through the foramen spinosum.

Miscellaneous
Ophthalmology, ENT, CSF, Microbiology, Endocrinology, Immunology

DIRECTIONS: Each question below contains five suggested answers. Choose the **one best** response to each question.

242. The fast — or kickback — phase of caloric or optokinetic nystagmus is thought to depend on

(A) efferent brain stem connections from the frontal eye fields
(B) ascending connections from the proprioceptors in the neck
(C) integrity of the cerebellar vermis
(D) impulses originating in the retina
(E) the dorsal longitudinal fasciculus

243. The anteroposterior diameter of the skull is mainly determined by growth along

(A) the sagittal suture
(B) the coronal suture
(C) the metopic suture
(D) the basilar synchondrosis
(E) none of the above

244. A patient exhibits a whitish patch extending from the margin of the optic disk. The patch has a roughly triangular shape with the apex pointing dorsolateral. The retina is otherwise unremarkable. The patient has no visual complaint. The most likely diagnosis is

(A) optic nerve hypoplasia
(B) primary optic atrophy
(C) acute papillitis
(D) medullated nerve fibers
(E) hypertensive retinopathy

245. Ptosis is most severe as a consequence of which of the following forms of denervation?

(A) Parasympathetic denervation
(B) Sympathetic denervation
(C) Vidian nerve lesions
(D) VIIth nerve lesions
(E) IIIrd nerve lesions

246. A 10-month-old infant presents with slight lethargy, slightly convex fontanelle, and mild cardiomegaly. A distinct, loud bruit is heard over the entire calvarium but is absent over the heart or neck vessels. The most likely diagnosis is

(A) glycogen storage disease
(B) cardiac myxoma with cerebral embolization
(C) butterfly glioblastoma of the corpus callosum
(D) aneurysm of the vein of Galen
(E) carotid-cavernous fistulae

247. To examine the contour of the anterior fontanelle of an infant for increased intracranial pressure, the examiner should place the infant in which of the following positions?

(A) Prone
(B) Supine
(C) Lateral recumbent
(D) Head down
(E) Vertical

248. The EMG finding that is most characteristic of chronic denervation and most reliably distinguishes it from other neuromuscular diseases is

(A) fibrillations
(B) giant polyphasic motor units
(C) low-amplitude motor units
(D) electrical silence during rest
(E) myotonia

249. A full interference pattern with low-amplitude potentials in the EMG is most characteristic of

(A) McArdle's disease
(B) muscular dystrophy
(C) myasthenia gravis
(D) acute denervation
(E) chronic denervation

250. In palpating the carotid arteries of a patient suspected of having occlusive cerebral vascular disease, the examiner should palpate

(A) both carotid arteries simultaneously, to compare directly the amplitude of the pulsations
(B) each artery separately to the point of occlusion, to test for syncope
(C) each artery separately and very lightly
(D) only with the patient's neck turned strongly to the side
(E) only with the patient's neck extended

251. Patients affected with the medial longitudinal fasciculus (MLF) syndrome, when attempting to look to one side, display

(A) nystagmus of the adducting eye and paresis of the abducting eye, with normal convergence during accommodation
(B) nystagmus of the abducting eye with paresis of the adducting eye, and adductor paresis during accommodation
(C) nystagmus of the abducting eye with paresis of the adducting eye, but adduction of the eyes during accommodation
(D) nystagmus of both adducting and abducting eyes, with paresis of vertical movements
(E) paresis of the abducting and adducting eyes, but adduction of the eyes during accommodation

252. If an infant's head exhibits transillumination, the best conclusion is that

(A) the skull is too thick
(B) the brain is too small for the skull
(C) some intracranial space or the scalp contains too much fluid
(D) the ventricles are enlarged and contain too much fluid
(E) the finding is normal up to 6 months of age in term infants

253. The typical hemorrhages that occur in the retina secondary to acute increased intracranial pressure occupy the

(A) choroid
(B) nerve fiber layer
(C) subhyaloid space
(D) vitreous body
(E) anterior chamber

254. The site of a restricted lesion that would selectively impair downward gaze is the

(A) superior colliculus
(B) cerebellar vermis
(C) region dorsomedial to the red nuclei
(D) bioccipital region
(E) internal capsule

255. A normal person looking at infinity will exhibit points of corneal light reflection that are located

(A) precisely in the geometric center of the corneas
(B) slightly lateral to the geometric center of the corneas
(C) slightly medial to the geometric center of the corneas
(D) slightly above the geometric center of the corneas
(E) slightly below the geometric center of the corneas

256. A patient who exhibits ocular deviation only when central vision is occluded and not at any other time has

(A) a central visual field defect
(B) paralytic strabismus
(C) IIIrd nerve palsy
(D) heterotropia
(E) heterophoria

257. In most normal persons, at maximum lateral gaze the limbus of the **ab**ducting eye reaches

(A) almost exactly to the apex of the external canthus
(B) 1 mm short of the external canthus angle
(C) 1 mm beyond the external canthus angle
(D) one-half of the distance from cornea to canthus
(E) none of the above positions

258. A patient has diplopia on left lateral gaze. Examination shows slight weakness of abduction of the left eye, but the right eye hyperadducts when the patient looks to the left. In this case, hyperadduction of the right eye is best explained by

(A) a lesion of the ipsilateral medial longitudinal fasciculus
(B) a supranuclear palsy of gaze from interruption of frontobulbar pathways
(C) preexisting ocular malalignment
(D) Hering's law of equal supranuclear innervation of yoke muscles
(E) a hysterical or malingering patient

259. To test for the integrity of the IVth cranial nerve in a patient with a IIIrd nerve palsy, the examiner requests the patient to look in which of the following directions?

(A) To the side opposite the IIIrd nerve palsy and down
(B) To the side ipsilateral to the IIIrd nerve palsy and up
(C) To the midline and up
(D) To the midline
(E) Upward

Questions 260-262

A previously well individual has been experiencing a gradual onset of weakness for two days, with some vague tingling in the extremities but no incontinence. He has generalized flaccid muscle weakness—perhaps worse proximally. Ocular movements, speaking, and swallowing are normal, but facial movements are questionably weak. On percussing the tendons, the examiner elicits no response, but the muscles do respond actively to direct percussion. Sensory examination discloses questionable loss of vibratory sensation in the toes. Laboratory values are as follows:

Serum electrolytes (mEq/L): Na^+ 137; K^+ 3.4; Cl^- 100; Ca^{++} 5
CPK normal

260. The most likely diagnosis is

(A) electrolyte imbalance
(B) acute myelitis
(C) acute polymyositis
(D) acute polyradiculitis (Landry-Guillain-Barré syndrome)
(E) familial periodic paralysis

261. On the third day of illness of the patient described above, a lumbar puncture is performed. Analysis of the CSF discloses these findings:

WBCs 5/mm³; glucose 65 mg/100 ml; protein 35 mg/100 ml; immunoelectrophoretic profile normal

The best interpretation of these results is which of the following?

(A) They argue most strongly for acute myelitis
(B) They are most compatible with electrolyte imbalance
(C) They argue against polymyositis
(D) They exclude the Landry-Guillain-Barré syndrome
(E) They are compatible with all the above diagnoses

262. The previously mentioned patient continued to have flaccid paralysis for a number of weeks and showed some slight recovery after 3 months, but then began to complain of headache and some blurred vision. Examination disclosed mild papilledema. The significance of this new finding is that it

(A) probably represents a new disease
(B) implies the presence of a brain tumor rather than a neuromuscular disease
(C) suggests impending renal failure
(D) raises the question of lead poisoning and lead neuropathy
(E) probably reflects chronically elevated CSF protein levels

263. To examine a patient who complains of blurred vision, the examiner swings a flashlight back and forth from one eye to the other. The pupils of both eyes dilate when the light shines in the left eye, but constrict normally when the light shines in the right. The pupils are of normal size and shape, and the fundi appear normal. These findings are indicative of

(A) an Argyll Robertson pupil
(B) an Adie's pupil
(C) parasympathetic denervation of the left eye
(D) sympathetic denervation of the left eye
(E) impaired conduction in the left optic nerve

264. A mother brings her 30-month-old child to be examined because she notices "crossed eyes," which have appeared intermittently during the last several months, especially toward the end of the day. Examination shows a mild esophoria and probable hyperopia. The examination is otherwise normal. The most appropriate management of this child is to order

(A) a CAT scan for causes of an intermittent VIth nerve palsy
(B) an edrophonium chloride (Tensilon) test for myasthenia gravis
(C) an electroretinogram
(D) an ocular muscle EMG
(E) corrective lenses

265. A vibrating tuning fork is placed on the vertex of a patient's skull (Weber's test). The patient consistently reports that the sound lateralizes to the right ear. Bone conduction of sound on the right is better than air conduction. Otoscopy discloses a normal ear drum on each side. The best conclusion is that the patient has

(A) right ear dominance for hearing
(B) neurosensory hearing loss on the right
(C) neurosensory hearing loss on the left
(D) conductive hearing loss on the right
(E) conductive hearing loss on the left

266. The best way to judge ocular malalignment is to

(A) compare the space between the canthi and the corneal limbus medially and laterally
(B) look for the corneal light reflections
(C) look for the relation of the eyes to the lower eyelids
(D) look for the relation of the eyes to the upper eyelids
(E) ask the patient about diplopia

267. The maximum upward excursion (elevation) of a normal eye from the primary position is approximately

(A) 15 mm
(B) 10 mm
(C) 7 mm
(D) 4 mm
(E) none of the above

268. The true vestibular component of caloric nystagmus is

(A) the slow, deviation phase
(B) the quick, kickback phase
(C) both quick and slow horizontal phases
(D) the vertical quick phase only
(E) both quick and slow vertical phases

269. Which of the following statements concerning the testing of a patient for alternating movements (dysdiadochokinesia) is true?

(A) The nondominant hand usually performs slightly better than the dominant
(B) The left hand performs best in both right and left-handed persons
(C) Both hands perform equally well
(D) Handedness is unimportant in judging the results
(E) None of the above

270. In performing a cold caloric irrigation of the ear of a patient sitting upright, an examiner should position the patient by

(A) leaving the patient's head vertical
(B) inclining the patient's head 60 degrees backward
(C) inclining the patient's head 30 degrees forward
(D) tilting the patient's head to the side of the irrigation
(E) bending the patient's trunk forward

DIRECTIONS: Each question below contains four suggested answers of which **one** or **more** is correct. Choose the answer

A	if	1, 2, and 3	are correct
B	if	1 and 3	are correct
C	if	2 and 4	are correct
D	if	4	is correct
E	if	1, 2, 3, and 4	are correct

271. Conclusive evidence that blood in a CSF sample originates from a pre-existing subarachnoid hemorrhage and not from a traumatic puncture is supplied by which of the following findings?

(1) Crenated red blood cells on microscopic examination
(2) Macrophages laden with red blood cells
(3) Large numbers of red blood cells in the spinal fluid
(4) Xanthochromia of the supernatant fluid after centrifugation

272. Diagnostic features that distinguish nonparalytic (concomitant) heterotropia from paralytic heterotropia include which of the following?

(1) The angle of the ocular malalignment remains the same during all directions of movement when both eyes are used
(2) Each eye shows a full range of movements when the other is covered
(3) Opacity of the media or severe refractive error may be present in one eye
(4) The patient complains of diplopia

273. Clinical characteristics of Adie's pupil include

(1) anisocoria
(2) irregular pupillary margin
(3) slow constriction and dilation
(4) frequent association with hyperactive stretch reflexes

274. An examiner places strong positive lenses (Frenzel lenses) over a patient's eyes to inspect for positional or caloric-induced nystagmus in order to

(1) produce pupilloconstriction
(2) occlude visual fixation
(3) prevent vertigo
(4) magnify the eye movements

275. A 6-month-old baby girl exhibits slow movements, rather firm, large muscles, sluggish but present muscle stretch reflexes, and percussion myoedema. Percussion myotonia is absent. The differential diagnosis should include

(1) glycogen storage disease
(2) infantile myotonic dystrophy
(3) hypothyroidism
(4) Duchenne's muscular dystrophy

276. Hyperthyroidism is frequently accompanied by which of the following motor system syndromes?

(1) Myasthenia gravis
(2) Periodic weakness with hypokalemia
(3) Ophthalmoplegia
(4) Enlarged, firm muscles

277. Correct statements concerning the syndrome of progressive ophthalmoplegia include which of the following?

(1) Historically, opinions have differed concerning its classification as a myopathic or a neurogenic disease
(2) It is frequently associated with retinitis pigmentosa
(3) It is characterized by ptosis and weakness of eye closing as well as by ophthalmoplegia
(4) Affected patients frequently present with diplopia

278. Amniocentesis may be an advisable procedure when an embryo is at risk for

(1) a karyotype abnormality
(2) myelomeningocele
(3) inborn error of metabolism
(4) Huntington's chorea

SUMMARY OF DIRECTIONS				
A	B	C	D	E
1, 2, 3 only	1, 3 only	2, 4 only	4 only	All are correct

279. Pseudopapilledema is distinguished from true papilledema by exhibiting

(1) maximum elevation of disk centrally
(2) preretinal branching of the vessels
(3) a normal sized blind spot
(4) frequent presence of drusen

280. Bruits may be heard over the head with some frequency in

(1) patients with carotid-cavernous fistulae
(2) normal infants
(3) young children with acute meningitis
(4) patients with chronic brain abscess

281. An EMG shows prominent electrical discharges in which of the following conditions?

(1) Myotonia
(2) Tetany
(3) Exercise-induced muscle cramps in normal individuals
(4) Muscle contraction in McArdle's disease

282. Myotonia may be identified by which of the following features?

(1) It increases with increasing contractions of the muscle
(2) It is demonstrable by percussion
(3) It is electrically silent in EMG
(4) It occurs after a single strong contraction

283. In comparison to small axons, large axons have which of the following characteristics?

(1) A slower rate of conduction
(2) A lower threshold for electrical stimulation
(3) More rapid response to local anesthetics
(4) More numerous myelin lamellae

DIRECTIONS: The groups of questions below consist of lettered choices followed by several numbered items. For each numbered item select the **one** lettered choice with which it is **most** closely associated. Each lettered choice may be used once, more than once, or not at all.

Questions 284-287

For each of the disorders listed below, choose the inheritance pattern with which it is most closely associated.

(A) Autosomal dominant
(B) Autosomal recessive
(C) Sex-linked recessive
(D) Hereditary influence without following a strict mendelian pattern
(E) No clear evidence of a hereditary predisposition

284. Duchenne's muscular dystrophy

285. Myotonic dystrophy

286. Pelizaeus-Merzbacher disease

287. Myelomeningocele

Questions 288-291

Match the following.

(A) Oxycephaly
(B) Plagiocephaly
(C) Scaphocephaly
(D) Acrobrachycephaly
(E) Trigonocephaly

288. A skull that is too short because of premature coronal suture closure

289. A skull that is too long because of premature sagittal suture closure

290. A skull that is too short and too narrow because of premature coronal and sagittal suture closure

291. A skull with a ridged forehead because of premature metopic suture closure

Questions 292-295

For each disorder listed below, choose the chromosomal condition with which it is most closely associated.

(A) 5 Deletion
(B) Trisomy 21
(C) Trisomy 13
(D) XXY
(E) No deletion or error of chromosome number is found

292. Holoprosencephaly/arhinencephalia

293. Cri du chat (cat's cry syndrome)

294. Neurofibromatosis

295. Klinefelter's syndrome

Miscellaneous
Ophthalmology, ENT, CSF, Microbiology, Endocrinology, Immunology
Answers

242. The answer is A. *(DeMyer, ed 3. p 287.)* The fast—or kickback—phase of caloric nystagmus depends in large part on the integrity of the efferent pathway from the frontal eye fields. Large hemispheric lesions that destroy the cortical projection system to the brain stem will abolish the kickback phase of nystagmus. In patients thus afflicted, the slow deviation phase (the vestibular or optokinetic phase) remains. Absence of the cerebral efferent pathway converts the response to merely deviation rather than to an organized nystagmus. Retinal receptors play no part in producing the fast phase of caloric nystagmus. In fact, voluntary fixation tends to inhibit caloric nystagmus. Integrity of the retinal receptors would be necessary for the pursuit phase of optokinetic nystagmus, but the fast—or kickback—phase is related to the integrity of the pathway from the frontal eye fields to the brain stem.

243. The answer is B. *(DeMyer, ed 3. p 23.)* The anteroposterior diameter of the skull is mainly determined by growth along the coronal suture, in accordance with Virchow's general law that the skull grows at right angles to the plane of the sutures. Premature closure of one of the sutures will restrict the growth of the head in a plane at right angles to that suture. The head then undergoes a characteristic deviation in contour that indicates the affected suture. From the characteristic alteration in head shape and from palpation of the ridged suture, the clinician can identify the prematurely closed suture or sutures. Plain skull radiographs aid in the evaluation. Premature suture closure should be detected in early infancy. Not only is the cosmetic result of craniectomy to create artificial sutures best achieved in young infants, but early surgery may prevent subsequent constriction of the brain during growth.

244. The answer is D. *(DeMyer, ed 3. p 123.)* Medullated nerve fibers characteristically are incidental findings during routine ophthalmoscopic examination. They are without specific clinical significance, produce no visual complaints, and differ from hypertensive retinopathy by the absence of any other changes in the vessels and the absence of exudates and hemorrhages. Medullated fibers, being opaque, increase the size of the blind spot.

245. The answer is E. *(DeMyer, ed 3. pp 104-106.)* A IIIrd nerve lesion causes the most severe ptosis of any form of denervation. The IIIrd nerve supplies the levator palpebrae muscle, which is the most important muscle for elevating the lid. VIIth nerve and vidian nerve interruption and parasympathetic denervation fail to cause ptosis.

246. The answer is D. *(Swaiman, pp 649-651.)* A vein of Galen aneurysm is associated with a massive arteriovenous shunting of blood. The shunt causes the intracranial bruit and leads to cardiac failure. The aneurysm compresses the underlying quadrigeminal plate and aqueduct, causing hydrocephalus and a bulging fontanelle. Carotid-cavernous fistulae are exceedingly rare in young infants, as are glioblastomas. Glycogen storage disease might cause cardiomegaly and some increased intracranial pressure, but would not cause a loud bruit. A cardiac myxoma might cause the cardiac failure, but any bruit heard over the head would have to be transmitted along the neck vessels and heard over them.

247. The answer is E. *(DeMyer, ed 3. pp 13-14.)*   To examine the contour of the anterior fontanelle, the examiner places the infant in the vertical position. With the infant vertical, gravity pulls the brain away from the vertex, allowing the fontanelle to assume its normal concave contour. When the infant is recumbent, or in the presence of increased intrathoracic pressure as when the infant cries or is bent forward at the waist, the fontanelle may fail to show its normal concave contour.

248. The answer is B. *(Adams, ed 2. p 879.)*   The EMG finding most indicative of chronic denervation is giant polyphasic motor units. These units are virtually pathognomonic and are absent in normal individuals or in patients with dystrophy. They are thought to represent enlargement of the motor units from regenerating nerve sprouts. In many disorders involved in the differential diagnosis of chronic denervation, the EMG will show fibrillations or low-amplitude motor units. Characteristically, patients with chronic denervation show fibrillations and slow positive waves in addition to the giant polyphasic units, but fibrillations also can occur in polymyositis and some dystrophies and lack the pathognomonic significance of the giant polyphasic units. Patients with muscular dystrophy and normal individuals show no electrical activity with the muscle at rest.

249. The answer is B. *(Adams, ed 2. p 879.)*   The characteristic EMG pattern of muscular dystrophy is a full interference pattern with low-amplitude potentials. The interference pattern depends on the number of motor units contracting and the number of muscle fibers responding. In dystrophies, the number of motor units remains the same, but the number of muscle fibers available to respond decreases as the disease advances. The reduced number of responding muscle fibers leads to the reduction in amplitude of the interference pattern. The full interference pattern with low-amplitude potentials, in combination with the absence of any of the EMG changes such as fibrillations and giant polyphasic units, lends support to a diagnosis of a primary muscle disease rather than neuronal disease.

250. The answer is C. *(DeMyer, ed 3. p 9.)*   In palpating the carotid arteries, the examiner palpates them separately and very lightly. If the examiner palpates too hard, blood flow through the vessel may be occluded. If the other carotid already has become occluded, as frequently happens, the patient may have symptoms of cerebral ischemia. For the same reason, the examiner should avoid palpating both arteries simultaneously, which may cause cerebral ischemia. Hard palpation also may dislodge an embolus from a plaque. In addition, hard palpation may cause syncope from a carotid sinus reflex. The patient's head should be straight during arterial palpation. Turning of the head may reduce blood flow through carotid or vertebral arteries by mechanical compression.

251. The answer is C. *(DeMyer, ed 3. pp 134-136.)*   In the medical longitudinal fasciculus (MLF) syndrome, the patient shows nystagmus of the **ab**ducting eye and paresis of the **ad**ducting eye. Both eyes adduct during accommodation. The medial longitudinal fasciculus conveys fibers from the region of the contralateral abducens nucleus to the lower motor neurons of the medial rectus muscle in the IIIrd nerve nucleus. These MLF fibers yoke the medial rectus of one eye with the lateral rectus of the opposite eye to mediate conjugate lateral gaze. Interruption of these MLF fibers causes paresis of adduction of the eye ipsilateral to the MLF lesion. During accommodation, the medial rectus is activated by pathways that run directly into the midbrain without traveling down into the pons and back through the MLF. The normal medial rectus action during convergence proves that the lower motor neurons of the medial rectus muscle remain intact in the MLF syndrome.

252. The answer is C. *(DeMyer, ed 3. pp 19-22.)* An infant's head that exhibits transillumination means that some tissue or space beneath the flashlight contains abnormal amounts of fluid. The head of a normal term infant does not exhibit transillumination. Some transillumination may occur in premature babies who have a very thin skull, but it is slight compared to the transillumination that may occur in infants with severe brain lesions. As the skull thickens during maturation, it blocks transillumination from intracranial lesions. The fluid displaying transillumination may be extracranial. Scalp edema, as from infiltration of intravenous fluid during feeding through a scalp vein, is the usual site of extracranial fluid that exhibits transillumination. The usual sites of **intra**cranial fluid displaying transillumination are the subdural space, subarachnoid space, enlarged ventricles, or in defects of the brain wall such as porencephaly. Large cysts in the posterior fossa also may show transillumination (Dandy-Walker syndrome).

253. The answer is C. *(Adams, ed 2. p 168.)* The retinal hemorrhage typical of acute increased intracranial pressure occupies the space between the internal limiting membrane of the retina and the hyaloid membrane. Therefore, it is a subhyaloid or preretinal hemorrhage. The blood apparently comes from rupture of the retinal arterioles. The ophthalmoscopic appearance of the various types of hemorrhage depends on the space into which the hemorrhage ruptures or upon the retinal layer into which it ruptures. Common conditions associated with subhyaloid hemorrhages include ruptured intracranial aneurysms and head injuries, often with acute epidural or acute subdural hemorrhage. Occasionally, severe coughing may induce a subhyaloid hemorrhage. The presence of subhyaloid hemorrhages, at least in a comatose patient, requires immediate investigation by CAT scan or angiography.

254. The answer is C. *(Adams, ed 2. pp 178-179.)* A restricted lesion of the region dorsomedial to the red nuclei will selectively impair downward gaze. At no other sites are lesions known to do so, whether in the cerebellum or cerebral cortex, or elsewhere in the brain stem. Several case reports now confirm this clinicopathologic correlation. At one time, the superior colliculi were thought to mediate vertical eye movements, a contention no longer accepted. Selective impairment of downward gaze indicates the presence of an intrinsic midbrain tegmental lesion that may be vascular, traumatic, demyelinating, or degenerative in type. External compressive lesions, particularly those that compress from the dorsal aspect of the midbrain, tend to impair upward rather than downward gaze.

255. The answer is C. *(DeMyer, ed 3. pp 35-38.)* When a person looks at infinity, the points of corneal light reflection fall slightly medial to the true geometric centers of the corneas. This phenomenon is explained by the fact that the visual axes of the eye and the geometric anteroposterior axes do not correspond exactly. The true anteroposterior axes diverge slightly. The points of corneal light reflection provide the best reference for deciding whether the eyes align properly. Reliance on the relation of the irises to the lid margins may lead to false conclusions about ocular alignment, because the size and shape of the palpebral fissures may vary in the presence of congenital malformations and neurologic diseases.

256. The answer is E. *(DeMyer, ed 3. pp 43-45.)* Ocular deviation occurring only with occlusion of central vision constitutes heterophoria. Normally, the eyes remain locked in alignment by the reflexes that underly fixation and fusion of the images of the two eyes. The eyes, once having achieved alignment during maturation, should remain aligned at all times in a normal, alert person. Deviation of an eye after occlusion of central vision during the cover-uncover test demonstrates that the patient's eyes must have central vision in order to maintain alignment. Restoration of central vision causes the deviant eye to snap back into alignment. If an eye does not snap back into alignment every time after restoration of central vision, the condition is called heterotropia.

257. The answer is A. *(DeMyer, ed 3. pp 2-3.)* At maximum abduction, in most normal persons the corneal limbus reaches almost exactly to the apex of the lateral canthus. This is a very precise and reproducible finding. Any departure suggests a disturbance of abduction—either weakness of the lateral rectus muscle action, a lid anomaly, enophthalmos, exophthalmos, or some anomaly of the eyeball itself. The examiner should check for the precision of this relationship every time a patient's range of eye movements is tested.

258. The answer is D. *(DeMyer, ed 3. p 55.)* Excessive action of an intact ocular muscle of one eye that normally is yoked to a paretic muscle of the opposite eye is explained by Hering's law. Hering's law states that the yoke muscles receive equal supranuclear innervation. A patient affected with a weak lateral rectus muscle overinnervates in an effort to activate the paretic muscle. The central connections of the nervous system, in obedience to Hering's law, send an equally strong innervation to the intact medial rectus. The paretic lateral rectus muscle underacts, and the intact medial rectus overacts, causing hyperadduction. The reverse occurs with a medial rectus palsy. When a patient with this deficit attempts to look to the side opposite the medial rectus palsy, the overaction of the intact lateral rectus muscles hyperabducts the eyeball.

259. The answer is D. *(Adams, ed 2. p 181.)* To test for an intact IVth nerve when the patient has a IIIrd nerve palsy, the examiner requests the patient to look to the side opposite the palsy and down. The examiner then watches for rotation of one of the conjunctival vessels. If the IVth nerve and superior oblique muscle are intact, the examiner will observe intorsion of the eye, although it will fail to adduct. With the eye laterally rotated from the pull of the intact VIth nerve and lateral rectus muscle, the eye is in the position in which the superior oblique muscle has its maximum strength as an intorter. The effort to look medially and down will activate the superior oblique muscle, but it will mainly display its action as an intorter of the eye.

260. The answer is D. *(Adams, ed 2. p 894.)* The patient described in the question has an acutely evolving, flaccid paralysis with areflexia and retention of percussion irritability of muscle. Sensation is only questionably involved, and the patient retains sphincter control. These features argue strongly against myelitis, which would manifest sensory loss and incontinence, even though flaccid paralysis may be present early in the course of the myelitis. Polymyositis usually has a much more indolent onset than occurred in this patient, and would not cause acute flaccid paralysis. The electrolytes values are slightly low, but not low enough to cause flaccid paralysis. Familial periodic paralysis of normokalemic type remains a possibility, but in terms of probability is much rarer and thus much less likely than the Landry-Guillain-Barré syndrome.

261. The answer is E. *(Adams, ed 2. pp 895, 912.)* Normal spinal fluid is compatible with any of the four diagnoses mentioned in the question. Acute myelitis may or may not show a significant change in the CSF; but very mild, acute electrolyte disturbances, polymyositis, and periodic paralysis characteristically would fail to show changes in the components ordinarily measured in a routine CSF examination. In Landry-Guillain-Barré syndrome, the protein level does increase, but occasionally the initial tap may show a normal protein content. The protein level then will increase, usually reaching a peak several weeks after the onset of the illness. Thus, a normal CSF during the acute stage of the illness does not exclude the Landry-Guillain-Barré syndrome.

262. The answer is E. *(DeMyer, ed 3. p 407.)*   A patient with a chronic flaccid paralysis, particularly in the presence of the Landry-Guillain-Barré syndrome, may have increased protein levels for prolonged periods of weeks to months. Such patients may develop papilledema. In the patient discussed in the question, the principle of parsimony in diagnosis calls for a **single** disease to explain the range of clinical manifestations of his illness. To invoke any diagnosis other than the original one of a neuromuscular disease violates this principle. The mechanism of the papilledema and increased pressure with prolonged elevation of CSF protein is probably a result of occlusion of the Pacchionian granulations by sludged protein.

263. The answer is E. *(Adams, ed 2. p 188.)*   If an examiner swings a flashlight in front of a patient from one eye to the other, normally the pupils should react equally. If both pupils dilate when the light shines in only one eye, the optic nerve on that side has impaired conduction, permitting pupillary escape from the influence of the light stimulus. In the patient presented in the question, the normal size of the pupils and reaction to light exclude an Argyll Robertson pupil. Absence of myotonia excludes an Adie's pupil. Unilateral sympathetic or parasympathetic denervation would cause anisocoria. Therefore, the lesion in this patient affects the optic nerve. The swinging flashlight test may remain positive after an attack of acute retrobulbar neuritis has undergone remission, even though the optic disk fails to show atrophy.

264. The answer is E. *(DeMyer, ed 3. pp 65-66.)*   Children with hyperopia tend to overuse their accommodation mechanism. Because the eyeball is too short relative to the eye's refracting power, the focal point falls behind the retina. Such children tend to accommodate all of the time to increase the focal power of the lens, which will bring the focal point forward onto the retina. Since convergence is an automatic part of the accommodation reflex, the eyes tend to cross. Phorias of this type generally are worse when the patient is tired. In the absence of any other findings suggestive of neurologic disease, further neurologic workup such as CAT scan, Tensilon test, EMG, or electroretinogram is unnecessary. The child should be fitted with corrective lenses and observed periodically.

265. The answer is D. *(DeMyer, ed 3. pp 279-280.)*   A person with normal hearing hears sound equally in both ears in response to Weber's test. Consistent referral of the vertex sound to one ear, with bone conduction better than air conduction in that ear, indicates a conductive hearing loss on that side. The test should be repeated several times to insure a consistent response. The cause of lateralization may be occlusion of the external auditory canal by wax or a foreign body, or a disturbance in the ear drum or ossicles. In other words, some factor impairs the conduction of sound through the external or middle ear to the inner ear.

266. The answer is B. *(DeMyer, ed 3. pp 37-38.)*   The best way to judge whether the eyes are aligned is to compare the corneal light reflections. The points of reflection of light from the two corneas should correspond. Any noncorrespondence indicates malalignment. Judging ocular alignment by the relation of the eyes to the lids may lead to error; several lid anomalies make the eyes appear malaligned when they are not. Lateral displacement of the medial canthi relative to the iris (as occurs in infants or in malformation syndromes), gives a spurious appearance of esotropia. Examiners cannot rely on a patient's reports of diplopia. Diplopia may be absent in congenital or early acquired ocular malalignments. Some mentally disturbed patients will report diplopia but do not have ocular malalignment.

267. The answer is C. *(Adams, ed 2. p 178.)*   A normal eye shows the least range of movement on upward gaze. From its primary position, the eye will rotate about 10 mm laterally or downward but only about 7 mm upward. In most disorders affecting the hemispheres diffusely—such as dementia, increased intracranial pressure, or aging—the range of upward eye movements generally will be impaired before restriction occurs in the other directions of gaze. As a rule, midbrain-diencephalic lesions affect upward gaze more frequently and more severely than downward gaze. A few specific exceptions to these general rules do occur. For example, in the syndrome of supranuclear palsy, downward gaze may be more severely affected, especially early in the course of the disease.

268. The answer is A. *(DeMyer, ed 3. p 287.)*   The vestibular component of caloric nystagmus is the slow, deviation phase and the nonvestibular component is the quick, kickback phase. The quick phase depends, in large part, on the cortical efferent system from the frontal eye fields. Interruption of this system will result in loss of the quick phase, but the slow, deviation phase in response to caloric irrigation remains. The direction of vestibular or caloric nystagmus unfortunately is named by the direction of the fast component, which is not the primary vestibular action.

269. The answer is E. *(DeMyer, ed 3. pp 250-251.)*   In testing a patient for dysdiadochokinesia, an examiner usually can distinguish the nondominant hand from the dominant by having the patient slap the thighs alternately with the fronts and backs of the hands. The examiner encourages the patient to perform this action as fast and as rhythmically as possible. By listening to the slapping sound and watching, the examiner can determine the hand that performs less well. The nondominant hand may be distinguished by its slightly slower rate and slightly irregular rhythm. Cerebral, cerebellar, and extrapyramidal dysfunction may be expressed in this test.

270. The answer is B. *(DeMyer, ed 3. pp 285-287.)*   Before performing a caloric irrigation test, an examiner has the patient sit erect, tilting the patient's head 60 degrees backward. The purpose of this maneuver is to place the lateral canal in the exact vertical plane. The lateral canal inclines 30 degrees above the horizontal, and the additional 60 degrees of inclination places it in a vertical position. With the lateral canal in the vertical plane, the effect of gravity plus the temperature effect of the irrigating fluid stimulates circulation of the fluid in the lateral semicircular canal, which in turn stimulates the vestibular receptors.

271. The answer is C (2, 4). *(DeMyer, ed 3. pp 414-416.)*   Evidence that blood in the CSF is not a result of a traumatic lumbar puncture is furnished by a demonstration either of red blood cell-laden macrophages in the CSF specimen, as obtained by sedimentation cytomorphology, or of xanthochromia of the supernatant fluid. Several hours are required for macrophages laden with red blood cells to appear, hence their presence is proof that blood existed in the CSF prior to the lumbar puncture. If the supernatant fluid appears xanthochromic after centrifugation, preexisting red blood cells have undergone lysis and released their hemoglobin into the CSF. Xanthochromia from lysis of the cells requires several hours to develop and, therefore, indicates preexisting bleeding. Centrifugation causes sedimentation of intact red blood cells, leaving the fluid clear if the blood cells are of recent origin. Neither crenation of red blood cells nor the number of red blood cells is evidence of their preexistence in the CSF. The greater osmolarity of CSF relative to red blood cells permits crenation to occur, whether the cells were recently introduced or were in the CSF to begin with.

272. The answer is A (1, 2, 3). *(DeMyer, ed 3. pp 61-62.)* Diagnostic features of nonparalytic (concomitant) heterotropia include the following: (1) the degree of deviation remains the same throughout all directions of movement when both eyes are used; (2) each eye shows a full range of movement when the other is covered; (3) one eye frequently will show an opacity of the media or a severe refractive error; and (4) the patient does not complain of diplopia. In contrast, in paralytic heterotropia from a nerve lesion, the degree of deviation of the eyes increases as the eyes move in the direction of pull of the paretic muscle; the affected eye shows the same restriction of movement when used alone as when both eyes are used together; and the patient **will** complain of diplopia (at least if the nerve lesion occurred after infancy and the patient does not have suppression amblyopia).

273. The answer is B (1, 3). *(DeMyer, ed 3. p 102.)* Adie's syndrome consists of anisocoria, myotonic constriction following response to light accommodation, regular pupillary margin, normal response to mydriatics, and frequent association with hypoactive or absent muscle stretch reflexes. This benign, fairly common syndrome is to be distinguished from other causes of anisocoria, especially the pupillary abnormalities in syphilis in which the Argyll Robertson pupil may be associated with tabes dorsalis and absence of the muscle stretch reflexes. Usually Adie's syndrome is discovered incidentally during an examination for some other complaint. Patients with this syndrome are free of symptoms or complaints despite the pupillary abnormality and hypoactive muscle stretch reflexes.

274. The answer is C (2, 4). *(DeMyer, ed 3. p 286.)* Frenzel lenses (strong positive lenses) are placed over a patient's eyes during caloric irrigation in order to occlude visual fixation and to magnify the eye movements for ease of inspection. The strong lenses abolish visual acuity and prevent visual fixation, which inhibits nystagmus. Blocking of fixation by the Frenzel lenses permits faint nystagmus to appear. The strong lenses magnify the eye movements, making it possible to observe faint, low-amplitude nystagmus. The lenses neither produce pupilloconstriction nor abolish the vertigo that may accompany caloric nystagmus.

275. The answer is B (1, 3). *(Adams, ed 2. pp 972-973.)* The differential diagnosis in an infant with firm, rather large muscles without myotonia include glycogen storage disease and hypothyroidism. The presence of myotonia would raise the additional possibility of myotonia congenita. Myotonic dystrophy may appear in infancy, but fails to present as enlarged muscles. Duchenne's dystrophy is an unlikely diagnosis because it rarely is clinically evident in young infants and is predominantly a disease of males. In evaluating an infant with firm, enlarged muscles, the clinician should perform thyroid function tests and an EMG. If the thyroid function test results are normal, further workup might include muscle biopsy or a biochemical study of the glycolytic pathway in tissue cultures of cells obtained from the patient.

276. The answer is A (1, 2, 3). *(Adams, ed 2. pp 990-991.)* Patients with hyperthyroidism may have myasthenic weakness with pathologic fatigability, periodic weakness with low blood levels of potassium, and ophthalmoplegia. Enlarged, firm muscles occur in **hypo**thyroidism. The possibility of thyroid dysfunction should be considered if a patient displays any of these four types of muscle disorders. Enlarged, firm muscles may occur prior to the stage of atrophy in several disorders, including Duchenne's dystrophy, some muscle disorders with myotonia, and glycogen storage disease. The variety of muscle disorders found in association with thyroid disease indicates the importance of testing for thyroid dysfunction in patients who have muscle disorders of obscure origin.

277. The answer is A (1, 2, 3). *(Adams, ed 2. pp 964-965.)* Progressive external ophthalmoplegia has been the subject of controversy for many years. At one time, it was considered to be an ocular form of progressive motor neuron degeneration, but now it is usually classed as a myopathy. The problem lies in interpreting neurogenic and myopathic changes in eye muscle biopsies. The disease does have an association with retinitis pigmentosa, far more so than do other forms of muscular dystrophy. Patients with progressive external ophthalmoplegia do not characteristically complain of, or present with, diplopia. The eyes may become completely immobile but generally remain in the primary position, because all muscles are equally involved. This fact, in conjunction with the extremely gradual evolution of the disease, make diplopia an uncommon complaint.

278. The answer is A (1, 2, 3). *(Swaiman, pp 300-301.)* In principle, amniocentesis is performed to identify a fetus with a neurologic or genetic defect. The mother may then elect either to carry the fetus to term or to undergo abortion. Amniocentesis can be used to identify fetuses having genetic diseases with known inborn errors of metabolism, with abnormal karyotypes, and fetuses with dysraphia. Inborn errors of metabolism can be detected by chemical tests on the amniotic fluid or on cells grown from it. Abnormal karyotypes are detected by growing cells obtained from the amniotic fluid. Dysraphic states are detected by demonstrating high levels of alpha fetoprotein. On the other hand, many diseases, even though genetic, lack a known or readily demonstrable metabolic error (such as Huntington's chorea), and currently cannot be detected by amniocentesis.

279. The answer is E (all). *(DeMyer, ed 3. pp 123-124.)* Pseudopapilledema is characterized by maximum elevation of the disk centrally, preretinal branching of the vessels, presence of drusen, and a normal blind spot, the opposite of the findings in true papilledema. An additional distinguishing feature of pseudopapilledema is a strong association with hyperopic, blond Caucasians. Pseudopapilledema is a nonpathologic condition, recognition of which will obviate unnecessary diagnostic procedures. Because pseudopapilledema frequently is familial, relatives of affected individuals should be examined for the condition.

280. The answer is A (1, 2, 3). *(DeMyer, ed 3. p 9.)* Bruits may be heard over the head in any condition associated with large amounts of cerebral blood flow. Thus, bruits are common in normal infants, whose brains receive about 20 percent of the cardiac outflow. Carotid-cavernous fistulae characteristically cause bruits, and bruits also may occur in acute meningitis because of changes in cerebral blood flow. Bruits are not associated with chronic brain abscesses, because the encapsulated mass does not increase cerebral blood flow.

281. The answer is A (1, 2, 3). *(Adams, ed 2. pp 876-881.)* An EMG shows prominent electrical activity in myotonia, tetany, and exercise-induced muscle cramps in normal individuals. No electrical activity is generated by muscle contraction in the exercise intolerance syndromes allied to McArdle's disease. In the first three conditions listed in the question, some active mechanism, either in the nervous system or muscle, drives the active contraction of the muscle. In the contraction of exercise intolerance, the defect—at least in some instances—rather than involving a mechanism that drives contraction, may involve the inability of the muscle to relax. Relaxation itself is an active process that requires energy.

282. The answer is C (2, 4). *(Adams, ed 2. p 880.)* Myotonia usually decreases with increasing use of the involved muscle, is demonstrable by percussion, causes a distinctive EMG pattern, and occurs after a single contraction. These criteria serve to differentiate it from other types of cramps and contractures of the muscle. It is important to have positive criteria by which to identify myotonia, because there are many other causes of muscle cramps. In addition, myotonia may be associated with weak muscles (as in myotonia dystrophica) or with strong muscles (as in myotonia congenita).

283. The answer is C (2, 4). *(Cooper, ed 3. p 25.)* Large axons conduct more rapidly than small axons, have a lower threshold for electrical stimulation, but respond more slowly to local anesthetics. In fact, a low concentration of local anesthetics can be given that blocks conduction in small axons, particularly peripheral autonomic axons, without blocking the large axons. Large axons have more numerous myelin lamellae than do the smaller axons. As a generalization, it can be said that visceral functions in both central and peripheral nervous systems are mediated by small, poorly myelinated or unmyelinated axons, whereas somatic motor and sensory functions in both peripheral and central nervous systems are mediated by large myelinated axons. However, pain and temperature fibers, although classed with the somatic motor system, are small and poorly myelinated or unmyelinated.

284-287. The answers are: 284-C, 285-A, 286-C, 287-D. *(Swaiman, pp 269-270.)* Myelomeningocele shows some familial clustering, suggesting a hereditary influence but without a specific mendelian pattern.

Knowledge of the hereditary nature of a disease is imperative for genetic counseling and for identification of individuals at risk for the disorder. A woman who is a carrier for a sex-linked recessive disease can avoid bearing an affected male by choosing to abort all male fetuses. Half of her daughters, however, will be carriers; and the overproduction of carriers throughout several generations can significantly increase the risk of the disease, as occurs in inbred populations.

Myotonic dystrophy exemplifies an autosomal dominant disorder, whereas Duchenne's dystrophy and Pelizaeus-Merzbacher disease exemplify sex-linked recessive disorders in which males are afflicted predominantly. In the autosomal dominant disorders, one parent of the affected patient should exhibit clinical evidence of the disease in order to establish the hereditary nature of the patient's disorder.

In the recessive syndromes characterized by inborn errors of metabolism, the parents of affected offspring may show no **clinical** evidence of the disorder, but frequently show **biochemical** changes. Appropriate biochemical tests can identify the parents as carriers of the disease trait in question and can be used to identify siblings or other relatives at risk as carriers of the disorder.

288-291. The answers are: 288-D, 289-C, 290-A, 291-E. *(DeMyer, ed 3. pp 24-26.)* Premature suture closure alters the skull shape, depending on which suture or sutures are involved. The head configuration is diagnostic of the involved suture. Too short a head is acrobrachycephaly, too long a head is scaphocephaly, too short and too narrow a head is oxycephaly, and a triangular, peaked forehead is trigonocephaly. Trigonocephalic individuals also exhibit orbital hypotelorism. Plagiocephaly indicates an asymmetrical skull due to unilateral suture closure.

Early recognition and diagnosis of these craniosynostotic head shapes is important because surgical correction during infancy produces the best cosmetic results and may possibly prevent some brain damage from the compressive effects of the unyielding skull. Craniosynostosis is evident at birth and should be diagnosed in the neonatal period.

The main problem in differential diagnosis is microcephaly. In infants with microcephaly, the small size of the brain results in a small-sized skull. Even though in microcephaly the fontanelles will be small, the examiner will still be able to palpate both the fontanelles and sutures. In case of any doubt, skull radiography will disclose the presence of the sutures and their patency. Patients with craniosynostosis also frequently have malformations of the extremities, such as syndactyly.

292-295. The answers are: 292-C, 293-A, 294-E, 295-D. *(Swaiman, p 389.)* Some disorders have well-established chromosomal anomalies and others, although unquestionably hereditary, have no obvious disorder in chromosome number or size. Trisomies and deletions are common disorders of chromosome number or size; of these, trisomies 13, 21, XXY syndrome, and the 5 deletion syndrome (cri du chat) constitute some of the best known. Neurofibromatosis fails to show a gross disturbance of chromosomal morphology. Holoprosencephaly may occur with a normal karyotype; but when a karyotype abnormality exists, it is usually trisomy 13, although other errors also occur.

By knowing which disorders have gross chromosomal errors, a clinician can offer amniocentesis to mothers at risk for producing infants with that disorder, allowing elective abortion of an affected fetus. Most gross errors of chromosome number or morphology are associated with an identifiable clinical syndrome of malformations. Not only do the affected individuals exhibit a clinically recognizable set of external malformations; they often have visceral malformations as well. The majority of patients with gross abnormalities of chromosome number or morphology have some degree of mental deficiency. Thus, a chromosome deviation may produce a defective brain, but no chromosomal abnormalities are known to be associated with superior intelligence.

Psychiatry Questions for Neurologists

DIRECTIONS: Each question below contains five suggested answers. Choose the **one best** response to each question.

296. In helping a nonpsychotic, basically rational, but emotionally troubled patient, a physician who follows traditional principles of psychotherapy would choose which of the following approaches?

(A) Provide direct advice on management of the patient's interpersonal relationships
(B) Help the patient to seek acceptable alternative plans of action and allow the patient to select the particular option to be followed
(C) Intervene by directly contacting persons of emotional significance in the patient's life
(D) Make the patient feel secure by much touching and active, demonstrative expressions of sympathy
(E) Prescribe appropriate psychotropic medication and urge the patient to seek diversion from the source of emotional conflict

297. The production of motor stereotypies by chronic amphetamine use in humans and animals is thought to involve which of the following mechanisms?

(A) Stimulation of the cholinergic mechanism of the reticular activating system
(B) Inhibition of the inhibitory outflow from the Purkinje cells to the dentate nuclei
(C) Direct stimulation of neurons in the motor cortex
(D) Activation of the substantia nigra neurons
(E) Activation of the dopaminergic systems

298. Psychomotor seizure patients as a group are best characterized sexually as

(A) being hyposexual
(B) being hypersexual
(C) having a very high incidence of pedophilia
(D) having the same incidence of sexual problems as a random sample of the general population
(E) not having sexual sensations and orgasm as part of their seizure

299. The first sign of an evolving parkinsonian syndrome induced by neuroleptic drugs is usually

(A) bradykinesia
(B) akathisia
(C) pill-rolling tremor
(D) cogwheel rigidity
(E) retropulsive gait

300. Current knowledge of the effect of bifrontal lesions (sparing the motor cortex) on human behavior is best described by which of the following statements?

(A) Bifrontal lesions are characterized by inappropriate joking (witzelsucht), but an absence of overactivity, driven behavior, or inappropriate sexuality
(B) Bifrontal lesions may cause profound effects on behavior or personality, frequently with little effect on standard IQ tests
(C) Bifrontal lesions produce behavioral and personality alterations that cannot be produced by lesions elsewhere in the cerebrum
(D) Bifrontal lesions heighten self-awareness of bodily dysfunction
(E) A specific frontal lobe syndrome exists that can be recognized by characteristic neurologic signs

301. A patient who is found to have Parkinson's disease and to be depressed would, at least in theory, be most helped by treatment with

(A) caffeine
(B) lithium
(C) benztropine
(D) imipramine
(E) L-dopa

302. Delirium is distinguished from dementia chiefly by the presence of

(A) loss of memory
(B) hyperemotionality
(C) apathy and withdrawal
(D) episodes of hallucinations
(E) clouding of consciousness

303. The differential diagnosis in a 61-year-old patient involves mild depression, early presenile dementia, and pseudodementia. Which of the following test results would argue most strongly against an organic disorder?

(A) A mild degree of EEG slowing in the temporal regions
(B) Normal Halstead-Reitan neuropsychological battery
(C) Normal routine lumbar puncture
(D) Normal radioactive brain scan
(E) CAT scan showing slight increase in sulcal markings

304. Pick's disease is most readily distinguished from other presenile dementias by which of the following histologic findings?

(A) Granulovacuolar degeneration of the hippocampus
(B) Neurofibrillary tangles
(C) Rounded or pear-shaped pallid cortical neurons
(D) Absence of gliosis
(E) Senile plaques

305. The effect on sleep opposite to that caused by destruction of the median raphe of the pontine tegmentum would be produced by which of the following substances?

(A) p-Chlorophenylalanine
(B) Tryptophan
(C) Amphetamine
(D) Caffeine
(E) Picrotoxin

306. The transient global amnesia syndrome may be explained on which of the following pathoanatomic bases?

(A) Infarction of the dentate gyrus
(B) Destruction of the mamillary bodies
(C) Lacunar state of the thalamus
(D) Degeneration of the hippocampal pyramidal cells
(E) None of the above

307. Fluent aphasic patients lose the ability to

(A) correct their own speech errors
(B) speak with prosody
(C) communicate by gesturing
(D) understand pantomime or gesture
(E) understand any spoken or written commands

308. The so-called paradoxical effect of medication in hyperactive children refers to which one of the following responses?

(A) Calming effect of drugs classed as stimulants
(B) Calming effect of phenobarbital
(C) Reduction in hyperactivity from benzodiazepines
(D) Proven adverse response to salicylates and red dyes
(E) Minimal response to alcohol as adults

309. The psychosis associated with chronic use of amphetamines resembles naturally occurring schizophrenia in every way EXCEPT for the absence of

(A) paranoia
(B) hallucinations
(C) withdrawal and apathy
(D) affective flattening and disordered thought associations
(E) stereotyped movements, repetitive behaviors, and grimacing

310. Akathisia most resembles

(A) athetosis
(B) dystonia
(C) Gilles de la Tourette's syndrome
(D) restless legs syndrome
(E) sleep myoclonia

311. The nature of the hyperkinesias in schizophrenic patients who have not been treated with psychotropic drugs is best described by which of the following statements?

(A) Prior to the psychotropic drug era, hyperkinesias were commonly described in association with schizophrenia
(B) The hyperkinesias of schizophrenia closely resemble the standard syndromes of chorea, athetosis, dystonia, and ballismus
(C) The hyperkinesias are associated with a relatively good prognosis
(D) The hyperkinetic patients evolve graceful, skilled movement patterns
(E) The hyperkinesias tend to disappear when the patient walks

312. A man with the recent onset of slightly slurred speech and some questionable difficulty in naming objects failed to protrude his tongue on command, but licked his lips a few minutes later. This observation is best explained on the basis of

(A) negativism
(B) hysterical overlay
(C) apraxia
(D) temporal disorientation
(E) corticobulbar tract interruption

313. A 50-year-old patient complains of increasing weakness of extremity and trunk muscles of several months duration, with sparing of the cranial nerve muscles. Examination reveals proximal weakness and possibly atrophy, with preserved muscle stretch reflexes. EMG and muscle biopsy are normal. Screening tests for collagen-vascular disease are negative. Serum enzyme levels are normal. Results of a toxicology screen for heavy metals are negative. These findings warrant which of the following conclusions?

(A) Organic disease of the neuromuscular system is excluded
(B) A lumbar puncture should be performed
(C) A myelogram should be performed
(D) A psychiatric consultation is required
(E) Thyroid function tests should be performed

314. A 21-year-old man detained because of assaultive behavior is tall, acne-scarred, and has minimal cerebellar signs. His IQ is 82. The study most likely to provide a diagnosis is which of the following?

(A) Extensive neuropsychologic testing
(B) CAT scan
(C) EEG
(D) Karyotype
(E) Urinary amino acid screen

315. A sensory modality is defined as

(A) any one of the special senses mediated through cranial nerves
(B) any one of the general senses
(C) any unique sensation not resolvable into elementary components
(D) any of the dorsal column modalities including light touch
(E) pain, temperature, and touch

316. Anosognosia is characteristic of which of the following conditions?

(A) Diffuse cerebral disease
(B) Frontal lobe lesions
(C) Right posterior parasylvian area lesions
(D) Right lateral occipital gyrus
(E) None of the above

317. A nondemented patient with a left homonymous hemianopia is unable to orient her clothes preparatory to dressing. This type of dressing apraxia suggests a lesion of

(A) the right frontal lobe
(B) the left frontal lobe
(C) the left posterior parasylvian area
(D) the right posterior parasylvian area
(E) both cerebral hemispheres

318. A patient has a complete arm monoplegia of obscure origin. The muscle stretch reflexes are equivocally increased in the arm. It hangs loosely at the patient's side but flexes upon coughing. This action is evidence of

(A) a hysterical origin of the paralysis
(B) an associated movement of upper motor neuron lesions
(C) a pontine tegmental lesion involving the cough center
(D) a brachial plexus lesion
(E) a high spinal cord lesion

319. The movement patterns of manic-depressive patients are best characterized by which of the following statements?

(A) The manic phase closely resembles the tardive dyskinesias
(B) They usually take the form of bizarre stereotypies and mannerisms in the manic phase
(C) They often closely resemble parkinsonian hypokinesia in the depressive phase
(D) They usually are expressed as tremors
(E) They have distinctive patterns that are typical of manic-depressive illness

320. Patients with chorea usually will also exhibit which of the following muscle states?

(A) Hypotonia
(B) Dystonia
(C) Rigidity
(D) Spasticity
(E) Normal tone

321. A woman complains of patchy loss of feeling in her left arm and paralysis of the fingers 10 days after a fall in which she injured her left shoulder. The examination shows absence of voluntary movement of the left hand, questionable atrophy of the intrinsic muscles, and variable hypesthesia without a reproducible pattern. An EMG shows very rare polyphasic waves that may be fasciculations, but otherwise shows electrical silence. The patient becomes upset and refuses further electrical tests. In this context, the EMG findings have which of the following diagnostic implications?

(A) They support a diagnosis of malingering
(B) They support a diagnosis of brachial plexus injury
(C) They suggest a spinal cord injury
(D) They argue neither for nor against a nerve or plexus injury
(E) They exclude a plexus or nerve injury as the cause of paralysis

322. The primary gain the hysterical patient is thought to achieve from a hysterical symptom is which of the following?

(A) Manipulative control over other persons
(B) Suppression of hallucinations
(C) Relief from anxiety
(D) Relief from pain
(E) Excuse from responsibilities

323. The correct formula for obtaining an IQ score is

(A) $\dfrac{\text{mental age}}{\text{chronological age}} \times 100$
(B) $\dfrac{\text{chronological age}}{\text{mental age}} \times 100$
(C) $\dfrac{\text{chronological age}}{\text{mental age} \times 100}$
(D) $\dfrac{\text{mental age}}{\text{chronological age} \times 100}$
(E) none of the above

324. Oscillopsia is best described as

(A) a patient's complaint that an object viewed appears to be moving
(B) an examiner's observation of the eye movements in nystagmus
(C) a rapid movement of the pupillary margins
(D) a shimmering scotoma of migraine
(E) none of the above

325. In Huntington's chorea, the most consistent biochemical abnormality in the basal ganglia is

(A) an increase in striatal dopamine and tyrosine hydroxylase
(B) an increase in substantia nigral dopamine and tyrosine hydroxylase
(C) a decrease in striatal GABA and glutamic acid decarboxylase
(D) a decrease in nigral serotonin and tryptophan hydroxylase
(E) none of the above

326. A patient who has a basilar skull fracture complains that sounds seem uncomfortably loud. This symptom most probably represents

(A) a conversion reaction
(B) a partial lesion of the VIIIth cranial nerve
(C) a lesion of the transverse temporal gyri
(D) interruption of the lateral lemniscus
(E) stapedius muscle paralysis

327. Hallucinations are defined as

(A) false beliefs that can be dispelled by reason
(B) false beliefs that cannot be dispelled by reason
(C) false sensory perceptions based on natural stimulation of a receptor
(D) false sensory perceptions not based on natural stimulation of a receptor
(E) any abnormal sensations from a neurologic lesion

328. A 4-year-old previously normal girl begins to display personality changes. Her parents feel that she does not walk as well as previously. The examination discloses slight clumsiness without overt motor signs. Stretch reflexes are somewhat hypoactive. The history and examination are otherwise noncontributory. The procedure most likely to yield a specific diagnosis is which of the following?

(A) CAT scan with contrast
(B) Neuropsychological test battery
(C) Determination of karyotype
(D) Lysosomal enzyme battery
(E) Urinary amino acid screen

329. According to *DSM-III*, the single criterion or symptom indispensable to the initial diagnosis of schizophrenia is

(A) hallucinations and delusions
(B) disorders of perception
(C) ideas of reference
(D) deterioration of mental function for at least 6 months
(E) depersonalization and separation of thought from self

DIRECTIONS: Each question below contains four suggested answers of which **one** or **more** is correct. Choose the answer

A	if	1, 2, and 3	are correct
B	if	1 and 3	are correct
C	if	2 and 4	are correct
D	if	4	is correct
E	if	1, 2, 3, and 4	are correct

330. Patients who are very likely to produce excessive countertransference in male physicians include which of the following?

(1) Patients with manic-depressive personalities
(2) Patients with antisocial personality disorders
(3) Middle-aged, overweight women who are given to complaining .
(4) Attractive young women

331. Use of the major antipsychotic drugs is contraindicated in

(1) acute anxiety states
(2) reactive depression
(3) recurrent unipolar depression
(4) psychotic depression

332. Advantages of benzodiazepines as antianxiety agents include which of the following?

(1) Wide gap between effective doses and lethal doses
(2) Relatively low activation of hepatic microsomal enzymes
(3) Long duration of action
(4) Relatively low risk of producing physical tolerance

333. In an effort to determine whether patients with psychomotor seizures have a greater tendency to criminal behavior than those with other types of epilepsy, a study was made of all epileptic patients who had attended a university outpatient epilepsy clinic for more than 3 years. Methodologically superior and more efficient ways to seek any such correlation would include

(1) drawing random samples from the population at large
(2) studying all patients with epilepsy seen at a large municipal hospital for 3 years
(3) studying only outpatients with psychomotor seizures
(4) studying a large number of prisoners with epilepsy

334. Correct statements concerning sudden jerks of the body when a person falls asleep include which of the following?

(1) They usually are associated with a spike in the EEG
(2) They frequently are associated with arousal from sleep
(3) They frequently occur in the deep stages of sleep
(4) They usually are benign

335. Pendular, jerky movements of the eyes when following a moving object are commonly found in 45 percent or more persons who have

(1) schizophrenia
(2) Parkinson's disease
(3) psychotic depression
(4) no disorder

336. Correct statements concerning behavior modification therapy include which of the following?

(1) It regards behavior disorders as maladaptive learning
(2) It excludes the use of extinction techniques
(3) It ignores psychodynamic formulations
(4) It dispenses with desensitization techniques

337. Operant conditioning may be described as

(1) requiring presentation of an unconditioned stimulus
(2) more useful in brain-impaired than normal individuals
(3) lacking application in conventional psychotherapy
(4) utilizing either positive or negative reinforcement

SUMMARY OF DIRECTIONS				
A	B	C	D	E
1, 2, 3 only	1, 3 only	2, 4 only	4 only	All are correct

338. Statements that accurately apply to the concept of body image include which of the following?

(1) A child's concept of its body image becomes an integral part of its personality
(2) Depersonalization may involve an extreme loss of body image
(3) The body image develops from sensory and motor experiences
(4) Neurotic persons usually have an undistorted body image

339. Rapid eye movement (REM) sleep has which of the following characteristics?

(1) It occurs cyclically throughout the night
(2) It exhibits low-voltage fast activity in the EEG
(3) It is associated with dreaming states
(4) It is useful in studying causes of impotence

340. Sites of lesions known to be associated with pathologic wakefulness include which of the following?

(1) Median raphe of the pontine tegmentum
(2) Reticular formation of the midbrain tegmentum
(3) Anterior hypothalamus and preoptic area
(4) Superior colliculi of the midbrain

341. Profound memory loss with little involvement of other mental functions is produced by bilateral damage to which of the following structures?

(1) Dorsomedial nuclei of the thalamus
(2) Ammon's horn and dentate gyrus
(3) Parahippocampal gyrus
(4) Fornix

342. Sleep paralysis is associated with which of the following characteristics?

(1) It occurs most commonly during transition to or from sleep
(2) It is usually associated with a strong feeling of fear
(3) It disappears when a person is called or touched
(4) It is associated with a shift of potassium into muscle

343. Statements that correctly describe the sexual consequences of neuroanatomic lesions include which of the following?

(1) Bilateral ventrolateral chordotomy usually causes loss of erection and ejaculation in males
(2) Destruction of the lumbar sympathetic ganglia causes loss of ejaculation but retention of erectile capacity
(3) Paraplegic males with complete cord transections may have intercourse and father children
(4) Destruction of the vulva or amputation of the penis prevents orgasm

344. The ego, as defined by classical psychoanalytic formulations, is described as

(1) incorporating the reality-testing and cognitive functions
(2) incorporating the solution-forming, defense-creating aspects of the personality
(3) bringing about a *modus operandi* for perceiving and relating to other persons
(4) containing the internalized ideal of what the person should be like

345. The narcolepsy syndrome typically includes which of the following?

(1) Irresistible sleep under inappropriate circumstances
(2) Cataplexy
(3) Hypnagogic hallucinations and sleep paralysis
(4) Episodic automatic behavior with amnesia

346. Statements that correctly describe the characteristics of the amnesia associated with head trauma and a period of unconsciousness include which of the following?

(1) The period of retrograde amnesia is usually shorter than the anterograde amnesia
(2) After recovering consciousness, a patient may seem rational and coherent for days or weeks yet fail to remember the period of unconsciousness
(3) Frequently, the period of retrograde amnesia shrinks during recovery
(4) The retrograde and anterograde aspects of amnesia differ greatly in comparing posttraumatic amnesia with amnesia associated with psychomotor seizures

347. Clinical features that help to establish a diagnosis of pseudodementia in elderly patients include a tendency on the part of such patients to

(1) complain greatly about loss of mental faculties
(2) exhibit low attention span and concentration
(3) exert little effort to perform on formal tests
(4) display behavior that is poor relative to mental function

348. Statements that describe acute dyskinesias induced by psychotropic medication include which of the following?

(1) They may occur within hours of a single dose
(2) They rarely manifest as dystonic movements
(3) They frequently affect the ocular, facial, and oropharyngeal muscles
(4) They frequently occur in response to reserpine

349. Altered mental states in combination with fiery red or scarlet skin may result from

(1) acetaldehyde syndrome of disulfiram
(2) carbon monoxide poisoning
(3) mercury intoxication
(4) hypoadrenocorticism

350. Psychedelic or hallucinogenic drugs are characterized by which of the following features?

(1) They produce heightened awareness of sensory input
(2) They have a strong tendency to cause addiction and continued use
(3) They are classified as indoleamines or phenyethylamines
(4) They are a common cause of auditory hallucinations

351. Correct statements concerning acute alcoholic inebriation include which of the following?

(1) The odor of the breath serves as a reliable diagnostic aid
(2) Forcing of oral fluids will reduce the blood alcohol level rapidly
(3) Hypothermia rules out alcoholic intoxication
(4) A blood alcohol level of 100 mg/100 ml constitutes legal drunkenness

352. The major antipsychotic drugs may produce adverse effects such as

(1) hypotension and hypothermia
(2) cardiac dysrhythmias
(3) coma
(4) seizures

353. Visual field defects that frequently occur in hysterical patients include which of the following?

(1) Spiral fields on confrontation testing or perimetry
(2) Paracentral scotomata as demonstrated on tangent screen
(3) Tubular vision
(4) Sector defects as demonstrated by tangent screen

SUMMARY OF DIRECTIONS

A	B	C	D	E
1, 2, 3 only	1, 3 only	2, 4 only	4 only	All are correct

354. True statements about sensory losses include which of the following?

(1) Patients with hysterical cutaneous anesthesia will flinch if the pain stimulus is made strong enough

(2) The hysterical patient has a sensory loss that conforms to the patient's mental image of the body parts

(3) In organic hemianesthesia, the loss of vibratory sensation stops abruptly at the midline when a tuning fork is applied to the forehead or sternum

(4) In hysterical paraplegia and anesthesia, the sensory loss extends horizontally around the waist, whereas in organic paraplegia, the sensory level slopes downward

355. As classically defined, the syndrome of Gerstmann includes

(1) right-left disorientation
(2) digital agnosia
(3) dyscalculia
(4) dysgraphia

DIRECTIONS: The groups of questions below consist of lettered choices followed by several numbered items. For each numbered item select the **one** lettered choice with which it is **most** closely associated. Each lettered choice may be used once, more than once, or not at all.

Questions 356-359

For each example of a mental defense mechanism, choose the term with which it is most closely associated.

(A) Fixation
(B) Regression
(C) Identification
(D) Projection
(E) Rationalization

356. A shy young man, formerly only moderately interested in athletics, begins to practice throwing a football and frequently organizes touch football games among acquaintances who then become friends. He has his hair cut in the style of Joe Namath and assumes that athlete's mannerisms. When he has a T-shirt imprinted with the great quarterback's number, his new friends nickname him Junior Joe.

357. A young woman with a large sexual appetite is married to a man whom she loves and with whom she feels basically compatible. While he is struggling to make a success of a business, she engages in a series of affairs with a variety of men. By most criteria, the husband does not neglect his wife, who nevertheless believes that her husband is more interested in his business than in her. She ascribes her many sexual affairs to traits in her husband rather than in herself.

358. A solder inflicts a wound on himself to escape front-line duty during a war. Later he feels guilty. To ward off the painful resultant anxiety, the soldier blames his physician for neglecting to treat the wound (which is slow to heal) and tries to kill him. The soldier is not consciously aware that, in trying to kill his physician, he is attempting to destroy his own actual deficiencies.

359. A 3-year-old child is fully toilet trained until a sibling is born, whereupon he starts to have toileting accidents and wet the bed at night.

Questions 360-363

For each of the definitions listed below, choose the term with which it is most closely associated.

(A) Instinct
(B) Drive
(C) Reflex
(D) Behavior
(E) Stimulus

360. Any relatively invariant, neurally mediated response of an organism to an identifiable change

361. Any innate, unlearned behavioral pattern triggered by a specific external stimulus

362. Any identifiable change capable of triggering a neurally mediated response

363. Any observable, neurally mediated change in an individual

Questions 364-367

For each definition below, choose the term with which it is most closely associated.

(A) Palinopsia
(B) Visual allesthesia
(C) Micropsia
(D) Simultagnosia
(E) Dyschromatopsia

364. Any defect in the perception of color

365. The persistence or recurrence of visual images after the stimulus object has been removed

366. Inability to organize a series of related pictures into the correct sequence or to understand the full meaning of a series of perceived parts

367. The displacement of a visual image from the visual field of perception into the opposite visual field

Questions 368-371

For each type of aphasia listed below, choose the lesion site with which it is most closely associated.

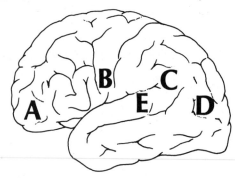

368. Dyslexia

369. Receptive or fluent aphasia (Wernicke's)

370. Auditory aphasia

371. Expressive (nonfluent) aphasia (Broca's)

Questions 372-375

For each clinical description given below, choose the term with which it is most closely associated.

(A) Negativism
(B) Catalepsy
(C) Gegenhalten
(D) Rigidity
(E) Catatonia

372. A patient sits quietly, mute and motionless, making no movement of body or face and showing little reaction to environmental events or stimuli, while the eyes remain fixed on a distant point, alternating with periods of overactivity

373. A patient shows slight resistance to movement but then maintains the body parts in any new position the examiner places them in

374. A patient shows plastic resistance to movement of the body parts in any direction, as if automatically resisting whatever movement the examiner imposes

375. A patient actively resists any effort to be moved or to move in response to command

Questions 376-379

For each clinical feature described below, choose the speech disorder with which it is most closely associated.

(A) Elective mutism
(B) Palilalia
(C) Cluttering
(D) Aphemia
(E) Perseveration

376. A patient repeats the last syllable of words or the last phrase

377. A patient runs words together, omitting sounds or entire words

378. A patient talks to selected individuals but, under certain circumstances, may fail to speak at all to others.

379. A patient suddenly loses the ability to say any words but remains alert and able to understand, read, and write

Questions 380-385

For each stage of sleep listed below, choose the EEG pattern with which it most nearly corresponds.

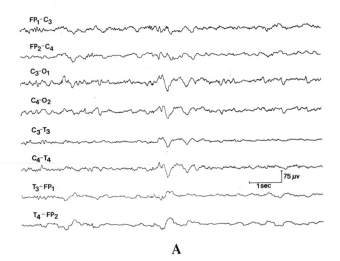

A

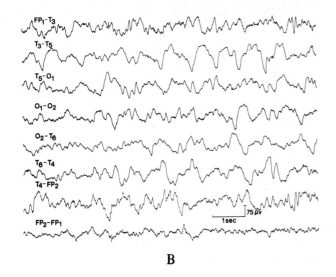

B

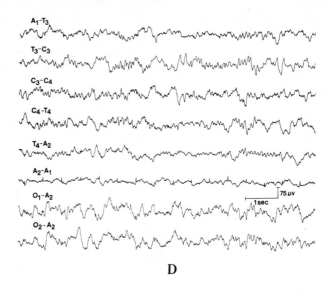

D

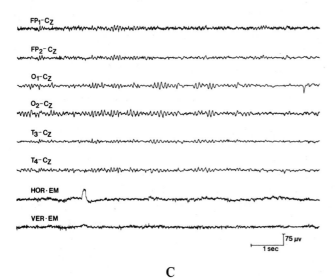

C

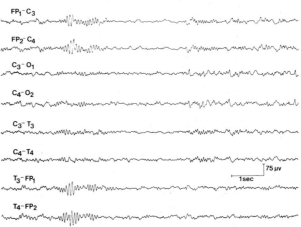

E

380. Normal waking record

381. Stage 1 sleep

382. Stage 2 sleep

383. Stage 3 sleep

384. Stage 4 sleep

385. REM sleep

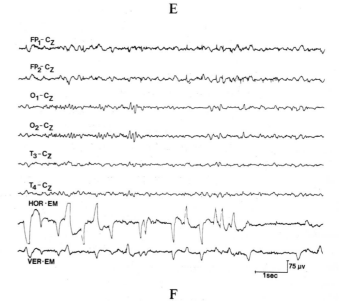

F

Psychiatry Questions for Neurologists Answers

296. The answer is B. *(Kolb, ed 9. p 788.)* In principle, the role of the physician in the physician-patient relationship is to help patients understand the options available and to provide the emotional support required to help them reach their own productive solutions. Paternalism, active advice, physical touching, and overly demonstrative sympathy only divert patients from finding their own solutions and direct patients' attention to characteristics of the physician rather than to the patients' own resources for selecting a healthy response. Thus, whether the object of the physician-patient encounter is strictly a medical problem such as the alternative ways to manage breast cancer, or an emotional problem such as how to work through a difficult divorce, the physician's role is to aid patients in reaching their own conclusions about the most productive option. Most nonpsychotic patients will work out their own solution if the physician provides the perspective from which such patients are able to recognize their own strengths and resources. The role of active touching in the psychiatrist-patient relationship remains controversial and is not part of ordinary psychotherapy.

297. The answer is E. *(Benson, pp 226-227.)* Chronic use of amphetamines in humans or experimental animals results in a motor syndrome characterized by repetitive, stereotyped behaviors. The production of stereotyped behaviors in this situation is believed to result from activation of the dopaminergic systems. These systems arise in either the zona compacta of the substantia nigra where they end in the striatum, or in the interpeduncular region where they play upon the medial basal olfactory and limbic structures. The amphetamine appears to act by increasing the release of dopamine and blocking its reuptake, making more of it available at the postsynaptic ending. L-dopa and methylphenidate produce a similar movement disorder.

298. The answer is A. *(Benson, pp 186-187.)* Patients with psychomotor seizures generally suffer from pervasive hyposexuality; males and females are equally affected. The hyposexuality occurs in patients whose seizures start early in life as well as those with onset during adulthood. However, some patients will have sexual feelings and even orgasm as part of the seizure. The hyposexuality tends to improve with seizure control. After medical or surgical treatment, patients may undergo a (rebound?) period of hypersexuality. While patients with psychomotor seizures do have a high incidence of mental illness, psychomotor seizures apparently fail to contribute significantly to the problem of the sexual offender; but some evidence indicates a relation to transvestism, exhibitionism, and disturbances in gender identity.

299. The answer is A. *(Benson, pp 229-230.)* In Parkinson's disease that evolves during treatment with a neuroleptic drug, the first sign usually is bradykinesia. A patient shows a lack of spontaneous movements, blank facies, absence of arm swinging, and a slowness in the initiation and execution of movements. The patient complains of weakness and fatigue. At this stage, the patient may lack the other classical signs, such as the 4-6 cps tremor, plateau speech, akathisia, and propulsive or retropulsive gait. While the pill-rolling tremor typical of naturally

124

occurring Parkinson's disease may appear in the drug-induced form, it occurs late and is relatively uncommon. The reported incidence of the parkinsonian state during neuroleptic therapy varies with the sensitivity of the method of ascertainment. The incidence may be as high as 90 percent when the most sensitive methods of measuring motor performance are used.

300. The answer is B. *(Benson, pp 151-159.)* While it has long been recognized that bifrontal lesions may profoundly alter behavior and personality, the type and specificity of change remain in question. Similar changes may follow diffuse brain disease or diencephalic lesions. Patients with bifrontal lesions tend to exhibit a syndrome of apathy and indifference that reduces their regard for and concern about bodily dysfunctions. Thus, after a prefrontal lobotomy, chronic cancer patients still report pain but seem to have an attitude of indifference toward it. Yet the results are not always predictable. Some patients with bifrontal lesions become hypomanic or even have a transient state of compulsive walking, and may become sexually overactive. In spite of the obvious clinical changes in behavior, patients with bifrontal lesions may score normally on IQ tests; indeed, the failure of routine IQ tests to show the specific effects of frontal lesions and frontal lobotomies was one of the historical reasons for the development of neuropsychology.

301. The answer is D. *(Benson, p 228.)* A drug that theoretically would be desirable for treating a depressed patient with parkinsonism would combine antidepressive action with central anticholinergic action. The tricyclic antidepressants, of which imipramine is a member, combine these qualities. The other drugs listed in the question would act against one or the other of the target symptoms, but not against both. The tricyclic antidepressants rarely produce extrapyramidal syndromes, but may cause a fine rapid tremor that appears to be an accentuation of physiologic tremor.

302. The answer is E. *(American Psychiatric Association, ed 3. pp 104-107.)* The essential symptomatic difference between delirium and dementia is that some degree of clouding of consciousness is associated with delirium. Most of the other symptoms listed in the question may overlap. If dementia and delirium coexist, the diagnosis of dementia will depend on the clearing of consciousness, leaving the dementia as the residual feature. The delirium usually lasts only a few days, or at most a few weeks. In general, then, delirium implies the probability of reversal. In the past, dementia has implied some inexorably progressive organic brain disorder, but *Diagnostic and Statistical Manual of Mental Disorders* (*DSM-III*) rejects any such connotation.

303. The answer is B. *(Adams, ed 2. pp 289-295. Reitan, p 229.)* In distinguishing between early presenile dementia, depression, and pseudodementia, many tests may show normal or nearly normal results yet fail to determine whether the patient has an organic or functional mental illness. Minimal slowing in the temporal regions in the EEG and a CAT scan that shows questionable ventricular and sulcal enlargement are unhelpful findings in the 61-year-old individual presented in the question. Radioactive brain scan may fail to show abnormalities in early dementias. Normal results on a routine examination of the cerebrospinal fluid would fail to rule out presenile dementia. On the other hand, a normal result on the Halstead-Reitan battery for this patient would, of all the tests discussed, provide the strongest evidence against organic brain disease. This particular battery involves a wide range of tasks devised to explore the organic condition of the brain, and patients with organic dementias, even in early stages, usually show measurable deficits.

304. The answer is C. *(Blackwood, ed 3. pp 817-821.)* The histologic feature most typical of Pick's disease is the presence of pear-shaped cortical neurons that stain pallidly with Nissl stains. The homogenous substance that appears to distend the neurons may have the appearance of a distinct body, but electron microscopy shows no distinct structure. The material consists of neurofilaments, tubules, and vesiculated endoplasmic reticulum. An intense gliosis accompanies the degenerative process in the cortical neurons. Neurofibrillar tangles and senile plaques, in contrast to their frequency in Alzheimer's disease and senile dementia, are infrequent or absent in Pick's disease. Granulovacuolar degeneration of hippocampal neurons occurs in both Alzheimer's and Pick's diseases.

305. The answer is B. *(Adams, ed 2. p 262.)* The destruction of the median raphe of the pontine tegmentum is well known to cause a state of increased wakefulness. The explanation for this phenomenon is that the lesion destroys the serotoninergic neurons of the nuclei of the raphe. Compatible with this hypothesis is the fact that administration of *p*-chlorophenylalanine, which inhibits the synthesis of serotonin, induces a wakeful state, while administration of tryptophan or 5-hydroxytryptophan, which promote serotonin synthesis, promotes sleep. While there are some inconsistencies in the theory of the relationship of serotonin to sleep, serotonin does play some role in sleep physiology. Agents such as amphetamines, caffeine, and picrotoxin cause hyperwakefulness, similar to that produced by destruction of the median raphe.

306. The answer is E. *(Adams, ed 2. p 293.)* Transient global amnesia occurs in middle-aged and elderly persons. The patient loses memory for a period of several hours, but retains consciousness and many cognitive abilities. Although the differential diagnosis of this condition includes psychomotor seizures, the pathologic substrate remains to be identified. The best surmise is that the syndrome represents a type of transient ischemic attack involving territories irrigated by the posterior cerebral artery, which supplies the inferomedial aspect of the temporal lobes and sends arcades to the hippocampus. The syndrome usually disappears.

307. The answer is A. *(Adams, ed 2. p 329. DeMyer, ed 3. pp 350-351.)* Among other speech deficits experienced by fluent aphasic patients is the inability to correct their own speech errors and, frequently, the failure even to perceive them. Such patients produce an excess of words that are often composed of unrelated syllables, constituting a word salad. The fluent aphasic patient retains the ability to speak with prosody—the normal inflections and rhythms—but loses the faculty to control **content** of speech. Also retained are the ability to understand certain written or spoken commands and a limited ability to communicate by gestures.

308. The answer is A. *(Adams, ed 2. pp 413-415.)* A paradox about hyperactive children (as has been stated in the past) is the observation that drugs classed as stimulants seemed to improve the cardinal symptoms of hyperactivity, impulsiveness, short attention span, and hyperexcitability. Contrarily, drugs that should have sedative action, such as the barbiturates, frequently worsen the target symptoms. One resolution of the paradox lies in the interpretation of the state of arousal. The hyperactivity might be interpreted as a reaction to a **hypo**-aroused nervous system. The stimulant drug normalizes the arousal and eliminates the compensating overactive behavior. Barbiturates would further reduce the state of arousal and cause the target symptoms to become correspondingly worse. This formulation might aid in selecting children who could benefit from stimulant medication by subjecting them to tests for hypoarousal.

309. The answer is D. *(Benson, pp 226-227.)* The chronic abuse of amphetamines may produce a paranoid psychosis that very closely resembles the naturally occurring disease. This psychosis is characterized by paranoid ideation, many stereotypies and mannerisms, hallucinations, and in the later stages, withdrawal and apathy. The major significant difference appears to be in the absence of affective flattening and absence of disorders of thought association, which characterize the naturally occurring disease. Amphetamine administration to other primates produces the same motor disturbances seen in humans.

310. The answer is D. *(DeMyer, ed 3. p 236.)* Akathisia, often a prominent feature of parkinsonism or drug-induced movement disorders, consists of an irresistible restlessness that compels a patient to shift position or to move around. It is a peculiar state, because the patient has an odd mixture of hypokinesia that is broken by compelling movement. Some patients pace incessantly, albeit displaying the parkinsonian gait. The restless legs syndrome, and perhaps to a lesser extent the hyperkinetic child syndrome, together with the manic phase of manic-depressive psychosis all offer parallels to akathisia. Thus, patients with the restless legs syndrome, in which the legs wander aimlessly around at night and prevent sleep, also describe the same irresistible need to move arising in the limbs or muscles that characterizes the parkinsonian patient with akathisia. Akathisia is the most common movement disorder associated with psychotropic medication, including the phenothiazines, butyrophenones, and reserpine.

311. The answer is A. *(Benson, pp 220-223.)* Even before the advent of psychotropic medications, movement disorders were frequently observed in schizophrenic patients. These usually take the form of stereotypies or mannerisms. These movements appear most frequently in catatonic schizophrenia and suggest a poor prognosis. The movements rarely take the form of skilled or graceful acts, rather appearing ungainly, clumsy, and awkward. The movement pattern of patients may deteriorate over time. The movements not only appear during walking, but often the walking itself involves stereotypies and mannerisms.

312. The answer is C. *(Adams, ed 2. pp 41-43.)* Characteristically, the apraxic patient is unable to execute a movement on command but may do so automatically. Thus, the patient described in the question was unable to protrude his tongue when asked but licked his lips automatically, indicating that the tongue was not actually paralyzed. Indeed, proof of the ability of a body part to act automatically or inadvertently is necessary to separate apraxia from paralysis. While this patient also could have been negative or hysterical, the dysarthria and possible dysphasia clearly suggest that he may have a lesion of the dominant hemisphere that would predispose to apraxia. Corticobulbar tract interruption would cause paralysis rather than apraxia.

313. The answer is E. *(Adams, ed 2. pp 971-973.)* A disease that may present with weakness but few other physical or laboratory signs is thyrotoxic myopathy. The affected patient may have none of the classical historical or physical findings of hyperthyroidism. Standard laboratory tests such as EMG and muscle biopsy may fail to show distinct abnormalities. All patients with chronic unexplained weakness should have thyroid function studies. This diagnosable and potentially treatable cause of weakness should not be overlooked. The blood tests for thyroid function are very inexpensive and carry no risk for the patient other than those associated with venipunctures. Since the threat to life arises from involvement of cardiac or respiratory muscles, the affected patient should be carefully followed by clinical examination and laboratory tests for cardiac and pulmonary complications of the disease.

314. The answer is D. *(Kaplan, ed 3. p 143.)* A tall, mentally dull, assaultive man displaying minimal cerebellar signs may have the XYY karyotype. The diagnosis can only be made by a chromosomal analysis. Extensive neuropsychologic studies may further document the relatively low mental capacity of the patient, but will fail to make the diagnosis. Similarly, the EEG may show nonspecific changes but none that are diagnostic; the amino acid screen also is nonspecific. The brain fails to show any characteristic lesion demonstrable by CAT scan, although mild cerebellar signs have been observed in some XYY patients. Although the XYY karyotype has been associated with antisocial behavior, many—perhaps most—individuals with that karyotype manage to live an extrainstitutional existence. A screening program to detect individuals with the XYY karyotype at birth was blocked on the grounds that foreknowledge would lead to a self-fulfilling prophecy that would adversely affect the lives of the individuals involved. Thus the issue was politicized before the scientific studies that might answer the question could be completed.

315. The answer is C. *(DeMyer, ed 3. pp 265-266.)* A sensory modality is any unique sensation not resolvable into elementary components. Thus, it may refer to any of the special or general sensations. The term is not confined to one grouping or one set of sensations, but is designed to recognize that some sensations are elementary and not resolvable into simpler components, such as pain. Other sensations, like perception of the form of a cube felt by the hand, may represent a blend of touch and position sense. It is sometimes presumed that cortical integration is necessary for all multimodality sensations like form sense (stereognosis), but that some modalities like pain might reach perception at a thalamic or brain stem level.

316. The answer is C. *(DeMyer, ed 3. p 322.)* Anosognosia is most characteristic in patients with right posterior parasylvian area lesions, in approximately the same zone that isolated lesions of the opposite hemisphere cause receptive aphasia, or Gerstmann's syndrome. Babinski coined the term to apply to a patient with a left hemiplegia who was unaware of the deficit. Clinicopathological correlation has repeatedly confirmed the association between posterior right parietal and parasylvian lesions and unawareness of either sensory stimuli or hemiplegia on the left side. This type of anosognosia does not occur with lesions elsewhere in the hemispheres. The term anosognosia sometimes is applied to any pathologic unawareness of disease, but in the context of Babinski's original description it implies a specific location of the lesion and a specific neurologic deficit.

317. The answer is D. *(DeMyer, ed 3. p 341.)* A type of dressing apraxia is characteristic in patients with right posterior parasylvian area lesions. Such patients cannot orient their clothes in preparation for dressing. For example, they may attempt to put a shirt or blouse on backwards. This type of dressing apraxia aids in localizing the site of the lesion to the right hemisphere and to the posterior parasylvian region of that hemisphere. Other signs of the lesion, such as a left homonymous hemianopia, usually appear. The dressing apraxia may be related to the inability of patients with a right hemisphere lesion to effect spatial concepts that permit them to relate the form and shape of their clothes to the form and shape of their own body. This particular syndrome of dressing apraxia is indicative of a lesion site rather than a lesion type. Any destructive lesion of the right posterior parasylvian area, whether infarct, hemorrhage, abscess, or neoplasm, may produce the same clinical deficit.

318. The answer is B. *(Adams, ed 2. p 39.)* Patients with upper motor neuron lesions may show associated or automatic movements (synkinesias) that activate the paralyzed part even though they are unable to move the part voluntarily. Thus, the paralyzed arm may flex when the affected patient coughs or yawns. When sitting up, the patient with an upper motor neuron paralysis of a leg may show an automatic flexion movement. These automatic movements in the presence of paralysis of volitional movements do not support a diagnosis of hysteria. Recognition of the nature of such associated movements helps to avoid a misdiagnosis of hysteria or even a lower motor neuron lesion as the cause for the paralysis. Lower motor neuron paralysis impairs all movements of the muscle whether of volitional, automatic, or reflex origin.

319. The answer is C. *(Benson, p 224.)*   Patients with manic-depressive illness exhibit no typical hyperkinesias. In the manic phase, the activities of daily living may increase in number and persistence, but such patients usually fail to exhibit the standard patterned types of hyperkinesias of other psychiatric and neurologic disorders. On the contrary, the differential diagnosis of parkinsonian hypokinesia and depression may offer many difficulties, particularly in dealing with a parkinsonian patient without tremor and who is also depressed, as many are. In such a case, one has to rely on the antecedent history, the pervading qualities of sadness and despair in the depressed patient, and the disappearance of the hypokinetic phase as the depression abates.

320. The answer is A. *(Adams, ed 2. p 58.)*   A patient with chorea usually shows loose, floppy extremities and slack movements that indicate hypotonicity. The state of the muscles resembles that seen in alcoholic intoxication or cerebellar disease. Clinicians should recognize the regular association of hypotonia with chorea because the hypotonia, as well as the excessive choreiform movements, contributes to the total motor disability of these patients. Recognition of the associated hypotonia helps to differentiate chorea from other involuntary movement disorders in which muscle tone is normal or increased.

321. The answer is D. *(DeMyer, ed 3. pp 204-205.)*   An electrically silent EMG or one showing a very rare fasciculation, when performed within 10 days of the injury, is evidence neither for nor against a nerve injury. With a muscle at rest, the EMG usually is electrically silent or may record a rare fasciculation in normal individuals who have no nerve injury. Fibrillations appear only days or weeks after denervation because some time must elapse before the muscle membranes become unstable. Thus, the absence of fibrillations at 10 days after injury is inconclusive. Moreover, since fibrillations are intermittent, they are not found with every needle insertion. The EMG in the patient described in the question failed to solve the clinical problem; in fact, the EMG supplied no clear evidence for or against either a functional or an organic diagnosis. Objective evidence of the integrity of the peripheral nervous system might have been obtained from nerve stimulation, sensory conduction studies, or somatosensory evoked responses, had the patient accepted further electrical tests.

322. The answer is C. *(DeMyer, ed 3. pp 449-451.)*   The primary gain that a hysterical person achieves from a hysterical symptom is generally thought to be the relief from anxiety, which the symptom serves to allay. Apparently such individuals feel more comfortable with the symptom than with the anxiety for which it is a substitute or mask. Indeed, this relative comfort on the part of such patients is presumed to account for the fact that they appear undisturbed by the symptom and rarely ask about its implication or the prognosis. Secondary gains for the patient include manipulative control over other people and an excuse from working and other responsibilities. The process that produces the hysterical symptom is thought to operate at an unconscious level, in contrast to malingering, which is regarded as conscious simulation of illness.

323. The answer is A. *(Adams, ed 2. p 285.)* The IQ score is obtained by dividing the mental age by the chronological age and multiplying by 100. The mental age is a statistical artifact of the test procedure. To develop an IQ test, an examiner gives test items to normal individuals of various ages. The average score achieved by the children at each age is then called the mental age. A mental age of five means that the individual made the same score on the test items as the 5-year-old individuals who previously took the test. If a patient scores comparably to other 5-year-olds, and has a chronological age of 5 years, the quotient is 5/5 x 100 or 100. If an individual scores like other 5-year-olds but is 6 years of age, the IQ becomes 5/6 x 100 or 83. Multiplying by 100 merely converts what could be a decimal to a more convenient number. The person with an impaired brain or less knowledge will score like younger persons and thus will have a lower "mental" age and a lower IQ. The person with a superior brain or more knowledge will score like older persons and thus have a higher IQ.

324. The answer is A. *(DeMyer, ed 3. p 140.)* Oscillopsia refers to a patient's complaint that the object viewed appears to move or to oscillate. It is one of the symptoms of nystagmus acquired after infancy. Patients with early acquired or congenital nystagmus do not complain of oscillopsia, even though they may have extreme and chaotic eye movements. Thus, the absence or presence of oscillopsia gives some evidence as to the time of onset of the nystagmus. Frequently, patients will fail to complain spontaneously of oscillopsia but will acknowledge it upon questioning.

325. The answer is C. *(Adams, ed 2. p 805.)* The most consistent biochemical abnormality in the basal ganglia in Huntington's chorea is a decrease in the γ-aminobutyric acid (GABA) content of the striatum. Accompanying the decrease in GABA is a decrease in glutamic acid decarboxylase, the enzyme responsible for the synthesis of GABA. Another frequent abnormality in the striatum is a decrease in acetylcholine and its synthetic enzyme, choline acetyl transferase, but this finding is less consistent than the loss of the GABA system. Thus, one would suppose that degeneration of the GABAergic neurons precedes the loss of the cholinergic neurons. These neurons are as yet inconclusively defined but they may consist of small interneurons in the striatum.

326. The answer is E. *(DeMyer, ed 3. p 275.)* A patient who complains of uncomfortable loudness of sounds (hyperacusis) may have paralysis of the stapedius muscle. This tiny muscle dampens the vibrations of the ossicles and may act as a protective mechanism or modulator of the amplitude of vibrations transmitted to the inner ear. The stapedius muscle receives its innervation from the VIIth nerve. Either the VIIth nerve or its stapedius branch may be damaged by a basilar skull fracture. Trauma may also affect hearing by disarticulating the ossicles, resulting in fuzzing or duplication of sound (diplacusis), which may also reflect damage to the inner ear.

327. The answer is C. *(DeMyer, ed 3. p 335.)* Hallucinations are false sensory perceptions not based on natural stimulation of a receptor. Hallucinations may, however, be triggered by a structural or biochemical lesion of the relevant areas of the brain. For example, an arteriovenous malformation of an occipital lobe may produce hallucinations of formed or unformed images. In alcoholic persons, the hyperexcitable state of the neurons following the withdrawal of the depressant action of alcohol may trigger hallucinations; auditory hallucinations may persist in such individuals. On the other hand, the hallucinations of schizophrenia (such as visions of God, or voices) cannot be explained on the basis of any known structural or biochemical lesion. Hallucinations contrast with illusions, which are false sensory perceptions based on natural stimulation of a receptor. For example, a line may appear longer than another line of equal length because of its relation to a background grid. In this case, the natural receptor functions normally; yet a perceptual error, an illusion, has occurred.

328. The answer is D. *(Adams, ed 2. pp 680-681.)* A child with personality changes, gait disturbance, and hypoactive stretch reflexes may be showing signs of a progressive degenerative disease. The combination of a possible central and peripheral nervous system disorder as evidenced by these clinical findings should, first of all, suggest metachromatic leukodystrophy. Because the child described in the question is a girl, Pelizaeus-Merzbacher disease and adrenoleukodystrophy are virtually excluded, both having a sex-linked recessive inheritance pattern. The child's age of 4 years excludes Krabbe's globoid leukodystrophy and her normal somatotype virtually rules out a mucopolysaccharidosis. The normal physical appearance of the child and the absence of malformations, along with the normal period of development, all virtually exclude the possibility of a chromosomal error. The normal retina argues against cerebromacular degeneration. Her previously normal mental state and lack of seizures exclude the usual amino acid disorders. The lysosomal enzyme battery will include tests for deficiency of aryl sulfatase A, which will lead to the specific diagnosis of metachromatic leukodystrophy.

329. The answer is D. *(American Psychiatric Association, ed 3. p 181.)* *DSM-III* lists deterioration of mental function as the one indispensable criterion for the diagnosis of schizophrenia. Other symptoms include disturbances in thought form and content, perception, affect, sense of self, and relation to the external world. Although schizophrenia almost always involves several of these symptoms, none is necessarily consistently present at the time of the initial diagnosis. Therefore, none is an indispensable criterion for the diagnosis of schizophrenia. *DSM-III* further states that the deterioration of mental function must have persisted for at least 6 months. The purpose of this stipulation is to exclude the schizophreniform disorders whose symptoms, although similar to schizophrenia, have different external correlates, such as the likelihood of recovery to premorbid levels and lack of a family history. The schizophreniform disorders run the gamut from prodromal through active and residual phases in time periods ranging from two weeks to six months. Illnesses that begin in older adults also are excluded from schizophrenia and are classified as atypical pyschoses.

330. The answer is E (all). *(Groves, N Engl J Med 298:883-887, 1978.)* Many patients will incite an excessive emotional response—countertransference, as Freud called it—in their physicians. The intensity of the response may then interfere with the physician's objectivity, professional judgment, and ability to treat the patient. Among these patients are those who suffer from manic-depressive psychosis. When manic, they may focus with unremitting zeal on generating antagonisms and difficulties. When depressed, they become mute and withdrawn, manifesting tenacious expressions of pain and anguish, powerless to help themselves or others. For male physicians, the nonpsychotic, overweight, complaining, pain-ridden woman in her forties offers a similar challenge because she is almost invariably depressed. A different problem is presented by the young, physically attractive sociopathic woman who, seemingly cheerful, rational, contrite, and cooperative while hospitalized, may excite the rescue fantasies of the physician who feels he has finally found a responsive patient. Deceived into placing undue trust in his patient, the physician unwisely grants her a weekend pass from the hospital, whereupon she resumes her sociopathic behavior. A similar countertransference may occur on the part of a physician for the attractive young woman who may excite his sexual fantasies, causing the physician to become entrapped in her seductive behavior.

331. The answer is A (1, 2, 3). *(Barchas, p 192.)* The major antipsychotic drugs should not be used in the treatment of anxiety states in patients who are nonpsychotic, or who suffer from reactive depressions, nor should they be employed as maintenance therapy in recurrent unipolar depression. In such situations the risk of causing tardive dyskinesias is too great; moreover, safer drugs, as well as safer forms of nondrug management, are available for treating the kinds of patients described. In some depressed patients with either psychotic symptoms or involutional melancholia, the use of antipsychotics is indicated either alone or in combination with tricyclic antidepressants. Acute anxiety that is not crippling and is based on real circumstances should be managed by traditional methods of psychotherapy rather than by drugs, when possible. Dealing with anxiety by utilizing a patient's own emotional strengths is far more valuable than transient relief of symptoms by chemical means, even if the drug chosen is relatively safe, let alone one of the major antipsychotic drugs.

332. The answer is E (all). *(Barchas, pp 234-235.)* Benzodiazepines have become the most frequently prescribed antianxiety medication. Although overused, they do have specific advantages when they are indicated. These advantages include a wide gap between the effective and lethal doses, low activation of hepatic microsomal enzymes, long duration of action (around 24 hours), and relatively low production of physical tolerance. The low activation of hepatic microsomal enzymes means that the benzodiazepines produce little alteration in the metabolism of drugs such as coumarin, antipsychotic agents, tricyclic antidepressants, and certain anticonvulsants, all of which are acted on by these enzymes. The benzodiazepines will, however, add to the pharmacologic effects of other medications, such as increasing the sedation caused by anticonvulsants or alcohol.

333. The answer is C (2, 4). *(Kolb, ed 9. p 301.)* Many attempts have been made to relate psychomotor seizures and other types of epilepsy to mental disorders and criminal behavior. Most of the studies have serious methodological defects. Attempting to draw random individuals from the general population would be too time-consuming and pose many difficulties in correlation. A study confined to patients who have attended a university clinic for 3 years would have the disadvantage that many of the patients who are stable or mentally ill, or who have criminal records, will have dropped out during this time, thus lessening the opportunity to establish any possible correlation. A better method to discover any relationship between types of epilepsies and mental disorders or criminal behavior would be to study a municipal hospital population, which always includes large numbers of indigent persons, mentally marginal individuals, and criminals. Probably the best method of all would be a study of **prisoners** with epilepsy, from which a direct answer to the question of the incidence of various seizure types could be obtained. To study only psychomotor seizures in outpatients or prisoners obviously would fail to supply baselines for comparison. A prison population, however, presents methodological difficulties owing to inaccuracies in patients' histories and the problem of ascertainment of seizures in individuals who are sociopathic. Therefore, this issue still remains controversial.

334. The answer is C (2, 4). *(Adams, ed 2. p 265.)* Sudden jerks of the body or of the extremities commonly occur in completely normal individuals during the early stage of sleep. Sometimes they follow an obvious stimulus, in which case the individual may awaken. Although they may be more frequent during times of emotional tension or stress, such movements usually are benign. They are unassociated with an EEG spike in most cases, although in epileptic individuals myoclonic jerks can occur in relation to sleep. Patients with myoclonic epilepsy usually have grossly abnormal EEGs, although the myoclonic jerks do not necessarily correspond with the occurrence of a spike.

335. The answer is A (1, 2, 3). *(Kaplan, ed 3. pp 1129-1130.)* One of the most significant findings in the physiology of schizophrenia is a disorder of smooth-pursuit eye movements. About 65 percent of schizophrenic persons untreated with psychoactive drugs and 45 percent of their first-degree relatives follow objects with jerky, pendular movements of the eyeball, as opposed to only 7 percent of the normal population. This finding was first reported by Holzman, et al. in 1973 and replicated by Shagass et al.. A large proportion of another group of psychiatric patients, those with psychotic depression, also possesses this defect. The fact that jerky eye-pursuit movements are associated with organic brain disorders like Parkinson's disease and cerebral arteriosclerosis suggests that many cases of schizophrenia and psychotic depression may have some form of brain dysfunction of undetermined nature. The pathophysiology of the abnormal eye-tracking movements is not well delineated.

336. The answer is B (1, 3). *(Kolb, ed 9. pp 788-790.)* Behavior modification is a system of therapy that regards maladaptive behavior as a type of learning disorder. It is assumed that the behavior is perpetuated by environmental contingencies that should be investigated. Behavior therapists attempt neither to formulate the psychodynamics of the behavior nor to rely on insight techniques. They do use extinction techniques (the ignoring by staff and family of unwanted behavior), although there is disagreement about their role. Behavior modification therapists also have tried to treat phobias by desensitization. After a therapist has determined the stimuli that elicit the unwanted behavior, patient and therapist construct a series of scenes that recapitulate the precipitating stimuli. After the patient has been taught deep muscular relaxation, the offending stimulus is conjured by means of mental images. The muscular relaxation is considered to be the means for deconditioning the anxiety initiated by the stimulus.

337. The answer is D (4). *(Kolb, ed 9. pp 51-53.)* Operant conditioning involves the linking of a behavior with either a reward (positive reinforcement), or punishment (negative reinforcement). To promote a behavior, the observer delivers a reward whenever that behavior appears. To extinguish a behavior, the experimenter metes out a punishment whenever that behavior appears. Operant conditioning thus differs from classical pavlovian conditioning, which is based on pairing an unconditioned stimulus (such as salivation in response to food) with a conditioned stimulus (such as the sound of a bell). Operant conditioning works best in non-brain-impaired individuals, a fact that limits its therapeutic usefulness. To the degree that the symptom depends on a damaged brain, it tends to persist. Thus, one cannot condition away spasticity or dystonia, although some minimal effects can be obtained by reduction of anxiety and by placebo effect. In a sense, traditional psychotherapy utilizes operant conditioning whenever a therapist reacts nonjudgmentally and nonpunitively to a patient's mistakes or problems. The patient thereby develops a healthier, more productive reaction to the implicit encouragement of the physician than to other authority figures, who may have reacted critically. Alexander called this type of psychotherapeutic operant conditioning "corrective emotional experience."

338. The answer is A (1, 2, 3). *(Kolb, ed 9. pp 73, 151, 393.)* A person's body image develops from the sensory and motor experiences during childhood and is modified by parental attitudes. The child may develop a pleasant, satisfying body image or a shameful, repellent one. In any event, that body image becomes an integral part of the mature personality of the individual and, in part, will determine both the reactions to life's stresses and the mental illnesses that may develop. The body image, or one's self-concept, is likely to be distorted in all kinds of psychiatric disorders, from the neuroses through the major psychoses. In extreme cases, affected patients may experience depersonalization—a feeling of estrangement or separation from one's personality and body. The distortion may reach such a degree that patients feel that their bodies fail even to exist.

339. The answer is E (all). *(Kolb, ed 9. pp 43-48.)*   Rapid eye movement (REM) sleep occurs in cycles of about 90 minutes throughout the night. The REM state of sleep is characterized by rapid eye movements, a low-voltage fast EEG pattern, irregular breathing and pulse, blood pressure elevation, and diminished muscle tone. Penile erection occurs automatically, a fact that can be used to distinguish functional from organic impotence by demonstrating the integrity of the neural and vascular apparatus for erection. When awakened during REM sleep, an individual usually reports dreaming, but does not report dreaming when awakened during non-REM sleep. REM sleep occupies a much greater percentage of sleep time in young infants than in adults. From the age of 3-5 years to senility, it occupies about 20 percent of sleep time. However, whether or not young infants dream remains a matter of conjecture.

340. The answer is B (1, 3). *(Adams, ed 2. pp 262-263.)*   Sites at which lesions may cause pathologic wakefulness include the median raphe of the pontine tegmentum and the anterior hypothalamus. The role of the anterior hypothalamus was suggested by von Economo from his studies of the neuropathology of encephalitis lethargica. In patients with this disorder who had stupor or coma, he found that the inflammatory changes tended to localize in the posterior hypothalamus and midbrain tegmentum, whereas in patients who tended to display pathologic wakefulness, the predominant changes occurred in the anterior hypothalamus and preoptic area. The median raphe of the pontine tegmentum contains serotonergic neurons that project to the forebrain. Destruction of this system causes insomnia.

341. The answer is A (1, 2, 3). *(Adams, ed 2. p 292.)*   Bilateral destruction of several sites in the cerebrum produces a relatively pure loss of memory but leaves cognitive functions relatively intact, including an ability to score in the normal range on IQ tests. Lesion sites that produce an amnestic syndrome include the dorsomedial nuclei of the thalamus, Ammon's horn and dentate gyrus, and the parahippocampal gyrus. Unilateral lesions cause only small or transient memory deficits. Since the fornix is an essential part of the circuitry connecting these structures, it is surprising that transection of the fornices, as has been performed in humans in an attempt to treat epilepsy, does not produce the amnestic syndrome. Although widespread bilateral loss of neurons in the cerebral cortex also causes memory loss, the affected patient will show overt signs of dementia in other areas of mental function. Thus, diffuse cerebral disease does not produce the relatively pure amnestic syndrome equated with lesions in the medial temporal lobes, hippocampal formation, or thalami.

342. The answer is A (1, 2, 3). *(Adams, ed 2. p 266.)*   Sleep paralysis occurs most commonly in the narcolepsy tetrad. It appears during the transition phases of wakefulness-to-sleep and of sleep-to-wakefulness. It is most frequent when a patient is falling asleep, and may be accompanied by fear-provoking visual or auditory hallucinations, the so-called hypnagogic hallucinations. The striking feature of sleep paralysis is its instantaneous disappearance when the patient is touched or hears a sound. This fact indicates that the disorder is related to a disturbance in the central nervous system rather than to a sudden potassium shift in muscle, which would be too slow to explain so rapid an arousal from sleep paralysis. However, patients with periodic paralysis who have a disturbance in potassium balance also may experience very severe fright and anxiety because of a similar feeling of helplessness during their muscular paralysis.

343. The answer is A (1, 2, 3). *(Adams, ed 2. pp 380-381. Benson, pp 200-203.)*   In the male, bilateral destruction of the lumbar sympathetic ganglia, particularly the second one, leads to loss of ejaculation but retention of erectile capacity. Erectile capacity requires the integrity of the parasympathetic fibers that travel from the sacral cord to dilate the arterioles of the penis, allowing the penis to fill with blood. In addition, the axons of the pudendal nerve innervate the periurethral muscles, which compress the draining veins of the penis. The fibers that convey sexual sensation and the suprasegmental fibers, which mediate the psychic and brain influences on the genitalia, travel in the ventrolateral quadrant of the spinal cord. Thus, ventrolateral chordotomy causes loss of erection and ejaculation in males and loss of orgasmic capacity in females. Even after vulvectomy or loss of the penis, patients may still experience sexual sensation and even orgasm. A different situation prevails following **complete** cord transection with paraplegia. As part of the exaggeration of certain reflexes after cord transection, erection may be produced by stimulation of the penis and, in fact, priapism may occur as a troublesome complication. Once the paraplegic patient has achieved erection, intercourse and ejaculation can take place.

344. The answer is A (1, 2, 3). *(Kolb, ed 9. pp 64-67.)* Freud, upon whose work much of classical psychoanalytic theory rests, divided the personality into the id, ego, and superego. The id consists of the instinctual drives (which reflect primary biological needs for food, sexuality, sleep) and the vegetative, homeostatic, and visceral functions. The primitive drives related to these functions produce states of emotion, aggression, fear, pleasure, and satisfaction. The ego is the reality-testing self that deals with the environment through conscious, cognitive processes. It brings about a *modus operandi* for psychosocial adaptation that establishes the manner in which individuals both perceive themselves in relation to other persons and relate towards them. The superego, on the other hand, incorporates the ego ideal—the internalized model of what individuals think they should be like, as established by childhood perceptions of the kind of person they perceive authority figures wanted them to be.

345. The answer is E (all). *(Adams, ed 2. p 269.)* In addition to the well-known narcolepsy tetrad of symptoms including pathologic sleep, cataplexy, hypnagogic hallucinations, and sleep paralysis, narcoleptic persons often may exhibit episodes of automatic behavior. These episodes might be interpreted as daytime somnambulism. Such individuals may remember the beginning of such an attack, then gradually lose awareness of surroundings but may continue to perform routine tasks. They may answer simple questions or may burst out with a series of irrelevant words or phrases. These episodes should be distinguished from fugue states, psychomotor seizures, and psychotic intervals. Such attacks of clouding of the sensorium, occurring in more than half of the affected patients, are more common than the better-known episodes of sleep paralysis and hypnagogic hallucinations. Moreover, the classical features of narcolepsy may appear asynchronously over a period of several years, making a diagnosis very difficult in patients with only partial expressions of the syndrome. The full expression of the four classical features occurs in only about 10 percent of narcoleptic patients.

346. The answer is A (1, 2, 3). *(Benson, pp 180-181.)* Amnesia following head injuries and amnesia following psychomotor seizures closely resemble each other in a qualitative sense. In either instance, patients show a period of ictal amnesia with retrograde and anterograde components. The retrograde amnesia is shorter than the anterograde and tends to shrink as the patient recovers. During the recovery phase, the patient will display a period of seemingly rational, responsive behavior and consciousness, but later may be unable to recall this period of time. For the post-traumatic patient, this period may last days or weeks, but lasts only briefly after the usual psychomotor seizure. The patient who has suffered epileptic status will have a memory deficit quantitatively and qualitatively like that of a post-traumatic patient.

347. The answer is B (1, 3). *(American Psychiatric Association, ed 3. p 111.)* Patients with pseudodementia may manifest many features that suggest an organic brain disorder, although their disorder is actually functional. While no absolute distinction can be made, several features suggest pseudodementia. These include a tendency of such patients to dwell upon their seeming mental incapacity, whereas the organic patient often lacks an appreciation of the degree of disability. The patient with pseudodementia displays little effort or interest in formal testing, preferring to respond with "I don't know," whereas the organic patient usually tries to perform well. In addition, patients with pseudodementia will have normal attention span and ability to concentrate and will retain a high level of general behavior in relation to the apparent loss of intellectual function.

348. The answer is B (1, 3). *(Benson, pp 231-232.)* Acute dyskinesias in response to psychotropic medication may appear within hours of a single dose of the drug. They usually affect ocular, facial, and oropharyngeal muscles as well as producing dystonic syndromes with spasmodic torticollis, dystonic trunk movements, and tortipelvis. The disorder consists of a mixture of hyperkinesias and spasms. The potent phenothiazines (including piperazines) and butyrophenones are the most frequent offenders, while reserpine apparently fails to cause acute dyskinesias. In contrast to the apparent predominance of parkinsonism in older women, the acute dystonias manifest more frequently in older men and in young adults and children.

349. The answer is A (1, 2, 3). *(Gilman, ed 6. p 387.)* Toxic states in which the skin turns red in association with the presence of mental aberrations include the disulfiram-alcohol syndrome, carbon monoxide poisoning, mercury intoxication, and atropine and nutmeg poisoning. If a person taking disulfiram ingests alcohol, the skin turns scarlet because of the dilating effect on peripheral blood vessels. In carbon monoxide poisoning, the binding of carbon monoxide to hemoglobin causes fiery red skin; a patient's disordered mental state may vary from mild obtundation to delirium or coma. In mercury poisoning, scarlet, painful extremities occur with an irritable, obtunded mental state. Hypoadrenocorticism causes changes in mental state, but produces a chronic brown rather than fiery red discoloration of the skin. The association in some patients of hypoadrenocorticism, brown skin, and a demyelinating encephalopathy led to the term bronze Schilder's disease.

350. The answer is B (1, 3). *(Gilman, ed 6. pp 563-567.)* Although the psychedelic drugs are difficult to define, they all act to produce a heightened awareness of sensory input, in many instances causing hallucinations affecting various senses. However, auditory hallucinations are rare in contrast to the state of auditory hallucinosis that follows prolonged use of alcohol. The psychedelic drugs, which, in general, are indoleamines or phenyethylamines, lack strong addictive properties, and recreational users eventually tend to lose interest in them. A high degree of tolerance develops for lysergic acid diethylamide (LSD). Withdrawal symptoms are absent or slight, and fatal intoxication is rare, although severe hallucinations while under the influence of LSD may lead to suicide.

351. The answer is D (4). *(Gilman, ed 6. pp 384-385.)* An alcohol blood level of 100 mg/100 ml constitutes legal drunkenness, while blood levels of 50-100 mg/100 ml together with behavioral evidence of inebriation may still support the diagnosis. Breath odor is an unreliable guide to the degree of acute alcoholic intoxication. Indeed, the offensive "drinker's breath" may result from products in the ingested fluid other than the alcohol. Even in an inebriated patient, the clinical state may result from another problem, like a subdural hematoma. Hypothermia is characteristic of a comatose patient with alcoholic intoxication, but also may be associated with other causes of coma. Since the metabolism of alcohol proceeds at a nearly constant rate, fluid ingestion fails to increase the rate of recovery from acute alcohol intoxication.

352. The answer is E (all). *(Barchas, p 141.)* Among the toxic effects common to the major antipsychotic drugs are hypotension and hypothermia, cardiac dysrhythmias, coma, and seizures. The cardiac dysrhythmias may, on rare occasions, result in unexpected death. The other adverse effects can be limited by avoiding an overdose of the drug, by reducing the dose if an adverse effect occurs, or by instituting appropriate remedial therapy. Hypotension is particularly bothersome in the aged patient or in a patient with cerebrovascular disease, because the hypotension may induce transient ischemic attacks or a frank stroke. In epileptic patients who may require antipsychotic medication, the anticonvulsant and antipsychotic medications when combined may produce an addictive sedative effect, but the anticonvulsant medication should be maintained.

353. The answer is B (1, 3). *(DeMyer, ed 3. pp 451-452.)* The visual field defects that are typical of hysteria consist of tubular vision and spiral fields. A patient with tubular vision has only a narrow central field of vision, as if looking through a tube. In the periphery of the visual field—which extends medially to 60 degrees from the midpoint and laterally to 80 degrees—the patient is blind. Geometrically, of course, the visual field of the normal person must expand as the visual target moves further away from the eye. In the hysterical patient with spiral fields, the size of the field diminishes as the probing of the periphery continues, causing a continually reducing spiral of vision. Paracentral scotomata, as demonstrated by tangent screen or sector defects, occur with retinal or optic nerve lesions and provide evidence for an organic type of visual disturbance.

354. The answer is C (2, 4). *(DeMyer, ed 3. pp 452-457.)* Certain patterns of sensory loss that recur regularly in hysterical patients are absent in patients with strictly organic lesions. Hysterical patients with an anesthetic level at the waist will usually show a horizontal boundary. However, the patient with an organic spinal cord lesion shows a border that slopes downward because the dermatomes slope downward, as do their nerves as they pass from the spinal cord. The hysterical patient has a mental image of the body as horizontal at the waist, rather than following the actual pattern of innervation. The principle that the hysterical patient loses sensation in the mental image of a body part rather than in the pattern of actual innervation serves to distinguish hysterical sensory losses from organic. Patients with hysterical hemianesthesia report abrupt loss of vibratory sensation at the midline, whereas the bone of the sternum or forehead in fact transmits the sensation to the normal side even **after** the tuning fork has passed some little distance onto the putatively anesthetic side. Thus, the border of sensory loss fades gradually in patients with an organic lesion. The amount of pain that the hysterical person can withstand offers no basis for differentiating a hysterical cutaneous anesthesia from organic; indeed, maximum pain stimuli should be avoided in any examination, whether or not hysteria may be present.

355. The answer is E (all). *(Adams, ed 2. p 311.)* Gerstmann's syndrome consists of right-left disorientation, digital agnosia, dyscalculia, and dysgraphia. The value of the syndrome is that it associates four elements that superficially seem to bear no necessary relationship to each other into a clinical entity that may indicate a structural lesion in a patient with a mature brain. (The syndrome also can be seen in part as a feature of the developing brain of the young child.) Patients with Gerstmann's syndrome most commonly have a lesion of the left posterior parasylvian area. Because of the location of the lesion, these patients in addition may show some element of dysphasia. If the lesion extends deep into the geniculocalcarine tract, a contralateral homonymous visual field defect may also be present. Gerstmann's syndrome, however, may occur with lesions distant from the posterior parasylvian area. Therefore, the coincidence of the four elements of the syndrome is suggestive, rather than pathognomonic, of a lesion in the posterior parasylvian area.

356-359. The answers are: 356-C, 357-E, 358-D, 359-B. *(Kolb, ed 9. pp 96-113.)* In 1896, Freud published his first work on defense mechanisms. Since that time, many other authors, chiefly psychoanalysts, have added to the literature. Kolb has listed 21 basic mental mechanisms and defensive processes. While all can be found in both mentally healthy and mentally ill individuals, some mechanisms are more commonly used by mentally ill people, e.g., unrealistic projection, denial, symbolization, and the acting out of conflicts. Also, the mentally ill person uses only a few defenses in a stereotyped nonadaptive way and possesses relatively few appropriately adaptive mechanisms. These include sublimation (the transfer of psychic energy to behavior beneficial to the self or society), altruism, conscious control, and ego-strengthening identification, as exemplified by the Joe Namath admirer described in the question.

In contrast, the soldier described in the question, who blamed the physician for his own defection from duty, was using a highly maladaptive, unrealistic projection to save himself from his own painful guilt. Such a projection can lead to murder and other dangerous and self-defeating behavior.

Rationalization is a common mental mechanism used by nearly everyone at some time or another. Frequently, the strongest motives for our behavior are based on greed, gluttony, anger, or other self-centered urges. We like to think, however, that we are rational and fair; therefore, we hide from ourselves the selfish nature of many of our acts and focus on a partial truth (or the semblance of truth) in a situation as the main reason for our behavior. Saving our self-image may cause more trouble than it is worth, for we fail to appreciate where our best interests lie. The young wife described in the question, who rationalized her promiscuity, failed to fully acknowledge a trait she felt guilty about and blamed her husband. This failure, in turn, blocked her search for other solutions that might have strengthened rather than jeopardized her marriage.

Regression is another common defense mechanism of everyday life and frequently occurs during stress. Reverting to a behavior pattern of an earlier developmental period represents an unconscious bid for another person to take care of the sufferer as a young child or infant. The regression, if temporary, can be used to gather strength to fight the battles of the real world on a later occasion. However, continued neglect of developmental problems will, in due course, lead to mental illness.

Mechanisms of defense are subjects for scrutiny in patients undergoing psychoanalysis or dynamic psychotherapy. The rationale behind such exploration is that patients will be able to bring their intelligence to bear on their problems rather than mindlessly engaging in repetitive, destructive behavior whose sole legacy is unhappiness and failure.

360-363. The answers are: 360-C, 361-A, 362-E, 363-D. *(Kolb, ed 9. pp 20-24.)* The development of neurology and psychiatry has required a new vocabulary of technical terms as well as the assignment of technical meanings to ordinary terms. For example, behavior—particularly to the behavioral therapist or psychologist—means any observable, neurally mediated change in an individual. The nervous system can produce behavior in only two ways—by changing the length of a muscle fiber or by causing the secretion of a fluid. No matter what we call the behavior—walking, crying, running, or murdering—the nervous system, operationally, can only do these two things. Pure behaviorists deal with behavior in terms of stimulus-response models, ignoring the internal circuitry concepts favored by the neuroanatomist or neurophysiologist on the one hand, and the realm of thoughts and feelings beloved by the psychiatrist on the other. Thinking is not observable; therefore, it is not a behavior.

A stimulus is any identifiable change capable of triggering a neurally mediated response. Such a change might be simply temperature or a sound or sight. The response might be a simple reflex that is a relatively invariant neurally mediated response to an identifiable change or a conditioned reflex, or an instinctual response.

An instinct is an innate, unlearned behavioral pattern triggered by a specific stimulus. The stimulus might be the appearance of a sexually attractive person, or the sight or smell of food. They key to the difference between a reflex and an instinctual response is the complexity of the latter, expressed by the term "behavioral pattern." The reflex is relatively simple and brief. The instinctual reaction is complicated and longer lasting.

A drive is a more general term for the motivational vectors presumed to arise from the primitive needs and expressing themselves in some sustained pattern of activity. No identifiable external stimulus elicits the drive, which would seem to arise from internal sources.

364-367. The answers are: 364-E, 365-A, 366-D, 367-B. *(Adams, ed 2. pp 174-175, 314-315.)* Dyschromatopsia refers to any disturbance in the perception of color. A defect in color perception will accompany virtually any defect of visual perception due to a cerebral lesion. Thus, color testing is a very sensitive test of visual function. The disorders in color perception may take the form of achromatopsia (lack of color vision), metachromatopsia (change in color perception so that green, for example, may appear as brown), and monochromatopsia (perception of all visual objects as having one color — for example cyanopsia, or blue vision).

Palinopsia refers to the persistence of visual images after removal of the visual stimulus. The object previously seen will persist, often in very vivid form, for minutes or hours. A single object may appear as a chain of many objects (polyopsia). The palinoptic image usually appears in visual fields that are only partially affected rather than completely blind. The causative brain lesions usually are severely destructive, such as infarcts or neoplasms, and will cause other visual and neurologic manifestations as well.

Simultagnosia refers to the inability to organize a series of related pictures into the correct sequence or to understand the meaning of a series of related parts. If given a series of pictures that tell a story, an affected patient is unable to order them into the story-telling sequence, but tends to perceive them as a series of independent events. In a series of dots that form a letter, the patient may see the dots but fail to perceive them as forming a letter. In other words, the patient fails to see the simultaneous relationship of visual sequences.

Visual allesthesia refers to the displacement of a visual image from the visual field of perception into the opposite field. The displacement occurs from the affected to the nonaffected field. Allesthesia also occurs in other sensory modalities, such as in the displacement of tactile stimuli.

368-371. The answers are: 368-E, 369-C, 370-E, 371-B. *(DeMyer, ed 3. pp 351-353.)* The zone in which lesions characteristically produce aphasia surrounds the horizontal ramus of the sylvian fissure. Thus, it is called the parasylvian area. Within this zone, the characteristic of the aphasia varies with the site of the lesion. The most posterior lesions (letter E in the figure accompanying the question) tend to cause dyslexia. Those at the anterior part of the zone (B) cause mainly a nonfluent type of expressive aphasia. Those in the parietal operculum and adjacent parieto-occipito-temporal confluence (C) tend to cause fluent aphasia. Those lesions toward the temporal lobe (D) tend to produce a more pure auditory aphasia. Lesions confined to (A) and (F) do not customarily produce aphasia.

Aphasia will occur not only after destruction of the cortex within the parasylvian area, but also after destruction of the underlying white matter. Such deeper lesions interrupt the thalamocortical and corticothalamic circuits. These axonal circuits connect the relevant areas of the cerebral cortex with thalamic nuclei. The largest thalamic nuclear mass connecting with the parasylvian area, particularly the posterior part of the aphasic zone, consists of nucleus pulvinaris. Lesions of the thalamus itself may result in aphasia by interrupting the thalamic end of the circuit. Lesions in structures caudal to the thalamus do not cause aphasia. As long as the lesion is destructive—a tumor, abscess, infarct, or laceration—the occurrence and type of aphasia depends more on the site of the lesion than its nature.

372-375. The answers are: 372-E, 373-B, 374-C, 375-A. *(Benson, p 223.)* Many terms are available to describe states of immobility or resistance to movement. The patient with catatonia remains mute and statuesque, showing little reaction to the usual environmental stimuli. Catatonia was described by Kahlbaum in 1874 as a component of the disorder newly termed dementia praecox, later to be supplanted by Bleuler's term schizophrenia. He noted that it was frequently associated with flexibilitas cerea or catalepsy.

Catalepsy refers to the condition in which patients maintain their body or limbs in whatever position, however uncomfortable, the examiner places them. While this feature is classically associated with schizophrenia, it also occurs in dementia and in the twilight states of disturbed consciousness of any origin, including seizures. Catatonia as such seems today to be a much less frequent finding in schizophrenia than formerly, judging by the older literature on the subject.

In gegenhalten (paratonia or motor negativism), patients show plastic resistance to any movement the examiner seeks to impose. The resistance, while relatively slight, remains nearly constant throughout the course of movement and will remain so regardless of where the movement starts or stops. The resistance will increase if the examiner tries to move the part too quickly, or will nearly disappear if the examiner moves the part very slowly. It may be unilateral. Gegenhalten occurs in the intact limbs of stroke victims while these patients have obtundation of consciousness, and under a variety of other conditions associated with altered consciousness.

Negativism is a general term for resistance by patients to any effort to move the parts, either passively by the examiner or in response to the examiner's command. This feature, often seen in the disturbed or retarded child, may totally defeat the parent when it pervades the whole behavior of the child. It may have partial expression in mutism, refusal to eat or dress or to go to school. The active opposition to the parental goal and the preservation of consciousness readily distinguish negativism from other resistances.

376-379. The answers are: 376-B, 377-C, 378-A, 379-D. *(Benson, pp 122-126.)* Disorders of verbal expression take many forms. One method of classifying them is to recognize the differences between disorders of speech, of language, and of thought. Among the disorders of speech are stuttering, cluttering, palilalia, and several varieties of mutism. Disorders of language include the aphasias, echolalia, and perseveration.

Among the speech disorders, palilalia consists of the repetition of the final word or phrase. There is an increased speed of repetition, but loss in volume of voice until the sound and lip movements fade away, with a patient then making only lip movements (aphonic palilalia). Sometimes, in exasperation at the repetitions, the patient may interrupt them by an expletive. Palilalia stands in contrast to stuttering, which involves the first sound of the word.

Cluttering consists of very rapid speech with the omission of entire sounds or words, resulting in incomprehensible speech in severe cases. Patients will say something like, "torow go toping" for "Tomorrow I want to go shopping." Asked to repeat the phrase, the patient says the same incomprehensible thing, but if cautioned to slow down, can produce the words individually. Nevertheless, the patient will revert to the cluttering upon making the next statement.

Among the many forms of mutism is elective mutism. In this disorder, a patient—usually a young child—consistently fails to speak to some persons or under certain conditions, but can talk normally or almost normally under other conditions. The child may fail to speak when introduced to anyone new or strange, or may not speak in the presence of a particular family member or other familiar person. Particular forms of mutism include akinetic mutism, due to a lesion of the brain stem or septal region, and aphemia.

Aphemia, or pure word mutism, is a particular type of aphasia. The patient suddenly loses all speech because of a lesion in the posterior inferior frontal region (Broca's area), but remains alert and able to write, read, and behave normally. Other terms for aphemia are pure word dumbness, cortical anarthria, and subcortical motor aphasia.

380-385. The answers are: 380-C, 381-A, 382-E, 383-D, 384-B, 385-F. *(Adams, ed 2. pp 258-263. Kaplan, ed 3. pp 166-167.)* The stages of normal sleep, while continuous, exhibit fairly characteristic EEG patterns that must be recognized and distinguished from patterns of abnormal sleep. It is particularly important not to interpret early drowsiness as pathologic slowing, or vertex sharp waves as spikes. The EEG of the normal, awake person shows an occipitally dominant alpha rhythm of 8-12 cps and low-voltage, mixed-frequency activity. As drowsiness evolves, the EEG shows some activity in the theta range, and in stage 1, the lightest stage of sleep, it shows low-voltage desynchronized activity and low-to-moderate amplitude waves in the theta range (4-6 cps). Such a person displays slow, roving eye movements during stage 1 sleep. The EEG pattern is similar during rapid eye movement (REM) sleep.

Stage 2 sleep features 12-15 cps sleep spindles and K-complexes. K-complexes consist of high-amplitude mixed sharp-slow waves, usually with a central or frontal dominance and often followed by sleep spindles. K-complexes will appear during attempts to arouse a sleeping individual, as well as spontaneously. The spindles and K-complexes appear against a background of low-voltage mixed-frequency waves.

Stage 3 sleep displays moderate amounts of high-amplitude, slow-wave activity. Some waves in the delta range (0.5-3 cps) appear. In stage 4 sleep, delta waves dominate the record.

The various stages of sleep alternate in cycles during the night, and although transitions occur between stages, the records can be scored as to how much of the night is spent in each stage. In young adults, stage 1 occupies 3-5 percent of the night; stage 2, 50-60 percent; stages 3 and 4, 10-20 percent; and REM, about 20-25 percent. The amount of time spent in the various stages of sleep varies with age. REM sleep occupies about 50 percent of the cycle in young infants. The elderly have very little stage 3 and 4 sleep.

The delta stage, stage 4, is generally interpreted as the deepest stage of sleep, in the sense that the person is least arousable during this stage. All of the first four stages taken together occupy the first 70-120 minutes of the night's sleep. Then, the first cycle of REM sleep occurs. The EEG resembles stage 1 sleep, but the person now undergoes a phase of dreaming. Although the REM stage is often thought of as a lighter stage of sleep, the person is not necessarily easier to arouse. It is also called paradoxical sleep because of the dreaming in conjunction with profound loss of muscle tone. It is not readily categorized as light or deep sleep, rather as a different **kind** of sleep. Repeat REM cycles occur at intervals of 90-100 minutes throughout the night. REM stages of sleep appear in all mammals and even in birds, and thus have some profound biologic significance. Daytime napping is associated with REM sleep that appears earlier and is of greater duration than in nocturnal sleep.

Psychiatry

Growth and Development

DIRECTIONS: Each question below contains five suggested answers. Choose the **one best** response to each question.

386. The development of earliest smiling in infancy depends most strongly on which of the following factors?

(A) The infant's ability to gain satiety through oral feeding
(B) The infant's biological timetable
(C) Reassuring sounds of the parent's voice
(D) Warmth and frequency of the parent's smile
(E) Amount of time the infant is held

387. The most important factor in establishing that a woman has suffered rape is

(A) absence of consent
(B) proof of physical violence
(C) damage to the woman's introitus
(D) physiologic evidence of postrape anxiety in the woman
(E) proof of nonpromiscuity by the woman

388. The symptoms of menopause are best described as which of the following?

(A) Great increase in the number of psycho-somatic complaints
(B) Increased vaginal secretions during sexual stimulation
(C) Increased incidence of depression in childless women
(D) Hot flashes, flushes, and perspiration
(E) Headaches

389. The relationship of mental status to the menstrual cycle is best described by which of the following statements?

(A) A relationship between mental status and the menstrual cycle has been hard to document clinically
(B) Menstruation is preceded by a feeling of calm for most women
(C) Women who report a disturbance in mental status prior to menstruation fail to experience relief when the flow of blood starts
(D) Daughters show little tendency to reproduce their mothers' menstrual pattern
(E) The majority of suicide attempts by women occur during the postmenstrual but pre-ovulatory phase of the cycle

390. Studies of life-changing or stressful events in relation to subsequent development of physical or emotional disorders indicate that

(A) a relation exists between life events and the subsequent development of both physical and mental illness
(B) a relation exists between life events and the subsequent development of mental illness but not of physical illness
(C) a relation exists between life events and the subsequent development of physical illness but not of mental illness
(D) life events cannot be adequately evaluated or scored to afford a valid correlation with the subsequent development of physical or mental illness
(E) no consistent results emerged because of methodological difficulties

391. The relationship between endocrine indexes of stress and life-threatening illnesses in individuals or their relatives is best expressed by which of the following statements?

(A) Patients and relatives who use defenses of denial, intellectualization, and avoidance of the prospect of death show little evidence of endocrine mobilization to stress
(B) Patients with myocardial infarction who use defenses of denial, intellectualization, and avoidance of their disorder have high indexes of endocrine mobilization to stress
(C) Endocrine responses to stress occur independently of the mental mechanisms deemed to be operative in response to stress
(D) Parents of leukemic children who use the mechanisms of denial, intellectualization, and avoidance of the subject of their children's illness show high indexes of endocrine mobilization
(E) Endocrine indexes of response to stress generally correlate inversely with the verbal and other overt expressions of anxiety and grief

392. In developmental theory, the concept of critical periods refers to

(A) a differential susceptibility of an individual to criticism during each stage of development
(B) a developmental event that must occur at a particular time or will be faulty or not occur at all
(C) certain mental forces that act to achieve an equilibrium in the face of a crisis
(D) crises that are necessary for personal development
(E) none of the above

393. Studies of feelings reported by mothers upon first holding their newborn infants show that

(A) virtually all mothers report strong positive feelings regardless of how the child develops
(B) mothers of children who become autistic usually feel very distant from their infant when first holding it
(C) mothers of infants who become autistic have feelings similar to those whose infants develop normally
(D) the majority of mothers of infants of unplanned pregnancies report negative feelings
(E) only a minority of mothers have any strong feelings of attachment until the infant is one week old

394. A previously normal 5-month-old infant begins to show the following behavior after eating a meal in the usual normal way: The infant's abdominal muscles contract persistently, followed by the appearance of milk from the stomach into the mouth. During this process, the infant's back is arched and the head held back. The infant then happily makes sucking and chewing movements on the regurgitated milk. This behavior characterizes which of the following conditions?

(A) Attachment disorder of infancy
(B) Bulimia
(C) Jejunal atresia
(D) Rumination (merycism)
(E) Seizures

DIRECTIONS: Each question below contains four suggested answers of which **one** or **more** is correct. Choose the answer

A	if	**1, 2, and 3**	are correct
B	if	**1 and 3**	are correct
C	if	**2 and 4**	are correct
D	if	**4**	is correct
E	if	**1, 2, 3, and 4**	are correct

395. Correct statements that reflect current knowledge about hysterectomy include which of the following?

(1)   The operation is performed much more often in the United States than in Britain
(2)   The conscious attitude of a woman toward the procedure will determine her postoperative reaction
(3)   Younger women are more susceptible than older women to adverse psychological effects of the operation
(4)   The operation is unlikely to affect significantly a woman's sexual performance and attitudes or those of her partner

396. Infantile autism, according to the original criteria of Leo Kanner, included which of the following?

(1)   Withdrawal from emotional contact
(2)   Desire for the preservation of sameness
(3)   Failure to use language for communication
(4)   Presence of hallucinations and delusions

397. Statements that accurately describe the relationship of work to mental and physical health include which of the following?

(1)   The most important factor in reducing the likelihood of new illnesses in a worker who is laid off is the availability of social support (e.g., unemployment compensation, job retraining programs)
(2)   Work satisfaction has no correlation with longevity
(3)   Workers in difficult or dangerous occupations who feel their work is useful and appreciated exhibit endocrine stress patterns similar to those of other workers
(4)   Individuals who retire from jobs that are gratifying are less likely to experience affective distress than those who retire from jobs that are less gratifying

398. True statements that apply to adolescent pregnancy include which of the following?

(1)   The recurrence rate is very high
(2)   A single, well-defined psychological profile describes the pregnant adolescent
(3)   The risk for both maternal and fetal complications during pregnancy is high
(4)   Most pregnant adolescents readily accept abortion as a solution

399. Statements that reflect current opinions about the development of sexuality and gender identity include which of the following?

(1)   Homosexual males have a lesser degree of identification with their mothers than do heterosexual males
(2)   Normal heterosexual identity depends on continuing contact with members of both sexes during growth
(3)   The family histories of confirmed lesbians and of matched heterosexual women are similar
(4)   Gender identity strongly depends on the psychological attitudes of the parents as reflected in their interactions with the child

400. Common splinter skills in autistic children include which of the following?

(1)   Exceptional skill in drawing
(2)   Ability to assemble puzzles
(3)   Exceptional skill in musical composition
(4)   Ability to recite sentences or words by rote

401. In comparing the characteristics of bipolar and unipolar depression, patients with bipolar depression show which of the following?

(1)   Earlier age of onset
(2)   Greater suicidal tendency
(3)   Retarded depressions
(4)   No family history of depression

402. Statements that reflect current knowledge about father-daughter incest include which of the following?

(1) The mother in the family frequently is aware of the sexual activity but fails to act
(2) Incest is a normally accepted practice in many cultures
(3) The father involved in incest is usually weak, ineffective, and often alcoholic
(4) The daughter in the relationship rarely becomes sexually promiscuous

403. Classical freudian psychoanalytic theory holds which of the following beliefs?

(1) Anxiety is regarded as a response to internal events; fear, to external
(2) One role of the ego is to keep the id strivings and superego controls unconscious
(3) Ego strength refers to the ability to use mature defenses such as anticipation and sublimation
(4) Anxiety is a signal to the ego to use stronger defense mechanisms

404. Characteristics of mentally healthy families include which of the following?

(1) Encouragement of the development of extra-family relationships
(2) Encouragement of the individual expression of emotions by its members
(3) Encouragement of a wide variety of approaches to problem solving
(4) Emphasis upon respect for authority

405. Statements that follow from the *tabula rasa* (clean slate) theory of personality, as espoused by a doctrinaire believer in the Watson behaviorist school of psychology, include which of the following?

(1) Innate drives and genetic predetermination have little to do with personality development
(2) If given sufficient control of environmental contingencies, the behaviorist could produce a child with any personality specified
(3) Mental illness is the result of faulty parenting or environment
(4) The theory of archetypes serves to explain many aspects of personality

406. The evidence supporting the concept of drives rests upon which of the following?

(1) Drives are subject to quantification in terms of physical units (centimeters, grams, and seconds)
(2) All normal individuals display behavior that seems goal-directed, such as striving for food and sexual expression
(3) Sexual drive can be demonstrated in the neonate
(4) Satiation reduces seeking (goal-directed) types of behavior

407. According to the epigenetic theory of personality development, which of the following statements are true?

(1) The earlier an adverse effect during infancy, the more serious the resulting impairment
(2) Each stage of development depends on the preceding one
(3) Proper environmental conditions must be available at critical periods of development
(4) Genetically predetermined stages of personality development drive the child into certain types of environmental interaction

408. The speech of autistic children is characterized by which of the following?

(1) Extreme richness of association and abstraction
(2) Absence of the normal echolalic speech patterns
(3) Correct use of the words "yes" and "no"
(4) Abnormalities of pitch and rhythm

409. In the first week of life, the behavior of a normal neonate includes

(1) orienting of the head to the human voice
(2) long latency between painful stimulus and crying
(3) a tendency to fix the eyes on a face
(4) absence of a grasp reflex

SUMMARY OF DIRECTIONS

A	B	C	D	E
1, 2, 3 only	1, 3 only	2, 4 only	4 only	All are correct

410. Statements that correctly compare older depressed patients with younger ones include which of the following?

(1) First depressions in persons over 40 years of age are associated with a positive family history less frequently than in persons whose first depressions appear at a younger age

(2) In contrast to early onset depression, late onset depression is more frequent in patients who had previously enjoyed relatively good physical and mental health

(3) Factors that precipitate depression in general are similar in kind and degree for both older and younger depressed patients

(4) Older, as opposed to younger, depressed patients show increased sensitivity to intravenous barbiturate sedation

411. Instinctual drives are characterized as

(1) arising from genetic determinants

(2) being elicited or heightened by environmental stimuli

(3) being subject to displacement to different behaviors or feelings

(4) forming the basis for conflicts that may lead to mental illness

412. A genetic (prenatal) origin of some aspects of behavior is strongly supported by which of the following established findings?

(1) Concordant behavior in identical twins separated at birth and raised separately

(2) Predictability of later personality traits from traits exhibited during the neonatal period

(3) Correlation between poor school performance and adverse events during prenatal life

(4) Increased incidence of schizophrenia in siblings raised by their natural parents

413. Which of the following statements concerning Freud's theory of personality development are true?

(1) Psychopathology is the result of failure of the individual to go through successive stages of psychosexual development

(2) Incomplete differentiation of infantile sexuality persists into adulthood, with adverse affects on the personality

(3) Infantile sexuality impulses that directly conflict with environmental demands can lead to neurosis and psychosis

(4) Motivational conflicts determine behavior, whether it is healthy or pathological

414. Pathological anxiety may have its roots in infancy and early childhood. Among the major determinants are

(1) constitutionally based differences in temperament

(2) parental teaching of a child to be overanxious

(3) a child's fears (realistic or unrealistic) of being abandoned

(4) parental anger at a child's incipient phobias

415. Developmental theory in psychiatry is emphasized for which of the following reasons?

(1) It attempts to reconcile the nature-versus-nurture controversy

(2) It reflects the importance of childhood memories as uncovered during psychoanalysis

(3) It recognizes that children pass through distinct stages of personality development

(4) It recognizes that the personality ceases to develop after young adulthood

416. Statements that accurately reflect the relationship of aging to mental illness include which of the following?

(1) The Goldstein catastrophic reaction occurs in the younger brain-impaired subject but is absent in the elderly subject

(2) The degree of mental decline closely parallels neuropathologic changes in the brain and in the CAT scan

(3) Conversion reactions fail to occur in the aged

(4) The need for psychiatric care increases with age

DIRECTIONS: The groups of questions below consist of lettered choices followed by several numbered items. For each numbered item select the **one** lettered choice with which it is **most** closely associated. Each lettered choice may be used once, more than once, or not at all.

Questions 417-420

For each of the following stages of psychosexual development as described by Freud, choose the age with which it is most closely associated.

    (A) One year
    (B) Two years
    (C) Three to six years
    (D) Six to twelve years
    (E) Thirteen to eighteen years

417. Latency period

418. Genital or phallic stage

419. Anal stage

420. Oral stage

Questions 421-424

For each of the following sets of essential diagnostic features relating to children, choose the diagnosis with which, according to *DSM-III*, it is most closely associated.

    (A) Oppositional disorder
    (B) Avoidant disorder
    (C) Overanxious disorder
    (D) Separation anxiety disorder
    (E) Generalized anxiety disorder

421. Great distress when either the parents or the child leave the home; persistent fears of danger to self or close relatives; phobias about monsters, death, being kidnapped; sleep disturbances and nightmares

422. Failure to involve self with unfamiliar peers; embarrassment, timidity, and lack of social contact even though it is desired; lack of motor activity and initiative; inarticulateness despite good language skills

423. Excessive worry and fear unrelated to stress or specifics of environment; excessive worry about possible injury, school tests, friendships; excessive worry about self-competence and criticism; sleep difficulties; psychophysiological symptoms

424. Resistance to authority even if contrary to self-interest; resistance to demands, causing more distress to self than to others; unresponsiveness to persuasion; provocativeness toward others, negativeness, stubbornness, procrastination, which block communication

Questions 425-430

For each clinical vignette that follows, choose the defense mechanism that best illustrates it.

    (A) Fixation
    (B) Resistance
    (C) Dissociation
    (D) Displacement
    (E) Restitution

425. An epileptic adult, with normal mentality, continually forgets to buy his anticonvulsant medication, loses it when he buys it, and forgets to take it when his wife brings it home for him

426. A juvenile male enters therapy because of an inordinate feeling of anger and hatred for policemen. He fears that he will attack or assault a policeman (or soldier) because he cannot stand the sight of the uniform or of a male wearing any uniform. The patient comes from a broken home with a harsh, punitive father whom, nevertheless, he claims to love.

427. An adult in psychoanalytic therapy is making satisfactory progress and then begins to arrive late at therapy sessions and seems disgruntled with the therapist

428. A 20-year-old woman who had recently become engaged experienced three episodes in which she wandered aimlessly on the street for 30-45 minutes; she did not injure or otherwise endanger herself. Although she recovered her self-awareness promptly after the first two episodes, she still seems withdrawn and confused following the third episode. The patient has complete amnesia for these episodes. Her neurological examination, including two EEGs, is normal

429. An 18-year-old woman enters therapy after having a child out of wedlock. The conception occurred several months after her younger sister died from rheumatic heart disease. The patient expresses strong feelings of guilt and responsibility for her sister's death and for the subsequent grief it caused her father

430. A 9-year-old boy is presented for therapy because of the mother's complaints of his excessive mouthing of objects, excessive appetite, and thumb-sucking. These have been lifelong behaviors. The child is dressed like—and acts like—a much younger individual and tends to use baby talk

Growth and Development Answers

386. The answer is B. *(Kolb, ed 9. p 69.)* The development of early smiling in an infant depends on its biological timetable, rather than on interactions with a parent. Deaf or blind babies who otherwise are neurologically normal will develop smiling at about the same time as infants without these sensory handicaps. Even neurologically normal babies with bowel disorders that require parenteral feeding will smile at about the same time as babies who obtain nutrition by mouth. This type of early smiling, which occurs around two weeks of age, has to be distinguished from social smiling, which is a later development; but even that tends to appear at about the same time in both sighted and visually handicapped babies, provided that the visually handicapped infant has no other brain disease.

387. The answer is A. *(Usdin, pp 492-493.)* The one essential factor in establishing that a woman has been raped is to ascertain that it occurred without her consent. Her previous sexual activity has no bearing on the issue, nor does evidence of either physical damage or a postrape mental state. Some rape victims appear outwardly calm, while others display the full postrape syndrome of acute disorganization with somatic and psychological symptoms. The postrape syndrome may include fears of encounters with men, a sense of betrayal, and disruptions such as nightmares and depression. A victim of rape has her fears of vulnerability and helplessness confirmed by the act, and may require much time to regain a sense of security and mastery over her own life and body.

388. The answer is D. *(Usdin, pp 486-488.)* The response of women to menopause varies. Although many changes in mental state have been related to the phenomenon, the most consistent complaints are hot flashes, flushes, and perspiration. The majority of women experience these complaints. The psychological response of the menopausal woman depends on many factors. She may look on menopause as a relief from childbearing, or if childbearing has been her way of proving herself, she may grieve the loss of this ability. Childless women, who may already have accommodated psychologically to their lack of children, tend to experience less depression than women who have borne children. Certainly not all women experience depression; some have the opposite reaction, feeling liberated and happier, particularly women in middle- and upper-class segments of society.

389. The answer is A. *(Usdin, pp 484-485.)* Menstruation is surrounded by much mythology and many impressions that are hard to document. Although premenstrual tension is blamed for some psychiatric disorders, objective verification of a premenstrual syndrome has been difficult to establish. Such a diagnosis should not deflect the physician's attention from alternative explanations for psychiatric disturbances. In those women who report it, premenstrual tension is generally relieved when the flow starts. The majority of suicide attempts associated with menstruation occur during the bleeding phase of the cycle. The degree, and even the presence, of the premenstrual syndrome may in large part be determined by expectations of the patient and the social context. However, psychologic explanations in the face of hormonal fluctuations that could affect brain function are to be regarded with suspicion.

151

390. The answer is A. *(Usdin, pp 260-621.)*   In the past two decades, the development of adequate methods of quantifying life stress has permitted a study of the relation of stressful life changes to the subsequent development of mental and physical illness. These studies consistently show that in the time preceding a physical or mental illness, such stressful events are more common than usual—life-changing events occur twice as often in individuals who subsequently develop psychiatric illnesses as in those who remain well. In patients who commit suicide, the life-changing events are four times greater than in controls. Frequently, patients who suffer cardiovascular disease or sudden death had previously experienced a sharp increase in life-changing events. Thus, if one compares a group of individuals who has a large number of life-changing events with a group who has a small number, the former group will display more illnesses. Attempts to refine the studies to permit a prediction of individual reactions, however, have been unsuccessful.

391. The answer is A. *(Usdin, pp 212-213.)*   The relationship of endocrine indexes of mobilization to stress in response to a life-threatening illness in oneself or close relative has been extensively studied. The results bring to mind the old James-Lange theory that emotion is the sensory awareness of the actual response to a situation; or, to put it in the form of a conundrum, does one feel fear because of running or does one run away because one feels fear? Those patients with myocardial infarction who use defenses of denial, intellectualization, and avoidance of the topic of death, show less evidence of endocrine mobilization to stress than those who react more overtly with fear and anxiety. Similarly, the parents of leukemic children who employ the same defense mechanisms show low indexes of endocrine mobilization.

392. The answer is B. *(Kolb, ed 9. pp 70-71.)*   The concept of critical periods in developmental theory rests on biological observations as well as psychiatric study. The theory holds that a developmental event must occur at a particular time or it will be faulty or will not occur at all. For example, if the human palate fails to close by 9 to 10 weeks of gestation, it will not close at all. Similarly, critical time periods develop for the child to see and hear. If a child is unable to see by a certain age because of cataracts, for example, the subsequent development of vision after cataract removal will be faulty. Similarly, the process of social bonding in infancy must occur at the correct times in order for the personality to develop. Still another example of a critical period occurs in the development of maximum physical or athletic skill, which can only be achieved if a person begins to develop that skill by a certain age. Thus, maximum skill in gymnastics or ballet dancing will accrue only to the individual who starts to practice early in life, prior to the end of the critical period. A person starting at the age of 20 years never achieves the skill of one starting at 10. On the other hand, too early an emphasis on skill achievement may place a ceiling on its development. In short, the concept of critical periods holds that there is an optimum time for everything.

393. The answer is C. *(DeMyer, pp 18-20.)*   Only about 90 percent of mothers report positive feelings toward their newborn infant when first holding it. Even among the mothers who did not initially want the infant or who had an unwanted pregnancy, the majority felt warmth on the first contact. The mothers of infants who later became autistic report the same kinds of feelings for their child upon first holding it as do mothers of children who develop normally. Even with children destined to become normal, however, around 10 percent of the mothers reported feeling distant until they had handled the infant for several days.

394. The answer is D. *(Kaplan, ed 3. pp 2603-2604.)* The persistent and pleasurable regurgitation of stomach contents is called rumination (merycism). A disorder rarely found after childhood, it was first described over two thousand years ago by Aristotle and later by Galen. According to *DSM-III*, it has four essential features: (1) After normal development, the affected infant starts to regurgitate food and fails to thrive; (2) without nausea or retching, the infant mouths, chews, or spits out food with no signs of disgust; (3) the back is arched and the head held back while the abdominal muscles strain; and (4) sucking movements give the impression that the child enjoys the process. Developmental delay frequently accompanies this condition, which has a mortality rate of about 25 percent. Rumination has been attributed to inadequate mothering. However, the condition may also occur in infants with good mothers who can become frustrated and alienated by an infant who rejects their feedings and who gives off a persistent foul odor. In both hiatus hernia and gastroesophageal reflux, the infant has uncomfortable dystonic or stiffening postures in response to feeding (Sandifer's syndrome). Jejunal atresia would produce symptoms soon after birth.

395. The answer is B (1, 3). *(Usdin, pp 488-489.)* Hysterectomy is performed far more often in the United States than in other countries. Posthysterectomy depression is a well-recognized entity and is more common than depression following other surgical procedures. A woman's conscious attitude toward hysterectomy is a poor guide to her postoperative reaction. The meaning of the uterus and the significance of its removal may have strong unconscious determinants. Younger women are more likely than those over 40 to have adverse psychological reactions. The procedure may adversely affect the sex life of the woman and her sexual partner, both of whom may feel that the operation has devalued her femininity and sexual attractiveness.

396. The answer is A (1, 2, 3). *(DeMyer, p 3.)* Kanner originally described autistic children as characterized by their withdrawal from emotional contact, desire for sameness, and failure to use language for communication. Because autistic children have little or very aberrant communicative language, the presence or absence of hallucinations and delusions cannot be readily determined and therefore has no part in diagnosis. Emotional withdrawal indicates an inability to make affective contact with other human beings, which often extends to the inability even to make eye-to-eye contact. The desire or need for the preservation of sameness is illustrated by the fact that changes in furniture placement or in a parent's attire may cause an autistic child to become very upset.

397. The answer is B (1, 3). *(Kolb, ed 9. pp 181-182. Usdin, p 212.)* Factory workers who are laid off experience fewer new illnesses if they have strong social supports such as unemployment compensation and an effective job retraining program. Workers in difficult or dangerous occupations may not show endocrine patterns of stress if they feel their work is useful and gratifying. Work satisfaction reduces the impact of life-stressing events on endocrine function. Work satisfaction, as opposed to work dissatisfaction, not only is related to lower mobilization of defenses against stress, but also correlates positively with longevity. On the other hand, workers who have derived gratification from their work will have greater affective distress upon retirement than will workers who have been indifferent to their work. The actual response of an individual will, of course, vary depending on personality and on the psychological needs that the job has fulfilled.

398. The answer is B (1, 3). *(Usdin, pp 482-483.)* The number of adolescent pregnancies continues to increase in the United States. It is a matter of concern because of the high rate of mental and physical problems caused by adolescent pregnancy, not only for the mother but also for the child. The younger the mother, the more likely she is to produce a brain-impaired child. The motivations to become pregnant in themselves frequently represent strong psychopathology. The risk of recurrence is high and may result in several children before the age of twenty, particularly in blacks. The problem offers no ready solution, least of all abortion. The psychological reasons for becoming pregnant may render abortion untenable, if the girl sees the delivery of the baby as establishing her womanhood or as a weapon of revenge against her parents.

399. The answer is C (2, 4). *(Kolb, ed 9. pp 620-621.)* The development of sexuality and gender identity depends on a mixture of biological and psychosocial variables. Normal heterosexual identity depends on continuing contact with members of both sexes during growth. Gender identity, the balance of femininity-masculinity in the personality, depends strongly on the psychological milieu. The establishment of gender identity appears to result from the attitudes and actions of the parent toward the child. Lesbians report a disturbance in their family backgrounds more often than do heterosexual women. They may have been subjected to abuses and poor affective contact and often are depressed. As a group, homosexual males have a stronger identification and attachment to their mothers than do heterosexual males.

400. The answer is C (2, 4). *(DeMyer, pp 49, 140.)* A splinter skill is a skill that is considerably more developed than the general performance or overall IQ of a child would indicate. The commonest splinter skills in autistic children are the ability to assemble puzzles or objects and the ability to recite words or sentences — or in some cases even long rhymes — by rote. Although an occasional autistic child has been reported to have exceptional ability to draw or to identify musical tunes or pitches, the skill is not put to **creative** use, such as producing original drawings or a musical composition. Not only do autistic children have splinter skills, but they also have splinter disabilities, one of which (by definition of the condition) involves inability to use language for communication.

401. The answer is A (1, 2, 3). *(Usdin, pp 571-573.)* The distinction between unipolar and bipolar depression has been widely accepted in psychiatry. Compared to the patient with unipolar depression, the patient with bipolar depression has (1) an earlier age of onset, (2) more severe and sudden depressions that often are of the retarded type with extreme psychomotor slowing, (3) definite manic-depressive cycles, and (4) a postpartum onset in females. The unipolar-depressed patient is much more likely to display agitation or anxiety with the depression than a bipolar-depressed patient, and lacks a history of manic cycles.

402. The answer is B (1, 3.) *(Kolb, ed 9. pp 174-175.)* Incest is prohibited in most cultures. The mother in a family of father-daughter incest usually was herself rejected as a child. She tends to abandon her role as homemaker to the daughter, who takes over the sexual as well as other roles of the ineffective mother. The mother is often aware of the incest but does nothing about it. The father, being weak and often alcoholic, plays upon the dependency and vulnerability of the female child. The daughter involved usually exhibits overt evidence of mental illness in the form of guilt, depression, psychosomatic disorders, masochism, and sexual promiscuity.

403. The answer is E (all). *(Usdin, pp 65-68.)*   According to classical psychoanalytic theory, anxiety is a state of unpleasant internal tension that appears when instinctual strivings threaten to overcome the internal controls. Fear is a response to external events. The ego functions to keep the id strivings and superego controls in the unconscious; if these forces remain in equilibrium, the conscious psyche suffers no discomfort. The mentally healthy person can use mature defenses such as sublimation and anticipation to defuse the anxiety that might otherwise produce psychic discomfort.

404. The answer is A (1, 2, 3). *(Usdin, pp 82-84.)*   The mentally healthy family as a group shows many traits that separate it from the mentally ill family. The healthy family fosters positive, caring relationships with other persons, which encourages reaching out. The healthy family encourages the development of personal autonomy of its members and avoids patterns of dominance and submissiveness. The latter pattern characterizes the situation in mentally ill "families," as epitomized by the Charles Manson and Reverend Jim Jones "families," in which the members of the sect became completely submissive to their leaders and completely distrusting of, and hostile to, all other groups or individuals. The healthy family has a variety of creative approaches to problem solving and encourages individual thought and self-expression of feelings and ideas.

405. The answer is A (1, 2, 3). *(Usdin, p 50.)*   The Watson school of behavioral psychology places little emphasis on genetic or prenatal influences on behavior, believing that parenting and the environment are prepotent in shaping it. Their theory is that an individual arrives at birth with a clean slate, which then receives indelible impressions from environmental influences that will determine the individual's personality structure. If the personality is undesirable, the parenting and environment were at fault. As yet, we lack evidence that behavioral psychologists raise better children than other parents; in fact, the doctrinaire views of early behaviorists are no longer held. The jungian theory of archetypes is diametrically opposed to behavioral theory.

406. The answer is C (2, 4). *(Kolb, ed 9. pp 20-22. Usdin, pp 45-46.)*   The concept of drives derives intuitively from clinical observation and the common experience that humans have of feeling needs. From a need for such things as oxygen or food, we recognize a periodic increase in seeking-activity and a reduction of that activity with satiation. These periodic changes in goal-directed behavior are called drives. While periodic chances of state in the infant might be interpreted as representing sexual drives, no operational criteria are available to establish this possibility. Therefore, infantile sexuality remains one of the controversial, unproved, accept-or-reject-on-faith principles of psychoanalysis. Drives, in the sense that they represent personality vectors rather than real entities, cannot be expressed in the language of physics—i.e., centimeters, grams, or seconds. Whether to regard the concept of a drive as any more or less subjective than the concept of number depends on one's philosophy of science.

407. The answer is E (all). *(Usdin, pp 42-43.)*   The epigenetic theory of personality development holds that development has successive, genetically programmed stages that lead to critical periods for the development of experiences and interactions. The developing child learns to cope with the psychosocial and biological crises of the successive stages of development, but each stage depends on the successful completion of the preceding stage. The epigenetic theory avers that disturbances in the completion of the early stages will preclude normal development in all of the successive stages. For this reason, it is proposed that the earlier the infant is exposed to disturbances in personality development, the more serious and tenacious will be the resulting impairment.

408. The answer is D (4). *(DeMyer, pp 39-49.)* One characteristic of the speech of autistic children is the poverty of vocabulary and absence of the richness of association and abstraction that develops in normal children. Autistic children do display echolalia, also a feature of normal children between the ages of 8 months and 2½-3 years. Parents of autistic offspring may remark that their children can repeat a number of words but are unable to use any of them creatively or to express their own thoughts and needs. Autistic children confuse words and often are unable to understand the concept of "yes" and "no" as applied to speech responses. The speech that autistic children manage to produce usually displays abnormalities of pitch and rhythm, a feature evident to many of the mothers in describing the early cries of their infants. However, the majority of mothers failed to report characteristic features in the cry of their autistic infants.

409. The answer is B (1, 3). *(Kolb, ed 9. pp 67-70.)* Neonates exhibit a number of innate responses that appear to promote infant-maternal interaction. A neonate will orient its head to the human voice and learns to respond preferentially to its own mother's voice. It will fix its eyes on the human face and may appear to "drink in" the object of visual regard. The grasp reflex, also present at birth, may represent a means for the human infant to cling to its mother; in arboreal primates, the utility of the grasp reflex is self-evident. The characteristics of an infant's cry also have strong implications for infant-maternal interaction. In normal infants, the cry occurs almost immediately—within a second or two of a painful stimulus—whereas in brain damaged infants, the latency period of the cry is significantly increased.

410. The answer is E (all). *(Benson, pp 110-117.)* First depressions beginning after 40 years of age are much less often associated with a positive family history of depression than those beginning earlier in life. Older patients are likely to have been physically and mentally competent, in contrast to younger depressed patients who tend to have a long history of poor adjustment. The factors that precipitate depression, such as bereavement or illness, seem to be present in both young and old patients to about the same degree, although in older men physical illness is significantly more important. Demented patients and temporarily depressed patients display an increased sensitivity to the sedative or soporific effects of intravenous sodium amytal. The threshold of the depressed patient to barbiturate sedation increases as the depression improves. This observation suggests that some change in the chemistry of the brain is associated with depression.

411. The answer is E (all). *(Kolb, ed 9. pp 20-24.)* Personality theory holds that the individual is born with certain genetically determined (inborn) behavioral patterns that are triggered by specific external stimuli, the so-called instincts. Instinctual drives arise that require some type of gratification. Setting aside the life-necessary drives for air, food, and water, the instinctual drives have a flexibility that allows them to become displaced or reattached to ends other than their original purposes. Thus, the sex drive, according to psychoanalytic theory, may motivate some creative effort only tenuously connected to the origin of the drive. Conflicts between the urges for gratification of instinctual drives on the one hand, and the forces of social circumstances and parental attitudes on the other, may lead to anxiety, which, if improperly allayed, can result in mental illness.

412. The answer is A (1, 2, 3). *(Usdin, pp 45, 50.)* The nature versus nurture controversy has been resolved by the recognition that some personality traits are determined predominantly by genetic or prenatal causes, and others by postnatal. Support for a genetic or prenatal cause for behavior comes from many sources. Concordant behavior in identical twins reared separately, such as preferences for the same color or type of clothing, occurs at a far higher rate than is explained by chance, a fact that suggests the possibility of a genetic determination. Recent studies have shown that certain temperamental qualities of the older individual are already apparent in the neonatal period. Several collaborative studies have shown the adverse effect of various pregnancy problems—such as low maternal weight gain—on the child's subsequent behavior and scholastic performance. On the other hand, the increased incidence of schizophrenia in siblings raised by their natural parents would not exclude the influence of parental environment in the genesis of schizophrenia. Thus, whether the disease is pre- or postnatal in origin is unresolved.

413. The answer is E (all). *(Kolb, ed 9. pp 18-20.)* The statements listed in the question are all part of Sigmund Freud's theory of human psychological development, which he constructed after engaging in a series of clinical observations during psychoanalytical therapy of adult patients. He believed that personality developed step-by-step as a result of a series of conflicts between the successive stages of infantile sexuality and the demands of the environment. The profound influence of infantile sexuality on the personality is disputed by many other theorists and practitioners who may, nevertheless, agree upon the pivotal role of intrapsychic conflict in determining both maladaptive and healthy human behavior.

414. The answer is E (all). *(Kaplan, ed 3. pp 2621, 2624.)* According to Thomas et al., various infants seem congenitally disposed to react differently to an event in the environment that may stimulate anxiety. For example, one infant may wait for a feeding without undue distress, while another infant may go into a frenzy of crying. However, the relationship of the parents to the child is also quite important in determining the child's feelings and expression of anxiety. Parents can teach overanxiety by inflating the importance of life's dangers. In our society, girls frequently are taught to be relatively helpless in the face of separation from sustaining adults or peers and are prone to develop separation anxiety. If a parent becomes intensely angry at childish fears, the child may react by becoming phobic about the object that originally was only mildly feared.

415. The answer is A (1, 2, 3). *(Kolb, ed 9. pp 63-70.)* Modern psychiatry believes that personality development is a dynamic process. Theories of personality development try to reconcile the notion of innate drives that must deal with environmental contingencies and the controlling and shaping forces of the parents who raise the individual. Developmental theory holds that the personality accrues by stages that have biological and environmental determinants. Arrest or distortion of development at one stage will be reflected in abnormal mental functioning and behavior in subsequent stages. Developmental theory incorporates the ideas of progressively higher levels of maturation, with the potential to regress to earlier stages under certain conditions of stress. It also recognizes that although major personality traits are displayed early, each stage of life displays different characteristics, and changes in personality continue through adulthood and senility.

416. The answer is D (4). *(DeMyer, ed 3. p 333. Usdin, pp 399-405.)* The need for psychiatric care increases dramatically with age. The aged show the gamut of mental illnesses displayed in the young, including neuroses and sometimes conversion reactions. Despite all wishes to the contrary, the aged brain fails to function as well as the young brain. Realistic recognition of this fact by the patient and physician will aid in making the proper adjustments. The degree of decline does not, however, closely match indexes of organic dysfunction such as histological changes and CAT scan evidence of atrophy, although a rough correlation does exist. The Goldstein catastrophic reaction occurs in the elderly as well as in the young brain-impaired person. It consists of the sudden appearance of irritability, anger, and anxiety that follows a trying situation, such as an insensitive mental status examination that machine-guns the patient with simplistic questions of dubious relevance.

417-420. The answers are: 417-D, 418-C, 419-B, 420-A. *(Usdin, pp 49-50.)* Freud based his concept of infantile sexuality and psychosexual development on material produced by patients during psychoanalysis. While he did not attribute adult sexual impulses to infants, he believed that adult eroticism and sexuality arose out of stimulation of the oral, anal, and genital regions at successive stages of development. He felt that sexuality represented a continuum throughout the individual's life. He believed that an elaborate mechanism of defenses developed to deal with the instinctual sexual drives, and that adults regressed to infantile or more primitive expressions of sexuality during the course of mental illness.

In Freud's view, oral sensations seemed to dominate the first year of life. This idea would be in keeping with the initial importance of the infant's mouth as the first source of rewarding contact with the environment, to provide satiation for the need for oxygen and food. The rostral-caudal order of development of reflexes in the fetus might also support this notion. The first movement that can be elicited in the human fetus (at about 7.5 weeks of age) is a bending of the neck in response to stimulation of the upper lip.

The anal stage, during the second year, was considered by Freud as a period in which the infant receives pleasurable stimulation from bowel and bladder, but which the infant also must learn to control or lose maternal love. Thus is the stage set for the genesis of a conflict that may remain throughout life.

Freud assumed that in the next stage of development, the genital or phallic phase, from three to six years of age, the individual's sexuality and center of pleasurable sensations centered on the genital region, assuming equal importance in males and females. To designate this shift to penis or clitoris, he spoke of phallic primacy. At this time, masturbatory play begins along with oedipal strivings.

During the latency period, from six to twelve years of age, the child's instinctual drives are channelled into work and social relations. During this time, the defense of sublimation originates. In the adolescent phase, the latent sexual strivings emerge into adult patterns of sexual expression.

421-424. The answers are: 421-D, 422-B, 423-C, 424-A. *(Kaplan, ed 3. pp 2618-2630.)* Anxiety disorders are an important category in the practice of child psychiatry. Anxiety-ridden children struggle with distorted ideas, terror-filled fantasies, and ruminations of dire events befalling themselves and close relatives.

Three chief symptom complexes appear in which such children are unable to displace their original anxiety to a symbolic object or situation. In other words, the anxiety is free-floating rather than phobic. The three conditions are called separation anxiety disorder, avoidant disorder, and overanxious disorder. In the first two entities, anxiety occurs when a child meets with specific life events, namely separation from home or parents (separation disorder) and contact with strange peers (avoidant disorder). In the third entity (overanxious disorder), the anxiety becomes a part of a child's life-style and is experienced in regard to many situations and people.

Under these three symptom complexes are subsumed many other types of anxiety symptoms, e.g., school refusal fears, some sleep disturbances, and many concomitant psychophysiological symptoms. Other childhood anxiety disorders can be placed in adult diagnostic categories, e.g., phobias, generalized anxiety disorders, and atypical anxiety disorder.

Oppositional disorder is the new term in *DSM-III* that replaces "passive-aggressive personality disorder," in which the child shows much underlying anger. A certain amount of oppositional behavior is normal, even necessary, to children in establishing their own identity; it occurs at all developmental stages. When oppositional behavior is prolonged or intense and inflexible, it becomes pathological and interferes with many other aspects of life, both social and academic. These children have a poor self-image that in turn contributes to social and school disability.

Anxiety disorders are more common in girls than in boys, whereas the converse is true concerning oppositional disorder. In separation disorder, the families generally are close-knit and overconcerned. Girls who have an overly close relationship with their mothers are prone to the disorder. The child who is susceptible to overanxious disorder frequently is the firstborn in a small, upper socioeconomic family who expects a great deal of the child. Avoidant children generally have at least one parent who is overanxious or shy. In contrast, the parents of oppositional children are likely to be preoccupied with issues of power and control and may not have wanted the child.

425-430. The answers are: 425-B, 426-D, 427-B, 428-C, 429-E, 430-A. *(Kolb, ed 9. pp 96-112. Usdin, pp 67-80.)* Various mental mechanisms attempt to achieve a balance between drives and the unrest or anxiety such drives induce when they cannot be met. The mechanisms permit some degree of stability or comfort, but they also may become warped and contribute to a mental illness.

Fixation refers to an undue persistence of an immature mode of coping. It has its origin in a stressful episode occurring in a developmental process, aborting, arresting, or interfering with its completion. The adult reverts to the mode of behavior and its affects that had been used earlier in life, a reversion that becomes extremely persistent or fixed. Therefore, we might recognize a type of pregenital fixation as oral fixation, in which the patient showed an undue interest in mouthing, sucking, and oral manipulation.

Resistance refers to opposition by a patient to the therapeutic process, whatever that process might be. In simplest form, it applies to the patient who refuses or "forgets" to take medication, a problem seen all too often in juvenile diabetic patients who fail to take their insulin and repeatedly return to the hospital with diabetic coma. To these individuals, the medication seems to symbolize the illness, and if they do not take the medication they believe that they do not have the illness. This association represents a prelogical or magical form of thinking. To the symbol of their illness (the medication) these patients attach a whole subsystem of illogical fantasies. They invest the medication with a tremendous amount of affect that represents the fear and resentment they have about their disease, as well as their resentment of the doctor as an authoritarian agent who makes them stick themselves with a needle. In psychoanalysis, resistances offer some of the most productive material for the analyst to work with.

In displacement, the affected patient transfers affect from one object to another, through which the patient can express the affect with less anxiety and spares himself the anguish of facing the real origin of the problem. Thus, a child's resentment of a harsh, punitive father may become unconsciously linked to some authority figures such as policemen, whose actions involve apprehension and punishment. Frequently, of course, the displacement is to something with much less obvious connection to the original source of difficulty.

In restitution, the patient relieves guilt by committing an act or adopting a life-style that atones for the perceived transgression. If a person wishes someone dead (who then dies), the person may feel responsible for the death. An act or acts of restitution, unconsciously determined, may then make reparation for the event. In the example given in question 429, the patient unconsciously replaced the dead sister with another child as a means of restitution. The situation also has oedipal implications.

In fixation, some of the psychic energy becomes abnormally attached to an earlier developmental stage. Behaviors appropriate to that stage continue. In the case of oral fixation, the patient may show various features of orality such as thumb-sucking, mouthing of objects, and smoking. Anal fixation is said to lead to the overly meticulous, obsessive-compulsive personality, whereas mother fixation may be related to homosexuality.

Psychopathology

DIRECTIONS: Each question below contains five suggested answers. Choose the **one best** response to each question.

431. The single best criterion indicating that a patient has become physically dependent on a drug is that

(A) the patient has used the drug at least six months
(B) the patient admits a craving for the drug
(C) the patient shows tolerance for the drug
(D) withdrawal symptoms occur upon discontinuing the drug
(E) the drug makes the patient overtly ill when ingested

432. Of the following terms commonly used in the past to diagnose depression, which do the editors of *DSM-III* consider obsolete?

(A) Affective disorders
(B) Melancholia
(C) Bioplar disorders
(D) Dysthymic disorders
(E) Endogenous depressions

433. The biogenic amine hypothesis (of Osmond and Smythies) proposes that schizophrenia may be caused by

(A) a deficiency of biogenic amine production
(B) a block in the synthesis of biogenic amines
(C) conversion of biogenic amines to aldehyde and acid end products
(D) production of amphetaminelike compounds from tryptophan
(E) production of aberrant methylated derivatives of biogenic amines

434. Characteristics of the Argyll Robertson pupil include

(A) enlargement, failure to react to light, but reaction in accommodation
(B) enlargement, reaction to light, but failure to react in accommodation
(C) miosis, reaction to light, but failure of reaction in accommodation
(D) miosis, failure to react to light, but reaction in accommodation
(E) miosis, failure to react to light or in accommodation

435. Studies of large numbers of patients with organic dementia show that the proportion of patients whose disorder is potentially reversible is about

(A) 1:5
(B) 1:10
(C) 1:50
(D) 1:100
(E) 1:500

436. A hysterical tremor is best distinguished from an organic tremor by its

(A) disappearance during sleep
(B) complete disappearance with psychiatric treatment
(C) reduction when patients are observed without their knowledge
(D) response to placebo
(E) intensification during times of emotional stress

437. Individuals who seek counseling for marital problems most frequently report experiencing

(A) envy
(B) remorse
(C) anger
(D) guilt
(E) sexual dissatisfaction

438. A pudgy 39-year-old spinster presents with depression. She has rounded shoulders and face, considerable facial hair, and acne. Photographs taken five years previously show a striking change in appearance. The test most likely to establish the diagnosis is which of the following?

(A) Urinary 17-hydroxycorticosteroid determination
(B) Urinary catecholamine screen
(C) Glucose tolerance test
(D) Lysosomal enzyme battery
(E) CAT scan

439. In the *DSM-III* diagnostic system, personality disorders are coded on which of the following axes?

(A) Axis I
(B) Axis II
(C) Axis III
(D) Axis IV
(E) Axis V

440. In clinical practice today, the type of schizophrenia most commonly seen is

(A) catatonic
(B) paranoid
(C) hebephrenic (disorganized)
(D) schizo-affective type
(E) schizoid disorder of childhood or adolescence

441. The demonstration of an increased incidence of schizophrenia in which of the following related persons would argue **against** the role of the intrauterine environment as a cause of schizophrenia?

(A) Identical twins
(B) Fraternal twins
(C) Non-twin siblings who are adopted
(D) Siblings adopted by and raised by other parents
(E) Paternal half-siblings

442. The most general working definition of drug addiction is

(A) reduction of personal flexibility owing to drug use
(B) drug use unsanctioned by the society at large
(C) craving or wishing for a drug
(D) recreational use of a drug
(E) required use of the drug for peer group acceptance

443. All of the following statements concerning conduct disorders of childhood are true EXCEPT that

(A) children without a permanent or stable home are particularly at risk for developing conduct disorders
(B) antisocial behavior may develop in a child who lacks a close relationship with a mother figure
(C) most children with conduct disorders have normal neurological examinations and average intelligence
(D) acting out, aggressive acts are more common in brain injured and epileptic children than in the general child population
(E) girls are more prone to conduct disorders than boys

444. In an emergency room, the immediate action on the part of the psychiatrist faced with a violent, assaultive patient should be which of the following?

(A) Quickly marshal sufficient force to subdue the patient
(B) Try to talk the patient into a calmer frame of mind
(C) Secure the patient in a calm, slow manner in the presence of other people
(D) Remain personally uninvolved and let emergency room attendants secure the patient
(E) None of the above

445. Depersonalization, psychogenic amnesia, fugue states, and multiple personalities are classified in *DSM-III* under which of the following general terms?

(A) Psychosexual disorders
(B) Dissociative disorders
(C) Traumatic neurosis
(D) Conversion disorders
(E) Factitious disorders

446. Prevalence rates of schizophrenia in various parts of the world vary by which of the following factors?

(A) 5
(B) 10
(C) 15
(D) 20
(E) 25

447. The cardinal clinical features of Sydenham's chorea, in addition to hyperkinesia, are

(A) peripheral neuropathy and paralysis
(B) transverse myelitis and urinary incontinence
(C) hypotonia and hyperemotionality
(D) spasticity and clonus
(E) seizures and cortical blindness

448. In an adult patient with a recent onset of generalized motor seizures, a normal interictal EEG argues most strongly AGAINST

(A) an acute destructive cerebral lesion
(B) delirium tremens
(C) falx meningioma
(D) a postconcussion syndrome
(E) hypoglycemic seizures

449. A patient has a history of vague loss of consciousness and possibly generalized jerking, but a clear description is unavailable. Her interictal EEG shows moderate amounts of symmetrical bitemporal theta activity. In this clinical context, which of the following statements about the patient's EEG is most nearly true?

(A) It strongly suggests a psychogenic or functional illness
(B) It is a diagnostic finding in 80 percent of patients with generalized motor seizures
(C) It virtually excludes an organic seizure disorder
(D) It fails to argue either for or against an organic seizure disorder
(E) It routinely requires a followup EEG with pentylenetetrazol (Metrazol)

450. All the following statements concerning health professionals participating in therapy training for sexually dysfunctional couples are true EXCEPT that

(A) changes in attitude toward sex must precede a trainee's participation
(B) participation aids a trainee in shedding inhibitions
(C) seeing explicit sex films involving sex therapy has instructional value
(D) curiosity, thinking, and feeling are stimulated
(E) a trainee learns some of the complexities underlying "interactional dynamics" of sexual adjustment symptoms

451. A 12-year-old patient suspected of having epilepsy has an EEG showing a large amount of moderately high-amplitude, 2-3 cps rhythmic slowing that begins shortly after hyperventilation starts, and stops about 10-15 seconds after hyperventilation ends. This finding suggests which of the following?

(A) A disease of gray matter
(B) A diencephalic tumor
(C) Epilepsy
(D) A systemic acid-base imbalance
(E) Normal finding for the age

DIRECTIONS: Each question below contains four suggested answers of which **one** or **more** is correct. Choose the answer

A	if	1, 2, and 3	are correct
B	if	1 and 3	are correct
C	if	2 and 4	are correct
D	if	4	is correct
E	if	1, 2, 3, and 4	are correct

452. True statements concerning biological risk factors for schizophrenia, as suggested by current research, include which of the following?

(1) Inadequacy of intrauterine blood supply rather than genetic factors may account for greater risk of schizophrenia among monozygotic twins than among dizygotic twins
(2) About 50 percent of the etiological variance of schizophrenia may be accounted for by genetic factors
(3) The increased risk that schizophrenic mothers impart to their children may be due to increased prenatal and perinatal, rather than genetic, factors
(4) Biological risk factors for schizophrenia, whatever their causal type, are now known to be expressed through lower than normal MAO platelet levels

453. Seventy percent or more of patients diagnosed as having schizophrenia by both computer and clinical methods exhibited which of the following symptoms?

(1) Lack of insight
(2) Auditory hallucinations
(3) Ideas of reference
(4) Thoughts spoken aloud

454. If the theory that epilepsy results from interference with the action of GABA is true, which of the following statements would also be true?

(1) Drugs that inhibit the degradation or removal of GABA at the synaptic cleft should be anticonvulsants
(2) Drugs that compete with GABA at presynaptic endings should cause seizures
(3) Deficiency of pyridoxine should cause seizures
(4) Oral or intravenous administration of GABA should block seizures

455. Depression in a geriatric population is characterized by which of the following statements?

(1) Death rates from causes other than suicide increase in untreated depressed patients
(2) Depression usually lifts in a spontaneous manner
(3) In the population over 60 years of age, the prevalence is 30 percent
(4) The symptoms are resistant to treatment in most cases

456. The third edition of the American Psychiatric Association's Diagnostic and Statistical Manual of Mental Disorders *(DSM-III)* differs from the second edition in that the third edition

(1) gives more explicit definitions of each disorder
(2) provides a biaxial diagnostic system
(3) defines schizophrenia more narrowly
(4) omits a definition of mental disorder

457. Elderly depressed patients differ from younger depressed patients by exhibiting

(1) more physical symptoms and complaints
(2) less mood disturbance
(3) more prominent apathy
(4) more frequent paranoid symptoms

458. Commonly held "myths" about suicide include which of the following?

(1) Religious beliefs protect against suicide
(2) Improvement after a period of great suicidal danger indicates that that danger is over
(3) A suicidal act is proof of psychiatric illness
(4) Suicide rates vary among socioeconomic classes

459. The usual symptoms of sleep terrors (pavor nocturnus) include which of the following?

(1) The episodes occur late in the night after several hours of sleep
(2) The onset is abrupt during the delta stage of sleep
(3) The patient has full recall the next morning
(4) The patient often screams and shows perseverative motor activity

460. The conditions necessary to produce tolerance for a drug include

(1) predisposing personality disorder
(2) severalfold increase in metabolism of the drug
(3) withdrawal symptoms on discontinuing the drug
(4) repeated administrations of the drug

461. Circumstances that may act to trigger seizures include which of the following?

(1) Laughter
(2) Sleep deprivation
(3) Overhydration
(4) Reading

462. If genetic predisposition or heredity played a role in the causation of seizures, which of the following statements should be true?

(1) If one twin has epilepsy, the incidence of seizures in the other twin, whether fraternal or identical, should be the same
(2) The seizure frequency in successive generations must show a definite mendelian ratio
(3) The incidence of migraine in families of patients with epilepsy would not be increased
(4) The "carrier" parents of epileptic children should have a greater incidence of abnormal EEGs than a control population, even if they lack overt seizures

463. Secondary depression commonly follows which of the following illnesses or physical conditions?

(1) Hypercalcemia
(2) Normal pressure hydrocephalus
(3) Parkinson's disease
(4) Brain tumors

464. Features that distinguish delirium from dementia include which of the following?

(1) Manifestations of widespread dysfunction of cerebral tissue
(2) No enduring lesion demonstrable
(3) Caused only by disorders exogenous to the CNS
(4) Duration relatively brief

465. The DSM-III Axis I classification of organic brain syndromes includes which of the following categories?

(1) Global cognitive impairment, either delirium or dementia
(2) Circumscribed cognitive impairment, amnestic syndromes, and hallucinosis
(3) Organic personality disorders
(4) Global mental retardation

466. Certain physical diseases commonly present with symptoms that may lead to a mistaken diagnosis of primary psychiatric illness. Disorders that may be misdiagnosed as anxiety states or attacks include which of the following?

(1) Hypothyroidism
(2) Hyperthyroidism
(3) Adenoma of islets of Langerhans
(4) Hypoparathyroidism

467. Findings that aid in distinguishing between functional depression and dementia in older patients include which of the following?

(1) Depressed patients tend to remain competent at work for a considerable period of time after the depression starts
(2) Quick changes from crying to laughter occur more often in the functionally depressed patient
(3) Near-miss answers and circumlocutions in response to questions are more frequent in organic illness
(4) Memory impairment occurs late in organic dementia

468. Factors that favor a diagnosis of psychomotor seizures over petit mal absences include which of the following?

(1) Presence of a definite aura
(2) Duration longer than 30 seconds
(3) Postictal confusion
(4) Automatic behavior such as undressing

469. Statements that characterize suicide or the potentially suicidal patient include which of the following?

(1) The period of greatest danger is usually short
(2) Many potentially suicidal patients are ambivalent about death
(3) The suicidal act has—at least in part—interpersonal implications
(4) All major psychiatric disorders carry higher than average suicidal risks

470. Typical features of Wernicke-Korsakoff psychosis include

(1) complete memory defect in registration of items
(2) severe memory defects in retention and recall
(3) severe impairment of cognitive functions and mild obtundation of consciousness
(4) confabulation

471. Correct statements concerning sexual relations in marriage include which of the following?

(1) Active sexual relations between partners are necessary for a happy marriage
(2) Unconsummated marriages usually result in early divorce
(3) Mutual orgasm is essential for sexual satisfaction
(4) Extramarital sexual activity is more dangerous for cardiac patients than marital sex

472. As described in *DSM-III,* disorders that are excluded from the category of schizophrenia include

(1) schizoaffective disorder
(2) residual type
(3) schizophreniform disorder
(4) hebephrenia

DIRECTIONS: The groups of questions below consist of lettered choices followed by several numbered items. For each numbered item select the **one** lettered choice with which it is **most** closely associated. Each lettered choice may be used once, more than once, or not at all.

Questions 473-476

For each of the case histories below, choose the disorder (according to *DSM-III* diagnostic criteria) with which it most closely corresponds.

(A) Schizotypal personality disorder
(B) Schizoid personality disorder
(C) Borderline personality disorder
(D) Paranoid personality disorder
(E) Avoidant personality disorder

473. A 39-year-old man reluctantly submits to a psychiatric examination at the urging of his siblings, whom he accuses of treachery in the family business and of plotting against him. Unable to relax, he is very guarded and totally humorless. He does not love his one woman friend but feels intensely jealous about any relationship she has with other men. He keeps the psychiatric appointment only to find out if his siblings are trying to "railroad" him into a mental institution. The psychiatrist detects no formal thought disorders

474. A 24-year-old college graduate submits to a psychiatric examination more in deference to her parents than from self-concern. The patient has obtained a degree in education, but is content with a job filing books in a library. She lacks friends and spends her leisure collecting recipes and cooking for herself. Less social than her siblings as a child, she has grown progressively asocial in adulthood. She seems indifferent to praise or criticism and has yet to form attachments to men.

475. A 46-year-old woman is referred to a psychiatrist by her 25-year-old daughter, who finds the mother antagonistic toward her and the few remaining people in her social life. The daughter remembers the patient as being different from other people, and as growing more eccentric and superstitious with the years. Her marriage ended, according to the daughter, because she became aloof, cold, and hypersensitive to the slightest hint of criticism. The patient's speech is odd without being incoherent or showing loose associations. The woman thinks she can summon **her** mother from the dead and claims clairvoyance and mental telepathy. She reports having no real friends except her daughter, whom she suspects of "doing things behind my back." The patient admits to anxiety about what others think of her, a symptom for which she wants medication; she declines psychotherapy, however

476. A 29-year-old man comes to a psychiatrist voluntarily, complaining of being unable to find friends who accept him as he is. In the interview, he appears sad and anxious, and expresses anger over his lack of friends. The psychiatrist encourages the patient to meet individuals of both sexes; however, he is so overconcerned with their opinions of him that he feels utterly belittled by the slightest hint of criticism. In turn, the patient berates them severely, thus aborting any hope of real friendship. He interprets the psychiatrist's remarks as hostile criticism that make him want to terminate therapy prematurely

Questions 477-481

For each of the physical findings listed below, choose the intoxicating agent with which it is most closely associated.

(A) Arsenic
(B) Copper
(C) Mercury
(D) Lead
(E) Bromide

477. Dark line along the gum margin

478. Pink, painful skin

479. White, transverse lines on the nails

480. Greenish brown ring at corneal limbus

481. Acneiform skin rash in adult with proliferative nodular lesions

Questions 482-487

For each of the case histories below, choose the disorder with which it is most closely associated.

(A) Migraine
(B) Islet cell adenoma of pancreas
(C) Porphyria
(D) Carcinoid syndrome
(E) Pheochromocytoma

482. A 23-year-old man complains of episodes of anxiety, pallor, sweating, and pounding bilateral headaches that occur several times per month and seem to be increasing in frequency. The attacks last from minutes to hours and are accompanied by weakness, dizziness, and often nausea without vomiting. The patient's skin exhibits multiple café au lait spots.

483. A garrulous and argumentative 23-year-old woman presents to the admitting room with numerous complaints. She feels that everyone has treated her badly, rambles on about abdominal pains and difficulty with bowel movements, and grimaces frequently. She has abdominal scars from three previous operations, but she is unable to state whether any definite diagnosis has been made. She has vague complaints of difficulty using her hands and gives inconsistent responses during the sensory examination

484. A 31-year-old woman begins to have attacks of anxiety, sweating, pallor, hunger, blurred vision, double vision, and difficulty thinking, accompanied by some slurring of speech. The attacks continue for several months. They tend to occur between 9 PM and breakfast, and sometimes after physical exertion. She occasionally loses track of time during the attacks. The physical examination is normal

485. A 7-year-old boy begins to have episodes of extreme irritability accompanied by nausea, abdominal pain, vomiting, and the desire to go into a quiet, dark room. He may go to sleep, at which time he may sweat excessively, and then feels better but seems drained out. He has some headache during the spells, but cannot localize it or describe it well. He does not lose consciousness. The neurological examination is normal

486. A 41-year-old man complains of episodes of hot flashes and flushing of the skin. He admits to moderately heavy use of alcohol and feels that the flushing may happen after alcohol ingestion, but claims it may happen at other times also. He suffers from chronic diarrhea and intermittent abdominal pain. He has telangiectases resembling acne rosacea over his facial skin, and an enlarged liver

487. A 26-year-old man presents with complaints of rapidly increasing weakness, beginning in the lower extremities and extending after several days to involve the hands. It now even has affected his face. He experiences constipation and some abdominal discomfort. He has mild hypertension and tachycardia. Neurologic examination shows decreased-to-absent muscle stretch reflexes and a mild stocking-glove sensory loss

Questions 488-491

For each of the case histories below, choose the eponym with which it is historically associated.

(A) Capgras
(B) De Clérambault
(C) Don Juan
(D) Briquet
(E) Ganser

488. A 29-year-old prisoner, accused of making a knife from a piece of metal, appears conscious and alert but gives bizarre answers to questions. When asked how the examiner is dressed, he may state that a male examiner is wearing a dress. When asked about the weather, he may reply that it is raining when the sun is shining. On the neurologic examination, he may give similar bizarre responses—for example, stating that his finger is up when it is down.

489. A 43-year-old man with long-standing feelings of persecution begins to claim he no longer knows his business partner and that his business partner has been replaced by a duplicate person. He believes that the duplicate of his partner is placed there to confuse him and affect his judgment

490. A 40-year-old psychiatrist is being sued for malpractice because of claims by a patient that he tried to seduce her. Fourteen of his other female patients make the same claim. Several report having had intercourse with him. He is known to constantly brush up against women and to make physical contact with them by hugging and touching. He jokes about spending the night with any new woman he meets, and will do so if permitted. He is a dapper dresser and speaks with an overly modulated, highly cultivated voice

491. A 30-year-old woman has a large collection of photographs of Robert Redford and articles about him. She sends herself gifts containing cards upon which she signs his name and writes herself love letters in his name

Questions 492-495

For each group of essential diagnostic features appearing below, choose the type of schizophrenia as listed in *DSM-III* or *International Classification of Diseases (ICD-9)* with which it is most closely associated.

(A) Catatonic
(B) Hebephrenic (disorganized)
(C) Undifferentiated
(D) Paranoid
(E) Simple

492. A person who meets the general schizophrenia diagnostic criteria of *DSM-III* and exhibits incoherence and flat, incongruous, or silly affect and fragmentary delusions or hallucinations (unsystematized)

493. A person who meets the general schizophrenia diagnostic criteria of *DSM-III* and exhibits stupor, rigidity, or excitement

494. A person who meets the general schizophrenia diagnostic criteria of *DSM-III* and exhibits persistent delusions of the persecutory, grandiose, or jealousy types and has hallucinations with themes of persecution or grandiosity

495. A person who has difficulty forming social relationships, i.e., few or no close friends, indifference to praise or criticism, insensitivity to others' feelings; such feature beginning during or after puberty. In addition, introgression, i.e., signs of being withdrawn, solitary, and absent-minded; bland affect, i.e., defective emotional expression, lack of a sense of humor, aloofness, absence of warm feelings; absence of eccentricities of behavior or communication

Psychopathology
Answers

431. The answer is D. *(Gilman, ed 6. p 536.)* The best evidence of physical dependence on a drug is the occurrence of withdrawal symptoms when the drug use is discontinued. Each drug may produce its own particular alterations of mental state and also may produce quite characteristic clinical features on withdrawal. For example, withdrawal from tobacco results in neither the heroin withdrawal syndrome nor the alcohol withdrawal syndrome. Dependence on a drug necessarily implies tolerance for the drug. Neither craving, nor even tolerance, for a drug proves physical dependence, which has as its operational definition the precipitation of physical signs and symptoms of an altered mental state and usually a period of rebound hyperexcitability.

432. The answer is E. *(American Psychiatric Association, ed 3. pp 205-221.)* "Affective disorders" is the main rubric for those disorders in which a mood disturbance is the basic feature. The editors of *DSM-III* state that a more accurately descriptive term would be "mood disorders," but that in the interest of "common usage" and "historical continuity," the term "affective disorders" has been retained. The various depressive disorders, manic disorders, and their combinations (bipolar disorders) comprise the major subclasses of the affective disorders. "Melancholia" is an old term deemed worthy of retention because it gives no false impressions. The term "endogenous depression" leads many people to believe that a precipitating event was not involved in the onset of depression, which, in many cases, is an erroneous assumption. Both "melancholia" and "endogenous depression" refer to a severe depression that responds favorably to some form of somatic therapy. "Dysthymic disorder" is the term used for mild depression, without hypomania, that fails to meet severity criteria for major depressive disorders.

433. The answer is E. *(Barchas, pp 100-102.)* Osmond and Smythies (1952) opened an era of biochemical research in schizophrenia by suggesting that the aberrant production of methylated amines might play a role in the pathogenesis of schizophrenia. Their theory suggested that schizophrenic individuals produce an endogenous psychotogenic chemical. Although no single biochemical hypothesis of schizophrenia has been established, the theory proposed by Osmond and Smythies has had a tremendous heuristic impact in schizophrenia research. The many false claims for a single biochemical error in schizophrenia are a warning that this is a difficult field of study in terms of biochemical competence and knowledge of experimental design.

434. The answer is D. *(DeMyer, ed 3. p 102.)* The Argyll Robertson pupil is miotic and reacts in accommodation, but fails to react to light. In addition, the pupil is irregular in outline and the iris is atrophic and fails to respond well to mydriatics. A pupil with all of these characteristics is almost pathognomonic of syphilis, but can be imitated by a few other conditions. These include diabetes, encephalitis, iris diseases, and some neuropathies affecting orbital nerves. A positive serologic test for syphilis and the presence of other signs of the active disease confirm the diagnosis indicated by the pupillary signs.

435. The answer is B. *(Wells, ed 2. p 250.)* Studies of large numbers of patients with organic dementia show that about 10-15 percent have potentially reversible disorders. This figure indicates the importance of a thorough medical workup for every patient with dementia in order to identify treatable causes. The intrusion of cost-effective schemes into medical practice may tend to suppress the range and scope of the workup. While unnecessary diagnostic procedures are to be condemned, those designed to save the patient's brain can hardly be contested in view of the salvage rate of around one patient in ten. Beyond the usual history and physical examination, the minimum workup of patients with organic dementia should include CAT scan, a serologic test for syphilis, CSF examination, and selected blood chemistry and endocrine function tests.

436. The answer is B. *(DeMyer, ed 3. pp 238-239, 451.)* Both organic and hysterical tremors and other involuntary movements disappear during sleep, are heightened by emotional tension, and may undergo reduction when the affected patients are observed without their knowledge. Both hysterical and organic disorders may respond to placebo. Thus, none of these features distinguishes hysterical from organic movement disorders. For example, a parkinsonian patient who may have been lying quietly in bed before ward rounds may begin to display the tremor prominently as the entourage of doctors, students, nurses, and social workers approaches the bedside. The presence of other people constitutes a form of stress, which may worsen organic as well as hysterical movement disorders. After the entourage moves on, the parkinsonian patient's tremor recedes. One of the classical criteria for distinguishing hysterical disorders from organic is the complete disappearance of the disorder with appropriate psychiatric treatment. This is the best and most conclusive link in the chain of evidence that establishes the correct diagnosis.

437. The answer is C. *(Usdin, pp 625-626.)* Individuals seeking marital counseling most commonly report experiencing anger. Their anger most often is expressed verbally, but also may commonly take the form of physical abuse, psychosomatic symptoms, or depression and neuroses. Anger commonly appears in a marital relationship that fails to supply the gratification desired yet whose intimacy evokes the expression of an individual's deepest needs. Such anger may not always be destructive if it mobilizes the individuals involved to recognize their problems before destructive reaction patterns in the relationship become irreversible.

438. The answer is A. *(Kolb, ed 9. pp 338-339.)* The round face and shoulders, facial hair, and acne described in the patient presented in the question suggest Cushing's syndrome. Depression is the most commonly encountered mental illness in Cushing's syndrome. These patients undergo a "Dorian Gray" transformation of appearance, as can be documented by looking at old photographs. A diagnosis of Cushing's syndrome would be supported by an increase in urinary 17-hydroxycorticosteroids. A glucose tolerance test may show abnormal elevation because of the gluconeogenetic effect of the steroids, but of itself would not be diagnostic. Cushing's syndrome occurs as a natural illness or as an iatrogenic disease secondary to steroid or ACTH therapy.

439. The answer is B. *(American Psychiatric Association, ed 3. pp 9, 23-25.)* The *DSM-III* recommends the use of five axes to evaluate mental conditions in order to give greater descriptive power over several dimensions of a psychiatric illness. The axes and their respective coded dimensions are as follows:

Axis I - (a) Psychiatric clinical syndromes (including mental retardation)
(b) Conditions not attributable to a mental disorder that are the focus of attention or treatment
Axis II - (a) Personality disorders
(b) Specific developmental disorders

Axis III - Physical diagnoses
Axis IV - Severity of psychosocial stresses
Axis V - Highest level of adaptive function in the past year
It is often necessary to code more than one diagnosis on the first three axes, but generally one diagnosis represents the condition that was the major one necessitating treatment or evaluation. This one is called the **principal diagnosis** and is usually on Axis I and needs no special notation when being coded. However, if the principal diagnosis is located on Axis II, then the phrase "Principal diagnosis" must be noted.
For example: Axis I: 303.93 Alcohol dependence in remission
                    Axis II: 301.81 Narcissistic personality disorder (Principal diagnosis).

440. The answer is B. *(Kaplan, ed 3. pp 1164-1165.)* Since Kraepelin (1869) first described three main types of dementia praecox, many other subtypes of schizophrenia have been delineated. For 30 years, the widespread use of neuroleptic medicines has blunted the diagnostic features of the various subtypes, not only by arresting the progress of the disease but also by blunting the initiative of schizophrenic patients. Diagnosticians now see proportionally more cases of undifferentiated and paranoid schizophrenia than they did before neuroleptics came into use. Khokhlov called this redistribution of incidence the pathomorphosis of schizophrenia.

441. The answer is E. *(Kolb, ed 9. pp 166-167.)* In assessing the causes of schizophrenia, investigators have tried to sort out genetic influences, the effects of the intrauterine environment provided by schizophrenic mothers, and the extrauterine environment. An increased incidence of schizophrenia occurs in identical twins, fraternal twins, and non-twin siblings of schizophrenic mothers—whether the children are adopted or raised by their natural mothers. An observation that diminishes any contribution to schizophrenia by the intrauterine environment of a schizophrenic mother is the finding that paternal half-siblings of schizophrenic adoptees also have a high risk for schizophrenia. This would argue for some direct, presumably genetic influence transmitted by the paternal gamete, independent of intrauterine influences from a schizophrenic mother.

442. The answer is A. *(Gilman, ed 6. pp 535-536.)* Drug addiction may generally be described as the need for or dependence on a drug to the point of limiting an addicted person's flexibility. Such individuals increasingly surrender more of their behavior to the drug. As the need for the drug gradually dominates both thought and behavior, these persons then enter the stage of compulsive drug seeking and drug taking. Perhaps "compulsive drug seeking and taking" is the best definition of all; it is general enough to include tobacco use as a drug-dependent state and it is as free of sociological connotations as possible. Requirement of a withdrawal syndrome on discontinuation of the drug provides an additional dimension for defining drug addiction on an operational-behavioral-biologic basis.

443. The answer is E. *(Barker, pp 48-51.)* Conduct disorders in children and adolescents comprise the largest category of psychiatric illnesses and are associated with many factors. The origins of the problem often lie in the home, e.g., parental attitudes of rejection, absence of a father figure, large family size, low socioeconomic status, inconsistent or harsh punishment. Nevertheless, factors inherent in the child also can increase the risk of conduct disorders. Boys are more prone to the disorder than girls. Neurologically and intellectually handicapped children are more likely to have conduct disorders than the general child population, although most children with conduct disorders are normal in these respects. Also, among the normal population are inborn temperamental factors that predispose to the development of conduct disorders. Children who are adaptable and easygoing develop conduct disorders less frequently than those who are volatile in temperament. Thus, the clinician assessing the origin of a conduct disorder must weigh not only the contribution of the family but also biological and temperamental attributes of the child.

444. The answer is A. *(Hackett, pp 402-403.)* While the violent and assaultive patient represents a highly difficult problem for emergency rooms of general hospitals, initial management of such persons is the unavoidable responsibility of the emergency room staff. According to W. Anderson, halfway measures are liable to create personal injuries and property damage. The best plan for the psychiatrist or other physician is to locate adequate physical help even before confronting a violent patient. Because emergency rooms generally have insufficient manpower for these emergencies, such help will have to be recruited from other sections of the hospital, such as security. The whole of the force should then be rapidly deployed in a concerted fashion, whereupon high-potency neuroleptics should be prescribed for immediate parenteral administration.

445. The answer is B. *(American Psychiatric Association, ed 3. pp 253, 255, 257, 259.)* A principal function of the ego is to integrate one's awareness of the self and bodily movement with respect to the environment. Arousal of too much anxiety by activation of inner conflicts may change this awareness of environment and self and result in dissociative disorders, of which memory loss is a core feature. In psychogenic amnesia, the basic feature is loss of memory for information concerning the self, such as name, occupation, and place of residence. When the person who has such a memory loss also moves to a different venue and assumes another role, such as a job, the phenomenon is called a psychogenic fugue state. In multiple personality, the self-identity disorder is manifested by two or more subpersonalities existing side by side but unrecognized by the original personality. The inclusion of depersonalization disorder under the rubric of dissociative disorders is controversial. Although the feeling of reality—and thus the person's sense of identity—is disturbed, memory loss is absent.

446. The answer is B. *(Kaplan, ed 3. p 1124.)* According to Herbert Weiner, prevalence rates of schizophrenia vary from 0.3 to 3 percent, a factor of 10. The median rate is 0.8 percent. Prevalence rates have been gathered by many investigators to determine the possible role of genetic factors in causing schizophrenia. Use of this method has thus far proved to be unsatisfactory because of inadequacies in application, i.e., unreliability of diagnosis, poor quality of records when hospitalized probands are used as subjects, and failure to control for socioeconomic class and experiential factors. Nevertheless, our understanding of schizophrenia would be enhanced by specific data concerning cultural or national differences in various rates of occurrence and the factors that cause these differences.

447. The answer is C. *(Swaiman, p 227.)* The cardinal features of rheumatic chorea are choreiform hyperkinesias, hypotonia, and hyperemotionality. Although a variety of neurologic and psychiatric disorders can occur in rheumatic fever, they do not include a paralytic peripheral neuropathy, transverse myelitis, spasticity, or urinary incontinence. Seizures may occur but are not among the cardinal features. Hypotonia is one of the more crippling aspects of the syndrome. Patients with hypotonia cannot maintain a voluntary contraction or postural set, and the sudden yielding of muscle tone causes them to drop objects and to fall. This sudden yielding of muscle tone may also be demonstrated during the clinical examination when testing a patient's strength. When asked to flex an arm and hold it flexed, the patient cannot sustain the muscular contraction. If the examiner attempts to pull on the arm, the resistance may yield abruptly.

448. The answer is A. *(Adams, ed 2. p 24.)* Most acute destructive lesions of the cerebrum cause unilateral delta activity. Thus, if a patient has seizures and a normal interictal EEG, in all probability the seizures are due to something other than an acute focal destructive lesion. Delirium tremens, meningiomas (which are chronic lesions and may be deep along the falx or base of the brain), postconcussion syndrome, and hypoglycemia frequently produce seizures in the presence of a normal interictal EEG. A delta focus may appear transiently after a seizure in a patient who lacks a demonstrable gross anatomic lesion. The focus will disappear within hours or days. Thus, a delta focus can reflect a transient physiologic change rather than an anatomic lesion.

449. The answer is D. *(Adams, ed 2. pp 22-23.)* A significant number of patients with generalized seizures, perhaps as many as 40 percent, fail to show significant epileptiform discharges in the interictal phase. The diagnosis rests on the clinical information rather than on the EEG. Pentylenetetrazol activation has little value in the differential diagnosis of seizure disorders and has no place as a routine activating procedure. Slight bitemporal slowing is too common a phenomenon to have any firm diagnostic value in seizure disorders.

450. The answer is A. *(Rosenzweig, pp 203-211.)* The psychiatric resident or other professional who participates in training for sex therapy achieves several personal advantages, according to various authors. The discomfort that assaults a neophyte in discussing sexuality with patients is largely dispelled. As a result, the therapist can more effectively obtain detailed histories of sexual dysfunction from both partners that reveal, in addition, the complex dynamics of the couple's nonsexual interactions. Much of the attitudinal change necessary for conducting sex therapy takes place not preparatory to, but in conjunction with, the learning process.

451. The answer is E. *(Adams, ed 2. p 22.)* Hyperventilation-induced rhythmic slowing is a customary EEG finding in normal children and may occur in normal adults. It bears a distinct time relationship, starting shortly after hyperventilation begins and lasting for some seconds after hyperventilation ceases. This normal activation of the EEG should not be confused with pathologic alterations indicating structural disease, a seizure disorder, or systemic disease affecting acid-base balance. Although hyperventilation may accentuate the slowing due to an underlying metabolic imbalance and can induce petit mal seizures, the normal slowing during hyperventilation must be distinguished from the slowing associated with these abnormal conditions.

452. The answer is B (1, 3). *(Kaplan, ed 3. pp 1128-1129.)* The research literature on critical biological factors in the genesis of schizophrenia is long, complex, and difficult to interpret. The role of genetics has been especially confusing. Wiener interprets the genetic data to mean that only about 25 percent of the etiological variance of schizophrenia may be explained solely by genetic factors. A key finding used by theorists to support the genetic hypothesis is that monozygotic twins (with identical genetic structure) are more at risk for schizophrenia than dizygotic twins (with differing genetic structure). However, the intrauterine environment of monozygotic twins, owing to 80 percent sharing of the same placenta (and thus a variable blood supply), is more hazardous than that of dizygotic twins. Research has failed to identify the biological defect that may be inherited but has pointed to several suspicious factors. For example, chronic schizophrenic subjects have lower platelet levels of monoamine oxidase (MAO) than either acute schizophrenic persons or members of the normal population. Evidence has also accrued that low or high levels of MAO may be inherited. Some theorists support the position that low levels of platelet MAO, therefore, are a genetic marker or risk factor for schizophrenia. Future studies will need to answer many questions about such a proposition.

453. The answer is A (1, 2, 3). *(Kaplan, ed 3. pp 1181-1182.)* The World Health Organization sponsored a research program encompassing several countries to elucidate reliable methods of diagnosing schizophrenia in a universally acceptable way. From a pool of 811 patients clinically diagnosed as schizophrenic, a second group of 306 patients emerged as schizophrenic from two computer methods as well as the original clinical method. Four different symptoms were highly specific to those 306 patients: lack of insight, found in 97 percent; auditory hallucinations, in 74 percent; verbal hallucinations and ideas of reference each found in 70 percent. Symptoms found in 50 to 66 percent of cases were (from most frequent to least) suspiciousness, flat affect, voices speaking to patient, delusional mood, delusions of persecution, inadequate description of problems, thought alienation, and thoughts spoken aloud.

454. The answer is A (1, 2, 3). *(Kolb, ed 9. p 294.)* GABA is presumed to be an inhibitory neurotransmitter. One theory of the origin of seizures and their propagation, perhaps including the action of convulsants and anticonvulsants, involves disturbances in the metabolism of GABA. If true, the theory would provide a unitary explanation for a variety of observations. Drugs that would inhibit the degradation or removal of GABA, by increasing its concentration in the synaptic cleft and so promoting its inhibitory action, should act as anticonvulsants and thus prevent the origin or propagation of the epileptic discharge. However, drugs like picrotoxin and bicuculline, which **produce** convulsions, act as receptor blockers for GABA. Pyridoxine is a requisite for pyridoxal phosphate, a coenzyme for the action of glutamic acid decarboxylase, which forms GABA from glutamic acid. Pyridoxine deficiency results in seizures. The administration of GABA orally or intravenously would not necessarily be expected to test the relation of GABA to seizures, inasmuch as the blood-brain barrier, in principle, excludes transmitters. Therefore, increasing the concentration of GABA in the blood might fail to alter its concentration in the central nervous system and thus would not be a crucial test of the GABA theory.

455. The answer is B (1, 3). *(Kaplan, pp 97, 104-105.)* Understanding depression in a geriatric population is important because of its prevalence in 30 percent of persons past 60 years of age. Among patients past the age of 65 who are admitted to mental hospitals, 45 percent are diagnosed as depressed. In elderly persons whose depression goes undiagnosed and untreated for two or more years, treatment is likely to be ineffective. If treated within that time, response in most cases is good. In contrast to depression in younger persons, depression in the elderly usually fails to improve spontaneously. Death from suicide has a high incidence in the geriatric depressed population, together with death from other causes.

456. The answer is B (1, 3). *(Spitzer, Am J Psychiatry 137:151-164, 1980.)* The content of *DSM-III* differs in many ways from its forerunners. After much debate in the task force, the authors gave, for the first time, a definition of mental disorder. This definition helped the task force to decide which disorders to include and how to characterize them. *DSM-III* provides more detailed definitions of mental disorders to improve diagnostic reliability, includes a multiaxial diagnostic system that should add to recorded information available for each patient, and revises the 17 major diagnostic classes. While the changes are too numerous to summarize here, they include: (1) the great increase in the number of diagnoses possible for children and adolescents, with provisions for giving children "adult" diagnoses and vice versa; (2) narrowing the concept of schizophrenia to identify a more homogeneous group, and (3) distinguishing between unipolar and bipolar depression.

457. The answer is E (all). *(Kaplan, pp 100-101.)* While the diagnostic criteria of *DSM-III* can be used to diagnose depression in a geriatric population, the diagnostician should be aware that symptom differences occur between older and younger populations. In addition to the differences listed in the question, the elderly have fewer feelings of guilt than younger persons. People over 65 have the full range of symptoms from mildly incapacitating to severe forms in which the patient needs help to meet such basic daily needs as eating and cleanliness.

458. The answer is E (all). *(Usdin, pp 469-470.)* There are many misapprehensions about suicide that may cloud the judgment of a physician who formulates disposition or treatment plans for the suicidal patient. Usdin and Lewis list 11 such prevalent mistaken beliefs, which they call "myths" or "fables." In addition to the misapprehensions listed in the question, the authors cite the fallacy that suicide occurs most frequently in people who don't talk about it or give a warning, and in those people who fully wish to die. Physicians must remember that eight of ten suicide victims have talked of suicide or clearly warned another person of their intentions. Many people weather the storm, never to try suicide again, especially if they are treated. No age or social class is immune. Ostensibly normal people, if despondent enough or intensely angry with persons who are important in their lives, may commit suicide. Clergymen of all denominations, including those whose beliefs strongly condemn the act, commit suicide. The time during which a physician should be most wary is in the 3-month period after a time of intense suicidal risk for the patient; this is the time in which such patients may recover the physical energy to commit the act for which they previously were unable to mobilize themselves.

459. The answer is C (2, 4). *(American Psychiatric Association, ed 3. pp 84-85.)* Sleep terrors usually occur during the early part of the night, while the EEG shows delta sleep (stage 3 or 4). A patient usually screams and sits up. Then the patient may display automatic motor acts, often of a perseverative type, like pounding or rocking. The patient shows all of the automatic signs of fright: pupillodilatation, sweating, tachycardia, tachypnea, and piloerection. The patient has little or no recall of the event the next morning. In contrast, nightmares are vivid, frightening dreams that appear during a REM sleep cycle later in the night, after the patient has slept several hours, and are subject to recall by the patient the next morning.

460. The answer is D (4). *(Gilman, ed 6. p 538.)* To produce tolerance for a drug, the drug has to be given repeatedly and in sufficient doses to challenge the function that is to become tolerant. Tolerance may develop with little physical dependence on the drug. Thus, the person who has few or no symptoms on withdrawal of the drug still may have developed tolerance. Tolerance may come about by a severalfold increase in the metabolism of a drug, but in many cases, as with the opiates, a great increase in the metabolism of the drug fails to occur. The development of tolerance may depend on many factors, such as changes in the enzyme levels of the target cells or increased rate of detoxification; the mechanism of tolerance may differ from drug to drug.

461. The answer is E (all). *(Kolb, ed 9. pp 294-295.)* A number of circumstances may act to trigger seizures. Physicians should be acquainted with the full range of precipitating agents and circumstances because of the difficulty often encountered clinically in separating seizures from other causes of disturbed consciousness. Unless there is recognition of the fact that a wide variety of events may precede and precipitate seizures, the seeming bizarreness of the circumstance may suggest a functional rather than organic disorder. The commonest methods of precipitating a seizure are hyperventilation and photic stimulation, which, along with sleep, are routinely used to bring out epileptic discharges during electroencephalography. A patient's medical history, however, may reveal that various events such as listening to music, reading, laughter, sleep deprivation, overhydration, and certain emotional states may either precede and precipitate the seizures or be a part of the seizure itself.

462. The answer is D (4). *(Kolb, ed 9. pp 297-298.)* Heredity has been shown to play a role in the causation of epilepsy, although strict mendelian patterns are not necessarily exhibited. However, some diseases of which seizures are one manifestation, such as phenylketonia and tuberous sclerosis, do show strict mendelian patterns. Compared with the normal population, the incidence of seizures will be increased in siblings (and very likely in other relatives) of a patient who has seizures but does **not** have one of the hereditary diseases with seizures as a feature; however, a strict mendelian pattern may not be apparent. The siblings and parents of a seizure patient, even if lacking clinical seizures themselves, do show an increased incidence of abnormal EEGs. This finding is consistent with current knowledge of carrier states in other diseases, in which some degree of the abnormality can be demonstrated, perhaps by chemical means, although carrier individuals exhibit no clinical signs of the disease. Since seizures and migraine both are hereditary and correlate with each other, families with one of the two disorders should exhibit an incidence of the other that exceeds chance expectations. A genetic factor for a trait is supported if identical twins have a greater concordance for that trait than do fraternal twins or siblings.

463. The answer is E (all). *(Kaplan, pp 113-117.)* Gerner lists 17 types of medical conditions leading to secondary depression that can exactly duplicate the symptoms of primary depression. Endocrine dysfunctions that can cause such depression include hyper- and hypothyroidism; other causes are menopause (from the lowering of blood levels of estrogen) and hypercalcemia. Disorders of the central nervous system that can present with depression as the first clinical sign are those due to head trauma, normal pressure hydrocephalus, Parkinson's disease, pernicious anemia ("megaloblastic madness"), encephalopathy due to virus infection, and dementias from any cause. Other miscellaneous causes of depression are alcoholism and drug addiction, various psychotropic and antihypertensive medications, and stimulants.

464. The answer is C (2, 4). *(American Psychiatric Association, ed 3. pp 103-112.)* Symptoms of delirium include a temporary state of clouding of consciousness, a disturbed sleep-wake cycle, and usually some perceptual distortion in the form of illusions or hallucinations. The affected patient may be agitated or withdrawn. The patient with delirium, like the demented patient, has signs of widespread dysfunction of cerebral tissue, but no enduring lesion can be demonstrated as the cause for the syndrome (although the aged or damaged brain is more susceptible to delirium). The cause of delirium often lies outside the central nervous system, such as liver failure, but it can arise from endogenous factors such as the postictal state or subarachnoid hemorrhage. When the primary process that causes the delirium resolves, the mental symptoms abate.

465. The answer is A (1, 2, 3). *(Kaplan, ed 3. pp 1362-1363.)* A fundamental provision of *DSM-III* is the classification of all mental illnesses into Axis I or Axis II. Axis II includes (1) all personality disorders that affect adults and some children, and (2) specific developmental disorders that appear before adulthood. These, of course, may carry through into adulthood. Axis I contains all of the remaining mental illnesses, including conditions that are not attributable to a mental illness but that become the focus of attention or treatment — for example, an interpersonal problem like a troubled love affair, for which an individual seeks professional help. Organic mental syndromes that cause global or circumscribed cognitive impairment, or organically related personality disturbances are classified under Axis I, but global mental retardation would be included in Axis II under specific developmental disorders.

466. The answer is E (all). *(Usdin, pp 337-351.)* Certain physical diseases are particularly prone to produce symptoms of emotional disturbance that may lead physicians to a misdiagnosis of mental illness. Hyperthyroidism and adenoma of the islets of Langerhans are commonly misdiagnosed as anxiety states, while hypo- and hyperparathyroidism may be mistakenly diagnosed as either anxiety states or depression. Other endocrine diseases that may masquerade as depression are hypothyroidism and hypoadrenalism (Addison's disease). In cases of severe hyperthyroidism and hyperadrenalism (Cushing's syndrome), the presence of deviant thinking and delusions may lead to a misdiagnosis of schizophrenia. Other illnesses commonly mistaken for mental disease are acute porphyria, pernicious anemia, hepatolenticular degeneration, intracranial tumors, pancreatic carcinoma, pheochromocytoma, myasthenia gravis, peripheral neuropathy, chronic organic brain syndrome, normal pressure hydrocephalus, multiple sclerosis, and lupus erythematosus. The psychiatrist must take a careful history and be sufficiently suspicious of all disorders passing for psychiatric illness to diagnose correctly any physical problems masquerading as psychiatric illness.

467. The answer is B (1, 3). *(Benson, pp 105-106.)* Both history and examination may provide information that helps to separate functional depression from progressive dementia. Depressed patients generally can function at work much longer than demented patients, whose early memory failure is reflected in poor job performance. Organically demented persons tend to switch more quickly from crying to joking (pseudobulbar affect) than do functionally depressed individuals. Organically demented patients tend to give near-miss answers and circumlocutions in response to questions, in contrast to depressed individuals who seek to avoid answering. Although an absolute distinction between depression and dementia is not possible, when taken in context the characteristics discussed provide significant evidence to support one or the other diagnosis.

468. The answer is E (all). *(Kolb, ed 9. pp 299-302.)* The distinction between psychomotor seizures and petit mal is important because of the differences in etiology, course, and treatment. Factors that favor a psychomotor seizure as the cause for the lapse of consciousness include a definite aura, duration longer than 30 seconds, postictal confusion, and the performance of automatic behaviors such as undressing. Patients with petit mal seizures have no aura, have seizures lasting less than 30 seconds (except for rare instances of petit mal status), do not have postictal confusion, and may smack their lips or continue walking but are unable to carry on complicated activities that appear goal-directed. The petit mal seizure is conceived of as a pure interruption of consciousness that comes and goes without warning or aftermath. These patients tend to stop what they are doing and to resume it immediately, often with no awareness of the occurrence of the seizure.

469. The answer is A (1, 2, 3). *(Usdin, pp 465-466.)* The first three statements listed in the question represent Shneidman's distillation of the important general factors operating in suicide. While some patients' peak potential for suicide lasts weeks or months, in most individuals the time of greatest danger is only minutes to days. Obviously, if the typical potential victim can be safely shepherded through this period, then a life can be saved and the basic forces driving the patient toward suicide can be dealt with therapeutically. Another factor, the patient's mixed feelings about death, can decrease future risk of suicide if the therapist can mobilize the patient's will to live. The underlying forces typically driving people to suicide involve their relationships with important persons, deep feelings of hopelessness, a sense of helpless dependency, guilt, loss of self-esteem, and lack of social supports. The diagnosis of a major mental disorder, with the one exception of schizophrenia in female patients, increases the risk of suicide. Depression was found by Guze and Robins to increase the suicide risk about 30 times over that of the general population, and depressed individuals represented the diagnostic group with the highest risk.

470. The answer is C (2, 4). *(Adams, ed 2. pp 704-711.)* The patient with Wernicke-Korsakoff psychosis shows defective retention and recall but has some temporary registration of memory and frequently confabulates, apparently to fill in memory gaps. In general, cognitive functions, alertness, attention span, the ability to read and comprehend, and consciousness per se are retained, leaving amnesia and confabulation as the outstanding features of Wernicke-Korsakoff psychosis. Such patients generally lack insight into their condition.

471. The answer is D (4). *(Usdin, pp 628-630.)* Two apparent myths about sexuality are that an active sexual relationship between the partners is necessary for a happy marriage and that mutual orgasm is essential to sexual satisfaction. While happy marriages and good sex relations are correlated, the role of sex and the frequency and expression of sex vary tremendously. Partners who are sexually compatible may find the rest of their relationship unrewarding, but dissatisfaction with other aspects of the marriage is likely to be reflected in poor sexual relations. Marriages in which the woman refuses consummation usually continue; she may become sexually active after psychotherapy. Extramarital sex apparently is more stressful than is marital sex. The male cardiac patient, while indulging in extramarital sex, is more likely to have blood pressure disturbances and to die than during marital sex.

472. The answer is B (1, 3). *(American Psychiatric Association, ed 3. p 181.)* Although nosologic boundaries of schizophrenia remain unclear, several disorders that stand near that boundary have been separated in *DSM-III*. These include schizoaffective disorder, brief reactive psychosis, atypical psychosis, and schizophreniform disorder. These are separated from schizophrenia because they fail to fulfill the basic criteria set forth regarding symptom complex, duration, prognosis, and historical antecedents for schizophrenia as the authors of the manual conceive it. Hebephrenia and residual type remain with schizophrenia. The distinctions clearly are provisional and will be subject to further revisions. One advantage of the *DSM-III* classification and justification for it is that it will stimulate efforts to derive conclusive data to reaffirm or deny the relationship of these syndromes.

473-476. The answers are: 473-D, 474-B, 475-A, 476-E. *(American Psychiatric Association, ed 3. pp 305-330.)* The symptoms of personality disorders usually become apparent by adolescence and are prominent features of an affected individual's life-style, often to the extent of severely interfering with work or social relationships. Each type of personality disorder has a group of symptoms that must be present in order to confirm the diagnosis.

The paranoid personality is characterized by extreme, unrealistic distrust and suspiciousness; exaggerated social hypersensitivity; and cold, restricted, humorless affect.

The schizoid personality displays such symptoms as the absence of tender feelings and indifference to others' opinions or feelings; coldness and aloofness; few friendships; however, oddities of speech, thoughts, or actions are not present.

The schizotypal personality must include any four of the following traits: oddities of thought, speech, or behavior (but not as severe as in schizophrenia); magical thinking; ideas of reference; absence of friendships; illusions; social distance; suspiciousness; and social hypersensitivity.

The avoidant personality is overly sensitive to even minor hints of rejection, and avoids relationships even though desiring them. Inadequate self-esteem also is a feature of this personality disorder.

A large admixture of depression, anxiety, and dissatisfaction with life is present in all types of personality disorders. In spite of the prevalence of these disorders and the frequency with which they appear in the practice of psychiatry, correct diagnosis is often difficult. It is to be hoped that the new guidelines as set forth by *DSM-III* will aid in discriminating one entity from another.

477-481. The answers are: 477-D, 478-C, 479-A, 480-B, 481-E. *(Adams, ed 2. pp 687-688, 775, 786-789. Kolb, ed 9. pp 358-362, 850.)* A number of toxic agents create a clinical picture of progressive dementia or psychosis and have some particular skin manifestation that offers a clue to the diagnosis. These skin clues should be sought in every patient with psychosis or dementia of unknown origin.

Lead intoxication in adults causes a visible dark line along the gum margin, more prominent along sites of pyorrhea. This line is rarely seen in children with lead intoxication. In adults, the major source of lead is from inhalation, whereas in children oral ingestion is the more common cause.

A dark, greenish brown (Kayser-Fleischer) ring appears at the corneal limbus in patients with Wilson's hepatolenticular degeneration, a disorder of copper metabolism. The associated dementia, often accompanied by extrapyramidal signs, begins in children or young adults and follows a progressive course. It is a treatable form of dementia and therefore important to recognize in its early stages.

In mercury intoxication, the patient may show "pink disease" (acrodynia). The skin has a vivid pink or dusky red color with desquamation and atrophic changes and tenderness to touch. Other features include gingivitis, tremors, albuminuria, gait ataxia, dysarthria, and changes in mood and behavior.

In bromide intoxication, the patient characteristically shows an acneiform skin eruption and, infrequently, proliferative nodular lesions. The condition is seen less frequently now that bromide is no longer an ingredient of over-the-counter proprietary drugs. The mental obtundation associated with the disorder is accompanied by depression of the stretch reflexes. Hence, bromidism is involved in the differential diagnosis of syndromes like mercury and arsenic intoxication, which also cause dementia and reduced stretch reflexes.

Arsenic ingestion inhibits nail and hair growth. The nails show a transverse white (Mees) line that advances from the lunula distally as the nail grows. The distance that separates the line from the lunula serves as a rough guide to the time of arsenic exposure. Also formerly present in proprietary remedies, arsenic is now an ingredient of insecticides and rodenticides.

482-487. The answers are: 482-E, 483-C, 484-B, 485-A, 486-D, 487-C. *(Adams, ed 2. pp 121-126. Bondy, ed 7. pp 1659-1664. Kolb, ed 9. pp 339-340, 342-348.)* Several organic disorders may give rise to periodic symptoms that commonly manifest in late childhood or early adulthood without necessarily any evidence of neurologic dysfunction on physical examination. The definitive diagnosis depends mainly on laboratory tests, although the clinical features should suggest the diagnosis. Included in this group of disorders are pheochromocytoma, islet cell adenomas of the pancreas, carcinoid tumors, porphyria, and migraine.

Pheochromocytoma is a catecholamine-secreting tumor that occurs in the adrenal gland or along the aorta, affecting children and adults. It may cause sustained hypertension or paroxysmal attacks of hypertension with the affective components of anxiety that accompany catecholamine release. All patients with periodic symptoms should be suspected of a pheochromocytoma. The lesion occurs with some frequency in neurofibromatosis, one manifestation of which is multiple café au lait spots. Diagnostic tests include urinary screen for catecholamines, the phentolamine and histamine provocative tests, and abdominal CAT scan.

Islet cell adenomas (insulinomas) occur in children and adults. They may give rise to periods of hypoglycemia due to excess insulin secretion. Affected patients manifest a variety of changes in mental status, from anxiety to coma. The attacks characteristically appear between 9 PM and breakfast or after heavy exercise, which reduces the available blood sugar. The patient may show organic neurologic signs during these attacks, varying from blurred vision and diplopia to convulsions. Diagnostic tests include glucose tolerance; provocative tests with tolbutamide, L-leucine, or glucagon; direct measurement of plasma insulin levels;

abdominal CAT scan; and, in some cases, aortography. The chemical tests should be selected and performed by an internist or neurologist, with proper precautions to prevent serious hypoglycemia.

The classical features of migraine may be absent early in the disorder, when it first manifests in a child. The standard stereotyped sequence of aura, visual disturbances, unilateral pain, nausea and vomiting, and a need to retire to a dark and quiet room, may take some time to evolve into the classical pattern. The headache may be vaguely described at first, particularly by children, and lacks the unilateral, throbbing character associated with migraine. Until the more typical pattern emerges that points to the correct diagnosis, the clinician may struggle with a variety of other explanations for periodic changes in mood and behavior.

Porphyria may present in diametrically opposite ways. On the one hand, the patient may have a psychiatric syndrome, or, on the other, a neurologic presentation with seizures and a chronic or acute peripheral neuropathy that may resemble Guillain-Barré syndrome. Psychiatrically, these patients present with agitation, depression, or psychoses of various types. There are usually bouts of unexplained abdominal pain, occurring spontaneously or after ingestion of barbiturates, alcohol, or other drugs. Although dark urine is a classical feature of porphyria, the urine reaches maximum color only after standing. Thus, patients, unaccustomed to inspecting their urine, may fail to notice this important feature of the disease. The diagnosis rests on spectroscopic demonstration of uroporphyrin in the urine.

The carcinoid syndrome is of particular interest to psychiatrists for two reasons. First, the carcinoid tumors release a number of substances related to neurohumors, including serotonin, bradykinin, and histamine. The carcinoid syndrome consists of intermittent episodic skin flushing, diarrhea, abdominal pain, asthmatic attacks, and weight loss. The major symptoms are related to intermittent release of the neurohumoral substances. Patients with carcinoid syndrome, unlike those with pheochromocytoma, do not have hypertension.

Secondly, the carcinoid syndrome is of interest to psychiatrists because ethanol ingestion may trigger attacks. This fact, together with the cutaneous telangiectases resembling acne rosacea, flushed red skin, and enlarged liver, is suggestive of alcoholism with cirrhosis as the basic diagnosis. The diagnosis of carcinoid syndrome depends on demonstration of excessive 5-hydroxyindoleacetic acid in the urine.

488-491. The answers are: 488-E, 489-A, 490-C, 491-B. *(Alexander, Neurology 29:334, 1979. Kolb, ed 9. pp 486, 511-512.)* Both men and women may have delusions that some famous person is in love with them. These individuals may describe very intimate conversations with the person, although they have never met. The whole life of the delusional patient may revolve around gathering information about the person and talking and fantasizing about the relationship. This particular form of paranoia in women is known as De Clérambault's syndrome.

A man with the Don Juan type of promiscuity compulsively tries to seduce almost any woman he meets. He may talk to her in seductive and well-modulated tones, often dressing modishly or stylishly and exhibiting numerous narcissistic mannerisms. With his own wife, he tends to be cold, distant, and frequently impotent. The behavior may serve several ends, such as to constantly reaffirm the existence of his penis, to ward off castration anxiety, or to establish dominance over women. The danger and thrill of the illicit relationship, which he may carry out in his office or under conditions that could lead to exposure, seem a prerequisite for the potency that he is unable to demonstrate with his wife.

In Ganser's syndrome, the affected patient gives approximate answers to the interviewer's questions. The answer shows, however, that the patient has understood the question and its context. Thus, the patient may describe the time as "6 o'clock" on a watch that shows 5 o'clock, or say "nickel" when presented with a quarter. In reply to the examiner's question as to whether the patient has eyes, the patient may reply, "I have no eyes." His responses are almost a caricature of a layman's concept of psychotic behavior. The syndrome usually appears in persons (often prisoners) who seek mitigation for some criminal act. How much of the syndrome represents simulation and how much is hysterical remains in question.

A patient with the Capgras syndrome has the delusion that some familiar person has been replaced by an imposter, a double who almost exactly duplicates the original person. Classically, this syndrome was described as part of a paranoid psychosis of functional origin; however, its description in many patients with a variety of brain disorders suggests that it is associated with structural damage to the brain, particularly bifrontal lesions with more extensive involvement of the right hemisphere than left. The Capgras syndrome borders on the reduplicative paramnesias, whose victims feel that a famous person or place has been duplicated.

492-495. The answers are: 492-B, 493-A, 494-D, 495-E. *(Kaplan, ed 3. pp 1165-1172.)* In a clinical entity with the protean manifestations of schizophrenia, it is to be expected that students of the condition will have described numerous types. In the 1980 editions of the two chief compilations of mental diseases (*DSM-III* and *ICD-9*), only a few of the many types of schizophrenia are officially recognized. While, for the most part, terms in *DSM-III* and *ICD-9* overlap, there are some differences. Notably, simple subtypes are no longer subsumed under the generic term schizophrenia in *DSM-III*, but are called "schizoid personality disorders," while *ICD-9* maintains the term "simple" and its association with schizophrenia. The basic reason *DSM-III* fails to recognize the "simple" subtype is because of its paucity of delusions and hallucinations. However, according to Lehman, "simple schizophrenia" and schizoid personality disorders should not be subsumed in the same category because of their differences in either onset or outcome. "Simple schizophrenia" commences during or after puberty and deteriorates, whereas schizoid personality disorder starts in early childhood and does not deteriorate.

The terms "disorganized" and "hebephrenic" schizophrenia are considered syndromes in *DSM-III*, both referring to a regressive course of silly and aimless but active behavior, with onset in adolescence or early adulthood. Unorganized delusions and hallucinations and extreme thought disorders also are strongly characteristic. This condition and catatonic schizophrenia, marked by psychomotor disorders as well as schizophrenic thoughts, often are called "nuclear schizophrenia." There are two subtypes of catatonia—stuporous and excited.

Paranoid schizophrenia patients who develop their illness later than most other schizophrenic victims also have more inner resources, such as good intelligence and emotional reactivity. Although the usual paranoid patients retain the superficial social graces, they typically react to others with suspicion, hostility, emotional reserve, and jealousy. Characteristic paranoid delusions concern persecution and grandiosity. *ICD-9* gives the term "paraphrenia" as a synonym for paranoid schizophrenia, whereas *DSM-III* fails to mention the term.

Another important subtype is "undifferentiated schizophrenia," which *ICD-9* and *DSM-III* use in different ways: the former, for a bout of acute schizophrenia; the latter, for grossly disorganized patients or for those with mixed subtypes.

Other subtypes commonly seen in adult populations include schizoaffective (carries a strong affective component), latent (the stage before onset of the full syndrome), residual (the symptom picture after a bout of the full syndrome), and schizophreniform disorder with schizotypal symptoms lasting a week or less. This latter condition is probably not true schizophrenia and is called by such other terms as *bouffeé délirante*, brief reactive psychosis, or hysterical psychosis.

Biological Psychiatry

DIRECTIONS: Each question below contains five suggested answers. Choose the **one best** response to each question.

496. The lesion site most consistently associated with severe impairment of memory in man and higher primates is which of the following?

(A) Mammillary bodies
(B) Fornix
(C) Polar regions of the frontal lobes
(D) Ventromedial quadrant of the temporal lobe
(E) Polar regions of the occipital lobe

497. A depressed patient receiving a tricyclic antidepressant is experiencing less depression, but begins to complain of constipation and difficulty urinating. Abdominal examination fails to disclose any abnormalities. The best management of this patient would be to

(A) order a gastrointestinal series and kidney, ureter, and bladder workup
(B) order a mild laxative and add a cholinergic drug
(C) reduce the dose of the tricyclic drug
(D) switch to another form of antidepressant therapy
(E) intensify psychotherapy because of somatic delusions

498. The liberation of an inhibitory transmitter at a synapse will cause the resting potential across the postsynaptic membrane to

(A) be locked at baseline level
(B) become more negative (hyperpolarized)
(C) reverse polarity
(D) become unrecordable
(E) do none of the above

499. When depression improves during electroconvulsive therapy, the ion that has been shown to decrease in body fluids is

(A) magnesium
(B) chloride
(C) phosphate
(D) calcium
(E) sodium

500. An acute schizophrenic patient who receives haloperidol and benztropine for several weeks begins to show orofacial movements and twitching of the head, but the schizophrenic symptoms are improved. The best management of this patient would be to

(A) stop the haloperidol
(B) stop the benztropine
(C) add trihexyphenidyl
(D) add lithium
(E) administer L-dopa

501. A severely depressed patient is started on 100 mg of imipramine per day and increased to 250 mg per day. The medication is given for a total period of two weeks, but there is no improvement. The best management would be to

(A) continue the same dose for two more weeks
(B) increase the dose by 100 mg per day
(C) add lithium
(D) switch to phenothiazine
(E) order shock treatment

502. The incidence of drug-induced parkinsonism is known to be

(A) sharply increased in patients over 40 years of age
(B) increased in adolescent males
(C) limited to adults
(D) equal in both males and females
(E) strongly related to a family history of parkinsonism

503. A prominent example of a disease that is mainly perpetuated by new mutations but subsequently acts as an autosomal dominant is

(A) Huntington's chorea
(B) Werdnig-Hoffmann's disease
(C) Tay-Sachs disease
(D) tuberous sclerosis
(E) myotonic dystrophy

504. The best genetic conclusion from the pedigree shown below, in which the children indicated by solid black all died before five years of age with a retrogressive neurologic illness, is which of the following?

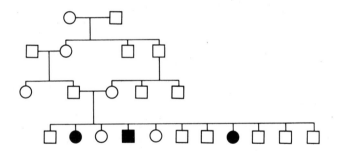

(A) Autosomal dominant disorder
(B) Sex-linked recessive disorder
(C) Autosomal recessive disorder
(D) Sex-linked dominant disorder
(E) Insufficient evidence to support a hereditary conclusion

505. Assuming that long-term lithium therapy is probably associated in some cases with renal damage, which of the following statements is true?

(A) Most patients should discontinue lithium after one year, because there is a clearly established correlation between duration of treatment and kidney dysfunction
(B) Because specific guidelines have been established for selecting patients and monitoring kidney function, it is possible to predict whom it is safe to treat and when to discontinue lithium for protection of the kidneys
(C) By increasing elimination of lithium through organs other than the kidneys, danger to the kidneys may be reduced
(D) The risk-benefit ratio should be determined for every patient being considered for lithium therapy and kidney function should be monitored periodically during treatment
(E) Lithium is so dangerous to the kidneys that all patients should discontinue the medication after two years, unless they are unresponsive to other forms of therapy

506. Aphasia implies a lesion in the left hemisphere in which of the following aphasic patients?

(A) Every patient, regardless of handedness
(B) Almost all right-handed but rarely left-handed patients
(C) Almost all right-handed and most left-handed patients
(D) Left-handed patients only
(E) Ambidextrous patients only

507. When prescribing lithium to a woman of child-bearing age, the physician should

(A) avoid any suggestion that lithium could affect a fetus
(B) advise that lithium might adversely affect a fetus
(C) forewarn the patient that lithium is strongly teratogenic
(D) restrict lithium only in the last trimester if the woman becomes pregnant
(E) advise breastfeeding if the woman has a baby

Questions 508-509

A disgruntled 62-year-old man who previously has seen many doctors complains of severe pain of several months duration in the neck, face, and shoulders. The pain is excruciating and migratory but may remain for days to weeks in one place, and is felt deep in the muscles. When present, it interferes with movement. The neurologic examination is normal. Joints are not red or swollen. During the examination, the patient complains of severe neck pain and will not permit movement in any direction. The strength, where it could be tested, was preserved.

508. The probable diagnosis in this patient is

(A) tabes dorsalis
(B) porphyria
(C) polymyalgia rheumatica
(D) polymyositis
(E) masked depression

509. In the patient presented above, the laboratory procedures most useful in providing a positive diagnosis are

(A) sedimentation rate and temporal artery biopsy
(B) CPK and muscle biopsy
(C) liver function tests and liver biopsy
(D) renal function tests and renal biopsy
(E) pulmonary function tests and lung biopsy

510. The most likely conclusion suggested by the following pedigree is that the disorder is

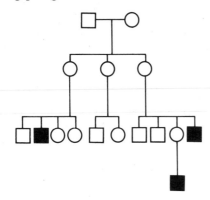

(A) nonhereditary
(B) autosomal dominant
(C) sex-linked recessive
(D) autosomal dominant with incomplete penetrance
(E) hereditary XXY karyotype

511. An acutely hallucinating young schizophrenic patient receives 200 mg of chlorpromazine for 4 days. The patient begins to pace around the ward and cannot sit still. Examination fails to reveal new findings except for the restlessness. The best conclusion is that

(A) the patient needs more chlorpromazine because the psychosis has failed to respond to the prescribed dose
(B) the restlessness suggests that chlorpromazine may be contributory and the dose should be reduced
(C) chlorpromazine characteristically produces agitation before sedation and the dose should be maintained
(D) the drug has unmasked an agitated depression
(E) the correct diagnosis should have been delirium tremens

512. A feeling of undue familiarity (*déjà vu*) in association with a hallucination of taste or smell suggests which of the following?

(A) An anterior temporal lobe lesion
(B) An olfactory bulb or tract lesion
(C) An insular cortex lesion
(D) Schizophrenia
(E) A feigned mental illness

513. The patient with gait apraxia generally has a lesion that involves the

(A) right parietal lobe only
(B) left parietal lobe only
(C) right frontal lobe only
(D) one hemisphere only
(E) cerebrum diffusely

514. The drug that consistently produces a paranoid psychosis that can be blocked by chlorpromazine is

(A) ethyl alcohol
(B) marihuana
(C) mescaline
(D) morphine
(E) amphetamine

Questions 515-516

A group of normal individuals and a group of patients each receives chlorpromazine. The results appear in the graph below.

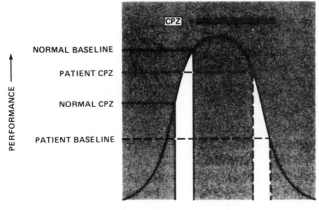

Used with permission of Oxford University Press, from *Psychopharmacology: From Theory to Practice* (p 73), by Barchas JD et al, © 1977.

515. The type of curve depicted above is called

(A) a bimodal distribution
(B) normal distribution
(C) a bar graph
(D) an inverted U-curve
(E) a cumulative frequency distribution

516. The figure appearing above indicates that the effect of chlorpromazine has been to

(A) improve the performance of both the patient and the normal subject
(B) decrease the performance of both the patient and the normal subject
(C) improve the performance of the patient but decrease the performance of the normal subject
(D) decrease the performance of the patient and improve the performance of the normal subject
(E) cause no difference in the performance of either the patient or normal subject

517. Which of the following statements best describes the behavioral depression that may occur after administration of reserpine?

(A) The depression lasts as long as the depletion of serotonin in the brain
(B) The depression is blocked by depleting the brain of serotonin by use of *p*-chlorophenylalanine before the reserpine is given
(C) The depression may be more closely related to depletion of catecholamines or to some other mechanism than serotonin depletion
(D) The depression is readily reversed by giving large amounts of tryptophan
(E) The depression is related to an increase in dopamine in the limbic cortex

518. In a patient suffering from an attack of severe mania, the preferred medication for initiating therapy would be

(A) a tricyclic
(B) a tetracyclic
(C) a benzodiazepine
(D) haloperidol
(E) lithium

DIRECTIONS: Each question below contains four suggested answers of which **one** or **more** is correct. Choose the answer

A	if	1, 2, and 3	are correct
B	if	1 and 3	are correct
C	if	2 and 4	are correct
D	if	4	is correct
E	if	1, 2, 3, and 4	are correct

519. The term apraxia may properly be used in describing a patient who meets which of the following preconditions?

(1) The patient's intellect must be relatively preserved
(2) The patient must have a relatively intact motor system
(3) The patient has an organic lesion as the basis for the deficit
(4) The patient has no delusions or hallucinations

520. In order to reduce the chance of assault by a violent patient on a psychiatric ward, a physician should

(1) force the patient to take an extra dose of medication
(2) assume control of the situation by threatening punishment for nonconformance
(3) insist on dealing with sensitive psychiatric material
(4) accede to as many of the patient's requests as are reasonable

521. The rationale for treating opioid addiction with methadone is that the drug produces

(1) cross-tolerance that blocks psychic effects of intravenous opioids
(2) opioid receptor blockade that prevents opioid action
(3) fewer withdrawal symptoms than opioids because of longer action
(4) distressing anxiety if opioids are used

522. The action of disulfiram in the treatment of alcoholism is correctly described by which of the following statements?

(1) It alters ethanol metabolism to produce acetaldehyde
(2) It causes hypotension and headache after alcohol ingestion
(3) It has little or no clinical effect unless alcohol is ingested
(4) It significantly increases phenytoin levels

523. Clinical disorders that typically appear during stage 4 sleep include which of the following?

(1) Somnambulism
(2) Sensation of paralysis
(3) Enuresis
(4) Restless legs syndrome

524. Sleep disorders that, in otherwise normal children, are quite common but that, in adults, frequently implicate a serious disorder include

(1) somnambulism
(2) enuresis
(3) night terrors
(4) fear of the dark

525. Common adverse effects of lithium therapy include which of the following?

(1) Polyuria-polydipsia
(2) Constipation
(3) Edema
(4) Pupillodilatation

526. Lithium has proved to be generally beneficial in the

(1) treatment of mania
(2) treatment of hypomania
(3) prophylaxis of depression
(4) treatment of depression

527. Tricyclic antidepressants produce relatively frequent side effects that include

(1)   cardiac arrhythmias
(2)   severe extrapyramidal movement disorders
(3)   anticholinergic action
(4)   agranulocytosis

528. Depressed patients who respond favorably to electroconvulsive therapy are likely to have which of the following symptoms?

(1)   Hysterical features
(2)   Severely depressed but labile mood
(3)   Overt psychologic precipitants of the depression
(4)   Paranoid delusions

529. Preparatory to treatment of a middle-aged patient with lithium, baseline studies should include

(1)   thyroid function tests
(2)   ECG
(3)   blood urea nitrogen determination
(4)   blood cell count

530. The choice of a major antipsychotic drug for treatment of a schizophrenic patient should be governed by which of the following principles?

(1)   A different drug should be used for each major target symptom
(2)   A previously used drug should be avoided even if it has been successful, because its reintroduction is likely to cause tardive dyskinesia
(3)   A major antipsychotic drug with a high loading dose should be given to produce an immediate reduction of the schizophrenic symptoms
(4)   Low potency, high sedative agents are preferable to low sedative agents in treating highly agitated patients

531. Marihuana effects that might especially impair automobile driving skills at night include which of the following?

(1)   Increased recovery time from glare
(2)   Impairment of performance on mental and motor tasks
(3)   A sensation of time distortion and drowsiness
(4)   Pupillodilatation

532. In patients with schizophrenia, a favorable response to electroconvulsive therapy is associated with which of the following features?

(1)   An illness of acute onset
(2)   Relatively good premorbid adjustment
(3)   A duration of illness of less than one year
(4)   A supportive social system

533. In prescribing methylphenidate for a hyperactive patient, a physician should observe which of the following guidelines?

(1)   Use the drug mainly for psychotic children less than six years of age
(2)   Monitor liver function with bimonthly bilirubin determinations
(3)   Discontinue anticonvulsant medication
(4)   Periodically check pulse and blood pressure

534. Marihuana, as compared to opioids, barbiturates, and alcohol, has which of the following characteristics?

(1)   It causes only minor physical dependence and withdrawal symptoms
(2)   It has no association with toxic psychosis
(3)   It displays a wide margin between psychoactive and lethal doses
(4)   It produces much greater development of tolerance

535. The pharmacologic effects of both amphetamines and cocaine may be characterized as

(1)   producing similar euphoric effects
(2)   acting as local anesthetics
(3)   tending to produce paranoid ideation
(4)   having a similar duration of action

536. Physiologic effects of nicotine include which of the following?

(1)   EEG alerting pattern with low-amplitude fast activity
(2)   Decrease in muscle tone and stretch reflexes
(3)   Peripheral vasoconstriction
(4)   Blockade of nausea and vomiting

537. Contraindications to the use of major antipsychotic drugs in the treatment of depression include their

(1) lack of beneficial effects
(2) tendency to cause tardive dyskinesia
(3) cholinergic action
(4) potential to worsen some endogenous depressions

538. The action of moderate amounts of ethyl alcohol includes which of the following?

(1) It increases the ability to perform fine motor tasks such as typing
(2) It acts as a convulsant as the blood alcohol level rises
(3) It conserves body heat during exposure to cold
(4) It raises the pain threshold

539. Compared with the general male population, tall, assaultive males in maximum security prisons or mental health facilities have a greater frequency of which of the following karyotypes?

(1) XO
(2) XYY
(3) Trisomy 13
(4) XXY

540. The standard karyotype is most likely to be abnormal when a mentally retarded patient presents with which of the following?

(1) Ambiguous genitalia
(2) An inborn error of metabolism
(3) Multiple extracephalic anomalies
(4) An autosomal dominant disorder

541. Studies attempting to relate specific effects to deprivation of sleep have produced which of the following conclusions?

(1) Objective tests show that distinct changes in mental function occur after loss of one-half of a single night's sleep
(2) Interruption of REM sleep produces a distinctive, recognizable clinical syndrome differing from interruption of deeper stages of sleep
(3) The effects of sleep deprivation are unrelated to the social, environmental, and emotional state of the individual
(4) Prolonged sleep deprivation may lead to a disorganized mental state with hallucinations and delusions

DIRECTIONS: The groups of questions below consist of lettered choices followed by several numbered items. For each numbered item select the **one** lettered choice with which it is **most** closely associated. Each lettered choice may be used once, more than once, or not at all.

Questions 542-545

For each end product that can be measured as an index of activity of the neurotransmitter pathway, choose the putative neurotransmitter with which it is most closely associated.

(A) Norepinephrine in the PNS
(B) Norepinephrine in the CNS
(C) Dopamine in the CNS
(D) Tryptamine in the CNS
(E) None of the above

542. Homovanillic acid (HVA) in the CSF

543. Dihydroxyphenylacetic acid (DOPAC) in the CSF

544. Vanillylmandelic acid (VMA) in the urine

545. Methoxyhydroxy phenylethyleneglycol (MHPG) in the CSF

Questions 546-550

For each psychotropic drug or drug group listed below, choose the pharmacologic mechanism by which it is thought to exert its psychotropic effect.

(A) Interferes with the uptake of catecholamines
(B) Stimulates dopamine receptors
(C) Blocks dopamine receptors
(D) Releases acetylcholine
(E) Inhibits synthesis of serotonin

546. Perphenazine and haloperidol

547. Reserpine and tetrabenazine

548. Apomorphine

549. Tricyclic antidepressants

550. Cocaine

Biological Psychiatry
Answers

496. The answer is D. *(Horell, Brain 101:434-436, 1978.)* The anatomic structures essential to memory have been the object of intensive investigation. While any disorder that diffusely affects the cerebrum can cause memory deficits, the minimum lesions that cause the maximum deficit of memory involve the ventromedial quadrant of the temporal lobe and its connections with nucleus medialis dorsalis of the thalamus via the inferior thalamic peduncle. Although completely critical evidence is still lacking, interruption of the fornix or its synaptic end station, the mammillary bodies, probably is not sufficient to cause gross memory deficits. The function of the hippocampus in relation to other structures of the ventromedial quadrant of the temporal lobe still requires elucidation. The temporal and occipital poles can be sacrificed without any clinically significant general impairment of memory functions.

497. The answer is B. *(Barchas, pp 196-197.)* Depressed patients on tricyclic antidepressant therapy may complain of constipation and dysuria. Assuming they are on a diet designed to minimize constipation, these patients should benefit from a mild laxative and a cholinergic medication such as bethanechol. Paralytic ileus and dysuria are common anticholinergic actions of the tricyclic drugs. In the absence of a history or physical findings of preexisting bowel or bladder disease, a full gastrointestinal and urologic workup is unnecessary. If the patient's depression is responding, the tricyclic drug should not be reduced or changed, unless the bowel and bladder problem becomes severe.

498. The answer is B. *(Cooper, ed 3. p 28.)* An inhibitory transmitter will hyperpolarize or increase the negativity of the resting potential across a cell membrane. Inhibitory transmitters appear to be able actively to increase the conductance of chloride. The chloride ion diffuses into the cell, increasing the negativity of the interior. The synaptic sites themselves are electrically inexcitable. The electrical equilibrium at synapses can be varied by applying current through intracellular electrodes and the effect of changes in ionic concentrations may then be determined. It is by this means that the relation of the mobile ionic species—such as chloride, sodium, and potassium—to membrane polarity can be studied.

499. The answer is D. *(Kaplan, p 114.)* Although the mechanism of action of electroconvulsive therapy (ECT) is still unknown, researchers have recently found some tantalizing clues. It has been shown that above-normal serum calcium levels can cause symptoms identical to those of depressive illness. Lowering calcium serum values to normal causes a lifting of depression. It has been found that when depression improves during a course of ECT therapy, serum and cerebrospinal fluid values of calcium also decrease. While calcium metabolism may not be primarily involved in the mechanism of action, these observations suggest an important role for calcium not only in the way ECT works but also in the pathogenesis of depression.

500. The answer is B. *(Barchas, pp 144-147.)* The clinical impression of the patient described in the question would be one of tardive dyskinesia. If a patient who receives a major psychotropic drug (haloperidol) in combination with an anticholinergic drug (benztropine) develops involuntary movements, the presumption is that a relative or actual cholinergic deficiency is present. For this reason, anticholinergics probably should not be given routinely with the major antipsychotic medications, although this issue remains controversial. Discontinuing the anticholinergic drug would help restore the dopamine-acetylcholine balance and might end the involuntary movements. In the patient described, the other alternatives listed in the question would be less desirable. Since the patient's psychosis was improving, it would probably be wise to continue the haloperidol. Adding trihexyphenidyl (Artane) would only worsen the patient's condition because, like benztropine (Cogentin), it is another anticholinergic drug. L-dopa most probably would worsen the movements. Presumably, haloperidol blocks the dopamine receptors and causes them to become hypersensitive to dopamine. Although lithium may improve the condition of some patients with tardive dyskinesias, adding a third medication in this case would only complicate the polypharmacy. The simplest management would be to discontinue the benztropine.

501. The answer is A. *(Barchas, p 193.)* The best management of a patient who fails to respond in two weeks to antidepressant medication is to continue the same medication for two more weeks. Even though pharmacologic actions of the drug can be demonstrated earlier, the depressed patient frequently fails to respond for 2-4 weeks, which is the trial period before changing therapy. The dose of 250 mg of imipramine is already high. Therefore, to increase the dose by 100 mg per day at the end of only two weeks would be unwarranted.

502. The answer is A. *(Benson, p 231.)* As generally reported in the literature, the incidence of drug-induced parkinsonism increases sharply in both men and women over 40 years of age. Females are reportedly affected twice as often as males, but dosages may differ as may the indications for the use of the drugs in the two sexes. Some evidence suggests that premenopausal women may be more susceptible than postmenopausal. Although the susceptibility to drug-induced parkinsonism generally increases with age, children and even neonates may occasionally be affected. Several other factors that might be suspected of influencing susceptibility to drug-induced parkinsonism (such as a family history of parkinsonism, the presence of subclinical parkinsonism, or preexisting brain damage) have not convincingly been shown to bear a relationship.

503. The answer is D. *(Swaiman, p 741.)* Tuberous sclerosis most often occurs as a new mutation. Affected individuals capable of reproducing transmit the disorder in an autosomal dominant pattern. It differs from autosomal dominant disorders like Huntington's chorea and myotonic dystrophy, in which most new cases are directly inherited from individuals affected by the disease, and from Werdnig-Hoffmann's disease and Tay-Sachs disease, which are autosomal recessives. Another autosomal dominant disorder maintained mainly by new mutations is achondroplastic dwarfism. If individuals with this disease reproduce, their children have a one-in-two chance of being afflicted. The body deformities produced by the condition do tend to lower the reproductive rate in achondroplastic dwarfs. Whether exposure to mutagenic chemicals or radiation may substantially increase the incidence of these disorders by increasing mutation is unknown.

504. The answer is C. *(Stanbury, ed 4. p 53.)*   The pedigree appearing in the question shows three of eleven children of a couple afflicted with a hereditary disorder. The pedigree would suggest a recessive disorder because all the affected children died in childhood, which is characteristic of recessive disorders, and there is no direct affected-to-affected transmission. Since males and females are both affected, the disorder is autosomal rather than sex linked. The presence of three affected individuals out of a total of 11 siblings is close enough to the expected ratio of one in four affected to support the conclusion of an autosomal recessive neurologic disorder. Most important of all, the children are the product of a consanguineous marriage, in this case between cousins. Most of the inborn errors of metabolism afflicting children, such as the aminoacidurias and lysosomal enzyme deficiencies, follow an autosomal recessive hereditary pattern.

505. The answer is D. *(Lippman, Psychiatr Ann 11:177-181, 1981.)*   While it is well established that lithium can cause damage to the kidneys, many aspects of the relationship between renal dysfunction and lithium therapy are unknown. The attitudes expressed in the literature concerning the relationship of lithium therapy and the risk of renal failure have undergone three major shifts. Until the mid-1970s, lithium therapy was generally thought to be safe if care was taken in selection of patients and monitoring kidney function. From 1977 to 1979, grave doubts were expressed about kidney safety. The most recent shift is toward more cautious monitoring of patients and, at the same time, adopting a more positive attitude toward lithium safety.

Nevertheless, several knotty problems face the practitioner in choosing patients and following kidney performance, mainly because of an absence of specific guidelines either for selecting patients or for monitoring kidneys. The physician must decide on a case-by-case basis whether lithium should be used and which monitoring procedure would be adequate. Since the kidneys are the only organs that eliminate lithium, obviously those patients with limited kidney function must receive the medication only if their psychiatric condition is unresponsive to any other form of treatment. It is possible to minimize lithium buildup by adequate sodium intake, but there is no way to divert its excretion to other organs.

All patients—regardless of their level of kidney function—must be advised of the risks, maintain good electrolyte balance through a balanced diet and adequate fluids, and avoid any reduction of sodium intake. Any factors that might change the amount of sodium available to the kidneys (e.g., thiazide diuretics, excessive perspiration, vomiting, diarrhea) must be discussed with patients under treatment, who in turn must communicate openly with the physician about all aspects of both lithium therapy and their general health.

506. The answer is C. *(DeMyer, ed 3. p 351.)*   Aphasia implies a lesion of the left hemisphere in almost all right-handed patients and in most left-handed patients. Thus, the left hemisphere is dominant for language and a lesion in that hemisphere will produce the language deficits recognized as aphasia. In some individuals, more frequently the left-handed than right-handed, the left hemisphere is dominant. Laterality of function in the brain is probably a biological property. The cerebrum has both anatomical and functional asymmetry. The left cerebral hemisphere is usually larger than the right and has a recognizably different pattern of vessels on angiography.

507. The answer is B. *(Barchas, pp 222-223.)*   A patient receiving lithium should probably be advised that lithium might adversely affect the fetus. Although its teratogenicity in humans has not been established, lithium is teratogenic in some animals and, in principle, any exposure of a pregnant woman to unusual chemicals is likely to have an adverse effect on the fetus. Teratogens are most damaging during the early stages of pregnancy, when histogenesis and organogenesis are in progress, and less damaging during the later stages when fetal growth is the main process. However, specific susceptibility to some teratogens does occur in the later stages of pregnancy. The milk produced by a mother taking lithium will contain about the same lithium concentration as her plasma. Therefore, breastfeeding is probably inadvisable as long as the medication is continued.

508. The answer is C. *(Adams, ed 2. pp 152, 583.)* Patients with polymyalgia rheumatica characteristically experience severe, incapacitating pain with few or no physical findings. They may become very disgruntled as they consult a series of doctors without having their malady diagnosed. The disorder characteristically affects middle-aged or older adults, who describe the pain as excruciating. Tabes dorsalis, while equally excruciating, is characteristically manifested in the lower extremities first, and the pain is lancinating rather than persistent. Polymyositis is not usually excruciatingly painful. Because patients with polymyalgia rheumatica have severe symptoms with few physical findings and almost always become depressed, they may be referred for psychiatric evaluation. The psychiatrist aware of this entity will not be misled by the depression into making a purely functional diagnosis.

509. The answer is A. *(Adams, ed 2. pp 130, 550.)* In the patient presented in the question, the limitation of movement and the migratory pains in the head, neck, and shoulders suggest a collagen-vascular disease—most probably polymyalgia rheumatica. Therefore, a determination of the erythrocyte sedimentation rate (ESR) and a temporal artery biopsy would provide the most relevant data. The ESR is elevated in polymyalgia rheumatica, and the syndrome is allied to temporal arteritis. Biopsy reveals a giant cell arteritis. The serum gamma globulin profile is frequently abnormal. Affected patients often exhibit mild leukocytosis and hypochromic anemia. The importance of establishing a correct diagnosis is that affected patients usually show a remarkable and gratifying response to steroid treatment. The pain subsides, systemic relief is provided, and blindness as a complication of the extension of the temporal arteritis to the ophthalmic artery is avoided.

510. The answer is C. *(Swaiman, p 271.)* The pedigree accompanying the question shows three males with a disease. Of the mothers of the affected males, two are sisters and the third is a daughter of one of them. The disorder would thus appear to be expressed in males and carried by females, the classical formula for a sex-linked recessive disease. Alternative genetic hypotheses cannot be excluded because of the small size of the pedigree, but the assumption of a sex-linked recessive is the most logical conclusion from the available information.

511. The answer is B. *(Barchas, p 142.)* In a psychotic patient who becomes restless and paces around, the possibility of a drug-induced akathisia should be considered. Increasing the dose of medication or even maintaining its levels may cause the involuntary movement disorder to worsen. In the patient described in the question, reducing the dose or perhaps adding an anticholinergic medication if the other symptoms are responding might be the best course of treatment. If the patient were affected with delirium tremens, the chlorpromazine should have improved the condition.

512. The answer is A. *(DeMyer, ed 3. p 269.)* A feeling of undue familiarity of something seen (*déjà vu*) or something thought (*déjà pensé*) in association with a hallucination of taste or smell may occur in patients with anterior temporal lobe lesions. When this combination of symptoms occurs as an aura of a seizure, it is called an **uncinate seizure**, referring to the uncus—the anteromedial aspect of the temporal lobe that is presumed to act as an integrating center for taste and smell. The combination of *déjà vu* or *déjà pensé* with the hallucination of taste or smell should prompt an investigation of the anterior temporal lobe for a structural lesion. An EEG, a CAT scan, radioisotope scan, or angiogram may be indicated in such patients. Careful visual field testing may disclose a homonymous contralateral superior quadrantic visual field defect due to involvement of Meyer's loop of the geniculocalcarine tract.

513. The answer is E. *(Adams, ed 2. p 85.)* The patient with gait apraxia has a lesion that affects the brain bilaterally or diffusely. Unlike some other apraxias that imply a relatively specific lesion site, gait apraxia does not result from lesions restricted to one locus in a hemisphere or even an entire hemisphere. Gait apraxia implies some degree of bilateral, diffuse involvement of the brain. Thus, gait apraxia may be seen in patients with such disorders as Alzheimer's disease and other cerebral degenerative diseases, general paresis, and senility. Affected patients show an inability to rise from a chair and initiate the sequence of leg movements that are required to walk, even though they are not paralyzed or completely demented.

514. The answer is E. *(Cooper, ed 3. p 178.)* Several drugs can produce psychosis, either during their active ingestion or after their withdrawal. These include mescaline, ethyl alcohol, marihuana, morphine, and amphetamines. Although each of these drugs may produce a psychosis of one type or another, amphetamine is the most likely to produce a paranoid state resembling paranoid schizophrenia. Although the paranoid state can be induced in adult human volunteers, where it can be reversed by chlorpromazine, the condition usually does not occur in children who receive amphetamines for treatment of hyperactivity.

515. The answer is D. *(Barchas, pp 66-75.)* In an inverted U-curve in pharmacology, a function that is measured (the dependent variable) improves or increases up to a peak with an increase in the experimental variable (the independent variable); then, after reaching the peak, the function decreases with an increase in the experimental variable. For example, a stimulant might increase endurance up to a certain point, but any further increase in the dose of the stimulant might then lead to a decrease in performance. When the measure of performance is plotted against the increasing dose of the stimulant, an inverted U-curve results.

516. The answer is C. *(Barchas, pp 72-75.)* The figure accompanying the question illustrates that chlorpromazine improved the performance of the patient but decreased the performance of the normal subject. The U-shaped curve offers an explanation for the seeming paradox that the drug improved the patient's performance and decreased the normal subject's performance. The performance measured depended on the degree of activation of the reticular activating system, which chlorpromazine decreases. In the normal subject, the decrease in the reticular activating system decreased the performance. In the patient, the reticular activating system was pathologically overactive, interfering with the performance measured. A decrease in the pathologically overactive reticular activating system thus improved the patient's performance.

517. The answer is C. *(Cooper, ed 3. pp 213-214.)* The behavioral depression that may occur after reserpine administration clears before the depleted levels of biogenic amines are restored. Reserpine sedation is more readily reversed by administration of dopa than of serotonin or its precursors. After administration of *p*-chlorophenylalanine, which depletes serotonin, reserpine will cause sedation—suggesting that the resultant fall in catecholamines is more closely allied to the reserpine effect than to the reduction in serotonin. Thus, reserpine sedation may be more closely related to catecholamine levels than to serotonin levels. On the other hand, the real mechanism may be neither the depletion of serotonin nor catecholamines, but something presently unrecognized.

518. The answer is D. *(Gordon, Psychiatr Ann 11:143-153, 1981. Reese, Psychiatr Ann 115:173-175, 1981.)* Although lithium is probably the most efficacious drug in maintenance and prophylaxis of all mania attacks, it has one drawback: its initial effect generally is delayed for 7-14 days. Thus, for severely disturbed manic patients whose symptoms may be life-threatening, medication with faster onset is preferable. Of those drugs listed in the question, haloperidol is the most effective in initiating therapy; other major tranquilizers, such as chlorpromazine, trifluoperazine, or thiothixene, also may be used. After manic symptoms are partially controlled, a switch can gradually be made to lithium. The tri- and tetracyclics are not commonly used to treat any kind of mania; in fact, they may stimulate mania if used to treat a patient with bipolar depression during an attack.

519. The answer is A (1, 2, 3). *(DeMyer, ed 3. pp 340-344.)* Patients with apraxia are unable to perform a voluntary act in spite of both comprehending the act — which requires a relatively preserved intellect — and having a motor system sufficiently intact to execute the act. The term apraxia is not meant to apply to the severely demented or retarded patient who cannot perform an act because of lack of comprehension. Neither does it apply to the patient whose paralyzed motor system prevents performance, nor to the hysterical, negativistic, or primarily mentally ill patient. Lack of an organic lesion excludes such individuals from the category of apraxia. However, the apraxic patient may have delusions or hallucinations in conjunction with the organic illness that causes the apraxia. Thus, although apraxic patients may not be entirely of sound mind, the intellect is sufficiently preserved that they can comprehend the act required.

520. The answer is D (4). *(Usdin, pp 445-446.)* In defusing a violent or homicidal patient, the physician should project an air of calm objectivity and avoid overreacting to the patient's agitated state. Medication should be presented as a helpful measure rather than a punitive one, because the threat of punishment usually is counterproductive. The psychiatrist should avoid dealing with sensitive psychiatric material. Approach to such patients should involve a team of individuals of both sexes. The presence of a female can reduce the aggressiveness of a male patient, and a team that is well staffed offers security to all. The team should set reasonable limits for the patient to follow and accede to as many of the patient's valid requests as is possible.

521. The answer is B (1, 3). *(Gilman, ed 6. pp 574-575.)* The rationale for methadone treatment of opioid addiction includes the production of cross-tolerance to intravenous opioids. Therefore, the injection of opioids fails to produce euphoric effects. This condition represents a state of blockade against the psychic effects of opioids, but is not an actual receptor blockade. Treatment with opioid antagonists like cyclazocine and naltrexone produces an opioid receptor blockade that prevents the euphoric effects of intravenous opioids. The opioid receptor blockers prevent physical dependence on opioids. The longer action of methadone is associated with fewer side effects than the opioids, theoretically allowing an easier withdrawal from all medication after the addict has been maintained on methadone for a period of time. Methadone does not cause any distressing symptoms such as nausea in a patient who combines its use with opioids. In this regard, methadone differs from disulfiram.

522. The answer is E (all). *(Gilman, ed 6. pp 387-388.)* Disulfiram increases the amount of acetaldehyde in the blood if the patient ingests alcohol, but otherwise has little pharmacologic action. Normally, the alcohol dehydrogenase in the liver oxidizes the ingested alcohol to acetaldehyde, which then passes through the citric acid cycle. Thus, acetaldehyde does not normally accumulate. Disulfiram is thought to compete for sites on the acetaldehyde metabolizing enzyme, acetaldehyde dehydrogenase, blocking its action. The resulting accumulation of acetaldehyde is thought to produce the distressing clinical effects that punish alcoholic individuals for violating their abstinence. Disulfiram, after itself undergoing metabolic conversion to diethyldithiocarbamate, inhibits dopamine β-hydroxylase, reducing the amount of norepinephrine at the sympathetic nerve terminals — which may explain the resulting vasodilatation with headache and hypotension. In a patient taking phenytoin, disulfiram may increase the phenytoin to toxic levels.

523. The answer is B (1, 3). *(Adams, ed 2. pp 264, 266-267, 271-272.)* Several clinical disorders of sleep typically occur during the deepest stage of sleep, stage 4. These include somnambulism, enuresis, and sleep terrors. The sensation of paralysis often occurs in association with a dream and appears during the REM stage of sleep. The restless legs syndrome consists of an uncontrollable urge to move the legs, which wander around incessantly while the patient attempts to fall asleep. Another disorder affecting the legs is nocturnal myoclonus, which occurs during the deeper stages of sleep. The violent leg movements may awaken these patients, who are unable to recall the leg movements and fail to understand the cause for the interruption of sleep. Usually, however, the patient's bedmate (if such there be) can give a complete history that establishes the diagnosis.

524. The answer is E (all). *(Adams, ed 2. pp 266-267.)* Many sleep disorders of children occur in the absence of serious psychiatric or neurologic disease. These include somnambulism, enuresis, nightmares, and fear of the dark. Children do tend to outgrow these disorders, but if these same disorders begin or persist prominently in adulthood, they generally implicate a significant underlying neurologic or psychiatric illness. In adults, frequent nightmares should arouse the suspicion of chronic alcohol abuse or barbiturate addiction and withdrawal. Some studies have shown that as many as 35 percent of young adult somnambulists are overtly schizophrenic, schizoid, or severely neurotic. Somnambulism, particularly in children, may occur with night terrors and enuresis. Persistence into adulthood of fear of the dark, a stage that most children pass through, indicates psychopathology generally based on the failure of resolution of some childhood problem. The persistence into adulthood of occasional frightening dreams (nightmares) is too common to be considered abnormal, but night terrors usually are limited to children.

525. The answer is B (1, 3). *(Barchas, pp 220-222.)* Common adverse effects of lithium therapy include polyuria-polydipsia, nausea, vomiting and diarrhea, tremor, muscular weakness, and edema. Constipation and pupillodilatation are seen with other psychotropic medications like the phenothiazines and the tricyclic antidepressants. Mild polyuria characteristically accompanies lithium treatment. If an affected patient has normal kidneys and a normal endocrine system, the polyuria, while annoying to the patient, will neither result in significant electrolyte disturbance, nor require a reduction in dosage. On the other hand, elderly individuals or patients who fail to maintain a normal diet or who have preexisting cardiac, renal, or endocrine disease, require careful monitoring of fluid and electrolyte balance during lithium therapy. Either fluid imbalance or lithium toxicity in the elderly patient may cause mental confusion, which must be differentiated from the underlying psychiatric disorder and be properly managed.

526. The answer is A (1, 2, 3). *(Reese, Psychiatr Ann 115:173-175, 1981.)* One of the primary uses of lithium is in the treatment and prophylaxis of mania and hypomania, as demonstrated by several well-controlled studies. While lithium is prophylactic for both bipolar depression and repeated bouts of unipolar depression, it is infrequently therapeutic for acute attacks of depression. Researchers continue to attempt to identify the clinical or biochemical features that might distinguish those few depressed subjects who could respond to lithium during a bout of depression.

527. The answer is B (1, 3). *(Barchas, pp 195-196.)* Relatively frequent side effects of tricyclic antidepressants include cardiac arrhythmias and symptoms of anticholinergic action, like a dry mouth and blurred vision. These drugs do not produce extrapyramidal involuntary movement disorders, such as result from the phenothiazines, although some tremor may occur. Agranulocytosis can occur but is a rare complication. Whether routine blood cell counts help in preventing serious hematologic complications remains doubtful, but they probably are indicated.

528. The answer is C (2, 4). *(Kolb, ed 9. p 859.)* Depressed patients who respond favorably to ECT, as contrasted to those who do not, exhibit a high incidence of somatic pain and physical illness. They often experience a sudden-onset depression but a labile mood, and nihilistic, somatic, and paranoid delusions. They tend to exhibit weight loss, a pyknic body build, and early morning awakening. The nonresponders to ECT tend to show evidence of anxiety, an accusatory nature, and hysterical features. While these distinctions are not absolute, they are helpful in selecting patients who are most likely to benefit from ECT therapy.

529. The answer is E (all). *(Barchas, pp 213-214.)* Baseline studies that should be executed before starting lithium treatment should include thyroid function tests, because lithium may cause goiter and hypothyroidism; ECG, because of the danger of cardiac toxicity; blood urea nitrogen determination, because the urine is the main route of excretion; and a blood cell count, because lithium may cause leukocytosis, which may be confused with an infection. An adequate series of normal baseline studies reduces the likelihood that lithium will produce serious or unanticipated adverse effects.

530. The answer is D (4). *(Barchas, pp 134-136.)* In selecting a major antipsychotic drug, the physician should choose a single medication rather than several drugs, each of which is reputed to be more effective in treating specific target symptoms. A previously used drug should be administered if it has been successful in a particular patient; it is probably no more likely to produce tardive dyskinesia than a new drug. Little evidence exists to support the "loading dose" concept in starting a major antipsychotic drug, but, in terms of avoiding adverse reactions, there are good reasons to start with a smaller dose. Generally, it is considered preferable to treat the highly agitated patient with an agent of lower potency but greater sedative action like thioridazine, than with a less sedative one, like fluphenazine.

531. The answer is A (1, 2, 3). *(Gilman, ed 6. pp 561-562.)* Marihuana produces many effects that may impair automobile driving skills, particularly at night. It may increase the time required for recovery from glare, cause drowsiness, and distort time sense. In general, it seems to impair performance on tests of vigilance, attention, and short-term memory. Marihuana lacks a clinically significant effect on pupillary size, although refined tests show a tendency to pupilloconstriction. Marihuana has an additive effect with alcohol and other depressants, as well as with medically prescribed psychoactive drugs, which may render the subject unfit to drive.

532. The answer is B (1, 3). *(Kaplan, ed 3. p 2340.)* According to Kalinowsky, the feature most often associated with a good response to electroconvulsive therapy (ECT) in schizophrenic patients is an illness of acute onset. Another favorable factor is an illness of less than one years duration, a consideration that underscores the importance of giving ECT as early as possible in the course of the illness. Still other clinical factors thought to portend a favorable response include catatonic excitement, acute paranoia, and the presence of affective features.

533. The answer is D (4). *(Gilman, ed 6. pp 589-590.)* In prescribing methylphenidate for hyperactivity, a physician should follow several rules. The medication appears to work best in nonpsychotic, hyperactive children. Its safety and efficacy for children under six years of age have not been established. Affected patients should have the pulse rate and blood pressure checked at intervals; methylphenidate tends to increase both. Methylphenidate does not produce significant clinical hepatotoxicity. Thus, regular monitoring of liver function is not required. Enzyme determinations such as SGOT, SGPT, and LDH are more sensitive than tests of bilirubin levels and would be indicated if pemoline were used for treatment of the hyperactivity instead of methylphenidate. When any of the stimulant drugs are given, the patient should continue on anticonvulsant medication because of the tendency of the stimulants to produce seizures.

534. The answer is B (1, 3). *(Gilman, ed 6. pp 561-563.)* Marihuana produces relatively little physical dependence and tolerance compared to opiates, barbiturates, and alcohol. The tolerance to marihuana is difficult to quantify, but it appears to be less than for the other drugs, although in certain cultures, chronic users consume high amounts. A wide margin exists between lethal and psychoactive doses of marihuana. Deaths attributable to marihuana, in comparison to the other drugs mentioned, are very rare. One danger of marihuana, toxic psychosis, may lead to bizarre behavior that can result in death or injury. Toxic psychosis can occur in chronic users as well as in naive individuals initially using marihuana.

535. The answer is B (1, 3). *(Gilman, ed 6. pp 553-556.)* Amphetamines and cocaine have similar central effects, producing anorexia and feelings of euphoria and energy. They both tend to produce toxic psychosis with paranoid ideation. The amphetamines act for considerably longer periods of time than does cocaine. The amphetamine-addicted person trying to produce a continuous state of euphoria injects the amphetamine every few hours, but a cocaine user trying to sustain such a state will have to take the drug every 30 to 40 minutes. Other pharmacological similarities of cocaine and amphetamines include potentiation of dopamine and partial blockade of their actions by dopaminergic blockers. Cocaine differs from amphetamines in its ability to act as a local anesthetic.

536. The answer is A (1, 2, 3). *(Gilman, ed 6. p 558.)* Nicotine causes an EEG pattern of low-amplitude fast activity. The stimulant effect of nicotine may be mediated through nicotinic and dopaminergic receptors. Nicotine reduces muscle tone and the muscle stretch reflexes, perhaps by stimulating the Renshaw cells, which inhibit the ventral motor neurons. It also produces peripheral vasoconstriction. Nicotine induces nausea and vomiting, perhaps by stimulating the chemoreceptor trigger zone in the medulla oblongata.

537. The answer is C (2, 4). *(Barchas, p 133.)* The major antipsychotic drugs apparently perform about as well as the tricyclic antidepressants in heterogenous groups of depressed patients. Despite their efficacy, however, major antipsychotic agents are not recommended for use in depressed persons because of their adverse effects; they produce tardive dyskinesias and may worsen some endogenous depressions. Like the tricyclics, they have an anticholinergic action rather than a cholinergic effect.

538. The answer is D (4). *(Gilman, ed 6. pp 376-378,553.)* Ethyl alcohol in general decreases the ability to perform fine motor tasks requiring attention and thought. Its consumption results in loss of body heat by causing vasodilation. Far from fortifying the drinker against the cold, alcohol promotes a feeling of warmth in the skin that may contribute to a false sense of security. Alcohol acts as an anticonvulsant as its blood level rises. Convulsions related to alcohol ingestion characteristically occur as the blood alcohol level is **dropping**, and in fact usually occur some time after a person has stopped drinking. Alcohol, which raises the pain threshold, is the oldest and best-known anodyne and euphoric.

539. The answer is C (2, 4). *(Kolb, ed 9. p 757.)* When all tall males incarcerated in maximum security prisons or mental health units are surveyed, the number with the XXY or XYY karyotype will greatly exceed that in the general population. This finding suggests that individuals with those karyotypes are more likely to commit serious criminal offenses **and** be apprehended than individuals without those karyotypes. One common denominator of patients with the two karyotypes, besides the characteristic physical stature, is a tendency to score low on IQ tests. Prison populations in general score lower on IQ tests than do citizens at large. The XXY individuals differ from the XYY in having gynecomastia and small, undeveloped testicles and to them is applied the eponym Klinefelter's syndrome. The XYY karyotype was once hailed in the press as the "criminal" chromosome, but individuals with this karyotype do not necessarily become antisocial. Patients with the XO karyotype, or Turner's syndrome, are phenotypically females and small in stature. Individuals with trisomy 13 frequently die in infancy, or if they survive are often small in stature and too retarded to bear responsibility for criminal behavior.

540. The answer is B (1, 3). *(Swaiman, pp 281-282.)* As a rule, the standard karyotype exhibits no abnormalities in the mendelian disorders like inborn errors of metabolism, which are recessives, or in the autosomal dominant disorders. The karyotype is most likely to be abnormal, and therefore clinically significant, when it is associated with ambiguous genitalia or multiple somatic anomalies along with mental retardation. Such persons show a high incidence of abnormal karyotypes. Thus, it is a general rule that mentally retarded persons with an abnormal somatotype are the most likely to have an abnormal karyotype, of which Down's syndrome is the best-known example.

541. The answer is D (4). *(Kaplan, ed 3. p 171.)* All studies of sleep deprivation show a striking difference in the subjective and objective effects. After even short deprivation of one-half of a single night's sleep, subjects report feeling tired, irritable, and out of sorts. On the other hand, measures of psychologic functions fail to show a corresponding decrement in mental abilities. Neither has it been possible by clinical or objective psychological measures to make any sharp distinctions between interruption of sleep in the REM and non-REM stages. The subjective effects of sleep loss are heavily dependent on the subjects' emotional states—whether normal or depressed—and on their motivation to perform tasks the next day. On the other hand, prolonged sleep deprivation does lead to some ego and personality disintegration in all subjects willing to submit to it.

542-545. The answers are: 542-C, 543-C, 544-A, 545-B. *(Cooper, ed 3. pp 170-173.)* Quantitatively, vanillylmandelic acid (VMA) is the major norepinephrine metabolite found in the urine as a product of activity of the sympathetic nervous system peripherally. The brain contains very little VMA. The norepinephrine in the brain is thought to produce mainly methoxyhydroxy phenylethyleneglycol (MHPG). Once formed, it enters the CSF, blood, and urine. The level of MHPG in CSF or urine thus is taken as a measure of the activity of the norepinephrinergic pathways of the brain. Even though MHPG is proportionately a small end product of peripheral norepinephrine metabolism, it still constitutes a considerable portion of the MHPG in the urine. This is one reason that it is difficult to use MHPG urinary assay as a measure of central catecholaminergic activity.

Important metabolites of dopamine are homovanillic acid (HVA) and dihydroxyphenylacetic acid (DOPAC). These substances accumulate in the brain and CSF, where they may be taken as evidence of activity in the dopaminergic pathways. Although such chemical measurement of metabolic end products in body fluids is still a crude measure of neurotransmitter function, these efforts represent the "state of the art" at the present time. It is difficult at present to see how a more intimate measure of neurotransmitter activity would be possible, particularly in the human brain.

546-550. The answers are: 546-C, 547-A, 548-B, 549-A, 550-A. *(Cooper, ed 3. pp 180-183.)* Although all the pharmacologic agents listed in the question have multiple effects, some effects are presently thought to be especially significant in explaining the psychotropic actions of the drugs. The phenothiazines and haloperidol, a butyrophenone, are thought to act by blocking dopamine receptors. Reserpine and tetrabenazine block the reuptake and storage mechanisms for catecholamines and serotonin. The effect of tetrabenazine on the storage granules is more readily reversible than that of reserpine. Apomorphine stimulates dopamine receptors.

The tricyclic antidepressants and cocaine block reuptake of the biogenic amines. One stumbling block in neuropharmacologic research has been the lack of a drug that selectively blocks the reuptake of the choline derived from acetylcholine hydrolysis. The reuptake of the biogenic amines, however, is blocked by many drugs and thus seems to be a mechanism that is much more sensitive or vulnerable to drug effects.

In spite of the common effect of blocking biogenic amine uptake shared by many drugs, their pharmacologic properties do not always correlate with this action. Thus cocaine, while blocking the uptake of biogenic amines, is less effective as an antidepressant than are the tricyclic antidepressants. The tricyclics, in contrast to cocaine, are potent anticholinergics. One tricyclic drug, iprindole, is an effective antidepressant but fails to block the uptake of biogenic amines. Thus, although one can demonstrate certain pharmacologic effects of the psychotropic drugs, the correlation between such effects and the mental changes that result remains speculative.

Psychosocial Psychiatry

DIRECTIONS: Each question below contains five suggested answers. Choose the **one best** response to each question.

551. The term "prestige suggestion" may be defined as

(A) a statement by a third party implanting the idea in a patient's mind that the patient's psychiatrist is highly regarded by other psychiatrists
(B) a therapist's suggestion to a patient that the therapist is highly trained and competent
(C) a suggestion by a treating psychiatrist that results in a restructuring of some aspect of a patient's personality
(D) a psychiatrist's suggestion, direct or indirect, that results in removal of a symptom
(E) none of the above

552. Flooding, graded exposure, and participant modeling all are involved in

(A) interpreting a patient's psychodynamics
(B) confronting a patient with the actual or imagined anxiety-producing event
(C) ascertaining the degree of psychopathology in the family
(D) employing tangible reward reinforcement in the form of a desired object
(E) eschewing the exercise of interpersonal influence on the part of the therapist

553. Hypnosis is least likely to succeed in which one of the following instances?

(A) Dental anesthesia
(B) Removal of conversion syndrome
(C) Recovery of functional amnestic deficits for recent events
(D) Age regression for recovery of childhood memories
(E) Enhancement of learning in mentally deficient subjects

554. Current opinion about the relationship of psychological factors to bronchial asthma is best described in which of the following statements?

(A) Asthmatic children have a recognizable personality profile that precedes and predicts the asthma
(B) Asthmatic persons have a childhood history of maternal neglect
(C) Emotional factors are unrelated to asthmatic attacks
(D) The significance of emotional factors in the etiology of asthma is poorly understood
(E) Bronchial asthma is solely an allergy-related disease

555. The type of patient most likely to have an adverse psychological reaction to surgery is a patient who

(A) is a young adult undergoing elective cosmetic surgery
(B) is depressed
(C) has a schizophrenic illness in remission
(D) has low preoperative anxiety
(E) has strong ties to the family

556. The role of biofeedback in current psychiatric practice is best summarized by which of the following statements?

(A) Biofeedback has yet to be established as the treatment of choice for any disorder
(B) The efficacy of biofeedback over placebo is established only for migraine headache
(C) Biofeedback is the treatment of choice for muscle tension headaches
(D) Biofeedback is established as having an adverse effect on cardiac dysrhythmias
(E) Biofeedback is established as the best method for producing relaxation

557. In using hypnosis to treat a patient who wishes to give up smoking, a therapist attempts to

(A) induce the patient to accept the therapist's authoritarian attitudes against smoking
(B) suggest to the patient that continuation of smoking will cause premature death
(C) give the posthypnotic suggestion that cigarettes will taste bad
(D) teach the patient to use self-hypnosis to reinforce an attitude of respect for the body
(E) reiterate the symptoms produced by smoking such as bad breath, cough, and shortness of breath

558. The use of dreams in psychoanalysis is best described by which of the following statements?

(A) The analyst should try to fit each dream into a known category that provides an automatic interpretation
(B) The dream represents the id undisguised by mental mechanisms such as symbolization and condensation
(C) The "dream work" refers to the somatic manifestations of the dream as shown in body movements and autonomic changes
(D) The manifest content of the dream is translated into the latent content by free association
(E) Dreams represent ancient memories and lack any trigger or component related to current events

559. The term "double-blind" as applied to the clinical study of drugs is best expressed by which of the following statements?

(A) The evaluator does not know whether the patient has received placebo or medication, but the patient knows
(B) The evaluator knows whether the patient is receiving medication or placebo but the patient does not know
(C) The family knows whether the patient has received medication or placebo, but the patient alone does not know
(D) Neither the patient nor the family knows whether the patient has received placebo or medication
(E) Neither the evaluator nor the patient knows whether the patient has received placebo or medication

560. The most common location for electrode placement to retrain for muscle tension in biofeedback is which of the following muscles or muscle groups?

(A) Gastrocnemius
(B) Vastus lateralis and medius
(C) Biceps
(D) Trapezius
(E) Frontalis

561. The chief function of the various mental defense mechanisms is to

(A) ward off fear
(B) ward off anxiety
(C) protect against neurosis
(D) protect against psychosis
(E) facilitate better social skills

562. The therapeutic technique of free association involves the use of all the following procedures EXCEPT

(A) frequently asking direct questions to expose distressing material
(B) encouraging the patient to verbalize every thought that occurs
(C) permitting the patient to discover the meaning of the material produced
(D) instructing the patient to describe the thoughts in the exact order in which they occur
(E) offering few direct interpretations

563. How many hours a week can a remitted schizophrenic patient generally be exposed to negative critical emotions without suffering a relapse?

(A) 5
(B) 20
(C) 35
(D) 50
(E) 65

DIRECTIONS: Each question below contains four suggested answers of which **one** or **more** is correct. Choose the answer

A	if	1, 2, and 3	are correct
B	if	1 and 3	are correct
C	if	2 and 4	are correct
D	if	4	is correct
E	if	1, 2, 3, and 4	are correct

564. In selecting individuals to participate in group psychotherapy, which of the following rules should generally be observed?

(1) Avoid group therapy with children
(2) Avoid acutely psychotic, severely paranoid, and manic patients
(3) Select patients who have a variety of problems such as alcoholism, criminal tendencies, and conversion hysteria
(4) Select patients of the same sex and roughly the same age and scholastic background

565. Statements that correctly apply to the doctrine of privileged information include which of the following?

(1) Psychiatrists under a subpoena may be held in contempt of court for failure to divulge information they consider privileged
(2) Patients may waive the privilege of confidentiality
(3) In general, courts respect the confidentiality of the patient-psychiatrist relationship even more than that of other physician-patient relationships
(4) The doctrine of confidentiality fails to apply to patients in a state hospital

566. Statements that currently reflect the best available opinions regarding the vitamin therapy of mental illness include which of the following?

(1) Vitamin B_{12} deficiency is definitely linked to a neuropsychiatric illness
(2) Advocates of megavitamin therapy have yet to demonstrate its efficacy by standard scientific methods of evaluation
(3) Gross deficiency of vitamins of the B group may cause psychosis
(4) There is no evidence that megadoses of any vitamin are harmful

567. Current problems of the community mental health movement include which of the following?

(1) Chronically mentally ill patients are neglected
(2) Traditionally underserved populations continue to be underserved
(3) Staff dissatisfaction, particularly among psychiatrists, is common
(4) Too few people in the catchment area are sufficiently well informed about available services

568. Correct statements about hypnosis include which of the following?

(1) Removal of a symptom by hypnosis is dangerous because of the possibility of substitution of another symptom
(2) Weak, passive individuals are easier to hypnotize than normal subjects
(3) Hypnosis is a form of sleep
(4) Normal subjects are easier to hypnotize than mentally ill individuals

569. Spontaneous cures of psychiatric illness may be explained by which of the following?

(1) Defenses that have become inadequate may be restored by reactivation of repressions
(2) A new philosophy of living may allow a reduction of mental turmoil
(3) Precipitating stresses in the environment may change due to fortuitous circumstances and facilitate regrouping of defenses
(4) Patients may experience reconditioning by a new environment that avoids the destructive aspects of the past

570. Established adverse medical effects of caffeine include which of the following?

(1) Insomnia
(2) Palpitation and tachycardia
(3) Restlessness and anxiety
(4) Withdrawal headaches

SUMMARY OF DIRECTIONS				
A	B	C	D	E
1, 2, 3 only	1, 3 only	2, 4 only	4 only	All are correct

571. True statements concerning anaclitic therapy include which of the following?

(1) The therapist assumes the role of caretaker
(2) The patient is encouraged to regress
(3) Mother-substitutes may be used to perform therapy
(4) It is appropriate only in patients who have undergone psychotherapy

572. Correct statements concerning the treatment of a rape victim in the emergency room include which of the following?

(1) The psychiatrist should make a judgement whether or not a rape has actually occurred
(2) If the patient was not using contraceptives, another method of pregnancy prevention should immediately be offered
(3) Before trying to deal with the woman's feelings about the rape, the psychiatrist should determine whether she has an underlying psychiatric problem
(4) Treatment for incubating syphilis and gonorrhea should be started after the patient has signed a written consent

573. True statements concerning the Masters and Johnson technique for sexual therapy include which of the following?

(1) It more closely resembles behavioral modification than traditional psychoanalytical techniques
(2) It advocates involving both partners in therapy
(3) It prohibits attempts at sexual intercourse during the early phase of therapy
(4) It encourages the partners to judge their sexual performance as it evolves

574. In research on the results of psychotherapy, errors that are commonly made in statistical analysis of the data include

(1) failure to determine the difference between statistical significance and magnitude of association
(2) inappropriate measurement of reliability
(3) failue to use statistical power analysis
(4) failure to consult a qualified statistician in devising the project

575. Psychoanalytic therapy, in contrast to intensive and exploratory psychotherapy, would probably include which of the following techniques?

(1) Establishing patient insight for identification of internalized conflicts
(2) Encouraging the development and resolution of a transference neurosis
(3) Assuming an active decision-making role (e.g., divorce, job change) on behalf of the patient
(4) Assuming a seated position behind the couch on which the patient reclines during the therapy session

576. Statements that reflect current opinions about homosexuality include which of the following?

(1) Homosexual males are consistently found to have lower testosterone levels than heterosexual males
(2) Female homosexuality is more prevalent than male homosexuality
(3) Homosexuals have a considerably higher incidence of mental illness than heterosexuals
(4) Rorschach test results fail to distinguish between homosexuals and heterosexuals

577. Marital therapy is indicated in situations in which

(1) other forms of therapy have failed to help an emotionally disturbed marital partner
(2) one marital partner has a narcissistic or paranoid personality
(3) the onset of symptoms in either marital partner is related to events within the marriage
(4) one marital partner has secrets that he or she is fearful of revealing

578. Patients generally consider Dr. X to be warm, perhaps even tender, whereas most patients describe Dr. Y as cool and detached. Assuming that the two physicians are about equal in medical competence, statements likely to be true concerning a diagnostic interview include which of the following?

(1) Most patients are likely to be reassured by Dr. X's warmth and be willing to give the specific information needed to make an accurate diagnosis

(2) Many patients interpret Dr. Y's distance as a lack of interest and will give the physician a less complete picture of their symptoms and life circumstances than they might give to Dr. X

(3) Some patients are made acutely uncomfortable by Dr. X's emotional warmth, which may cause the patient to feel too anxious to give a complete and accurate history

(4) If Dr. X is a man, patients are likely to see him as effeminate. If Dr. Y is a woman, patients may see her as too masculine. These perceived role reversals may cause patients to be anxious and to withhold vital information

579. The psychiatrist, in consultation with nonpsychiatric physicians, may recommend specific methods of handling "difficult" patients. In which of the following situations is the recommendation appropriate?

(1) Hostile or uncooperative patients—A physician makes a clear and definite request for cessation of any childlike behaviors, which dissipate most readily when the physician assumes a "parent" role

(2) Sexually seductive patients—If a mild flirtation is a patient's usual approach to other individuals, a doctor can limit this approach by failing to respond. Aggresssive seduction, however, may require an open and direct response

(3) Generally difficult patients—A physician who responds to difficult patients with undue anxiety should conceal such feelings and concentrate upon positive management

(4) The "crock"—The multiple and changing physical complaints presented by these individuals should be considered a sign of underlying anxiety or even psychiatric disorder, and treated as such

580. Hypersexuality frequently is a manifestation of

(1) Huntington's chorea
(2) hypomanic phase of manic-depressive illness
(3) Kleine-Levin syndrome
(4) prefrontal lobotomy

581. In a physically ill person, reactions that are considered to be normal responses include

(1) a feeling of alienation or disconnection from family and friends
(2) denial of physical symptoms, especially if severe
(3) irrationality about the illness
(4) feelings of profound helplessness and lack of control over personal matters

582. Which of the following statements appropriately apply to the treatment of patients with personality disorders?

(1) Most patients are so difficult to engage in outpatient psychotherapy that, from the outset, other forms of therapy should be employed
(2) Although the medication of choice must be found on a trial-and-error basis, the appropriate drug, once found, is likely to be quite effective
(3) Many patients who are unresponsive to medication or several forms of milieu therapy may respond well to ECT
(4) Severely affected hospitalized patients may respond favorably to long-term intensive milieu and individual types of therapy

583. The general living systems theory is characterized by which of the following critical subsystems?

(1) Information processing
(2) Matter-energy processing
(3) Reproduction
(4) Retrieval

584. Correct statements concerning the epidemiology of suicide include which of the following?

(1) Most countries reporting high suicide rates are characterized by some hardship condition such as extreme poverty, hostile climate, war, or repressive government
(2) In the United States, more men than women commit suicide, but more women than men attempt it
(3) The rate of suicide is consistent throughout most of the United States
(4) Of all the countries in the world, Hungary has the highest reported suicide rate

585. Statements that accurately describe the epidemiology of opioid drug use include which of the following?

(1) An addiction-prone premorbid personality pattern has been identified
(2) About 2-3 percent of persons 18-25 years old have tried heroin at one time or another
(3) An intelligent and knowledgeable individual rarely becomes addicted
(4) Usage has spread from large cities to small communities and rural areas

586. Characteristics of the hysterical personality include which of the following?

(1) Self-awareness
(2) Psychological dependency
(3) Conscious attention seeking
(4) Dramatization and overreaction

587. Patients with the Munchausen syndrome are usually described as having

(1) a strong need to fool medical professionals
(2) basically hostile, evasive personalities
(3) masochistic acceptance of painful procedures
(4) a satisfactory prognosis

588. Studies of battered women reveal that they

(1) have a high dropout rate from treatment
(2) usually are clinically depressed
(3) try to conceal the fact that they have been abused
(4) are involved with men who tend to be sociopathic

589. Which of the following types of impulses commonly generate phobic reactions?

(1) Aggressive
(2) Sexual
(3) Acquisitive
(4) Altruistic

590. Breath-holding spells in children are characterized by

(1) an absence of specific antecedent events
(2) an association with a high incidence of mental illness
(3) responsiveness to psychotherapy
(4) a distinct, stereotyped pattern of events

591. Statements that accurately describe dance therapy for mentally ill patients include which of the following?

(1) Dance therapy is limited in usefulness to neurotic patients of normal intellect
(2) Patients are taught set patterns of dance steps and movements
(3) The goal of dance therapy is to teach patients to control affective expression
(4) Patients' movement patterns reveal their psychic states

592. Contingency contracting, as applied to marital counseling, is characterized by

(1) changing the locus of therapy to the patient's natural environment
(2) recognizing that feelings and attitudes have to change before behavior may change
(3) seeking to replace a system of mutual punishment with one of mutual reward
(4) permitting the patients to change their behavior arbitrarily

593. Behavior therapy involves the use of which of the following techniques?

(1) Ignoring stuttering and rewarding fluency with rapt attention
(2) Desensitizing the patient to reduce anxiety
(3) Inducing a low-anxiety state by deep muscular relaxation
(4) Confronting the patient with the anxiety-producing situation in full intensity (flooding)

594. Client-centered psychotherapy recognizes which of the following principles?

(1) Clients are admonished to suppress feelings about the therapist
(2) Therapists cultivate a caring, unconditional regard for their clients
(3) Clients are encouraged to change their life style by changing certain aspects of their behavior
(4) Therapists communicate their own genuine feelings experienced during interaction with the patient

595. Correct statements concerning jogging as part of a program for mental and physical health include which of the following?

(1) It provides greater opportunity for fantasizing than almost any other sport
(2) It precludes physical injury
(3) It induces euphoria without the ingestion of chemical substances
(4) It produces a sense of fatigue that affects other daily activities

596. Individuals who are involved in automobile accidents tend to

(1) have an unconscious sense of guilt and need for atonement
(2) be victims of a critical phase of the biorhythm cycle
(3) use alcoholic beverages
(4) have a quiet, contemplative, daydreaming personality

DIRECTIONS: The groups of questions below consist of lettered choices followed by several numbered items. For each numbered item select the **one** lettered choice with which it is **most** closely associated. Each lettered choice may be used once, more than once, or not at all.

Questions 597-601

For each clinical sketch appearing below, choose the type of resistance to which it most closely corresponds.

    (A) Secondary gain resistance
    (B) Superego resistance
    (C) Id resistance
    (D) Transference resistance
    (E) Conscious resistance

597. During a session of free association, a patient thinks about describing having masturbated the night before, but does not tell the analyst because of feelings of shame and embarrassment

598. During a therapy hour, a patient begins by rather freely discussing his feelings about his father, using veiled criticism with no display of affect. The therapist listens quietly. The patient becomes silent for a period; then, somewhat inappropriately, with an edge on his voice he remarks, "Why don't you say something? You are just sitting there"

599. In discussing her repetitious hand-washing, a patient is unable to connect the act with the early desire she had to handle her older brother's genitals. On many occasions, the therapist had, by gentle interpretation, suggested to the patient the possibility of a connection when the hand-washing and the early fantasy had been repeatedly linked by the patient during free association

600. A patient struggling with an offer of a job far better than any held by his siblings or father is unable to make a decision to accept it. The analysis discloses strong feelings that the patient wants to be the most loved and successful member of the family, with much attendant guilt

601. A patient, after years of indulgence on the part of her husband for her headaches and infirmities, has improved in her ability to work and to complete household chores like grocery shopping, but cannot induce herself to learn to drive, insisting that her husband drive her wherever she goes

Questions 602-605

For each set of primary goals of psychotherapy listed below, select the originator with whom it is most closely identified.

    (A) Alfred Adler
    (B) Harry Stack Sullivan
    (C) Karen Horney
    (D) Jules Masserman
    (E) Eric Berne

602. To relieve immediate distress and guide the patient by any ethical means to more satisfactory ways of living and a new life philosophy

603. To increase a patient's social interest so that the patient can feel an equal among peers and abandon unrealistic views of life

604. To free patients from compulsions and resistance to change so that their creative forces can be expressed

605. To maintain and develop a patient's self-esteem and interpersonal security

Psychosocial Psychiatry
Answers

551. The answer is D. *(Wolberg, ed 3. pp 81-83.)* Suggestions, either direct or indirect, are part of most psychotherapy situations, even though the treating psychiatrist may endeavor to keep them to a minimum. However, in many patients for whom a symptom is very uncomfortable or embarrassing and for whom it binds minimal anxiety, good results may follow from a direct suggestion that the symptom disappear. Such symptom removal may then have important consequences for restructuring the patient's attitudes and even upon general functioning. Such "prestige suggestions," which depend on the esteem in which the patient holds the therapist, should not be overused or used prematurely to eliminate symptoms that the patient may be unprepared to relinquish.

552. The answer is B. *(Kaplan, ed 3. p 2147.)* Flooding, graded exposure, and participant modeling are behavioral techniques employed in exposing patients to the anxiety-producing event. In flooding, the real event is encountered, e.g., going to a high place for a patient who fears heights. Another method of exposing the patient to anxiety is "implosion," or reproducing the anxiety-provoking situation in the patient's imagination. Although the behaviorist method does not emphasize an exploration of the patient's psychodynamics or family psychopathology, the interpersonal influence of the therapist remains very much a part of the therapist-patient transaction in behavioral therapy.

553. The answer is E. *(Kaplan, ed 3. pp 2168-2170.)* Hypnosis can be successfully used for several purposes. By the use of posthypnotic suggestion, patients may be relieved of a conversion symptom or experience little or no pain during a dental procedure. Under hypnosis, a person may reveal additional details about a recent event or may undergo age regression to childhood to recover repressed memories or display childlike behavior. In mentally retarded persons, hypnosis has little application for two reasons—it cannot produce skills or behavior not already possessed, and such individuals have only a limited ability to enter a hypnotic trance.

554. The answer is D. *(Kaplan, ed 3. pp 2607-2608.)* Although bronchial asthma was once hailed as a prime example of psychosomatic disease, subsequent studies have failed to substantiate earlier claims. The contribution of emotional factors to the development of asthma is not clearly established. We cannot identify a specific personality pattern that correlates with asthma either in children with the disease or their mothers. The same statement applies to other diseases like rheumatoid arthritis and ulcerative colitis. In all these diseases, the interrelationship of heredity, environment, and parenting is of such complexity as to defy attempts to establish the priority of one factor over another.

555. The answer is B. *(Kaplan, ed 3. pp 2058-2059.)* The patients most likely to have the most severe psychological response to surgery are those who are depressed. The anesthesia and the symbolism of being put to sleep to undergo an assault are least accepted by depressed persons. Whenever possible, depressed patients should receive psychiatric help to achieve a remission prior to surgery. Surgery does not appear to cause a significant incidence of psychotic breaks in previously psychotic patients who are in remission at the time of surgery. Patients most likely to remain psychologically stable after surgery include young adults undergoing elective cosmetic operations (who have realistic expectations of what the surgery will accomplish), patients with low anxiety, and those who have strong ties with their families.

556. The answer is A. *(Kaplan, ed 3. pp 448-479.)* In spite of its publicity, biofeedback has not been clearly established as the treatment of choice for any disorder and remains an experimental and unproved technique. The studies of biofeedback are mostly case reports or uncontrolled experiments offering no evidence that the results of biofeedback exceed the placebo effect. On the other hand, no definite adverse effects have been associated with this technique. Even for producing relaxation, biofeedback lacks clear superiority over other methods. Although it may be permissible as an adjunct to a comprehensive program of treatment for disorders that have not responded to better-established methods, biofeedback should not be used to the neglect of other forms of treatment.

557. The answer is D. *(Kaplan, ed 3. pp 2175-2176.)* In using hypnosis for treating patients who wish to give up smoking, therapists should avoid authoritarian methods and aversive or scare tactics. These patients are already frightened or worried about their habit and generally need encouragement and not intimidation. Once patients have achieved a rational understanding of the dangers of smoking, such as its effect on the respiratory tract, reduction of longevity, and the adverse effects on a fetus, therapists should attempt to provide the conditions under which patients can withdraw from smoking by mobilizing their own strengths. Patients are encouraged to pursue the positive goal of regarding their bodies as worthy of respect rather than the negative goal of giving up smoking. Patients are taught to use their own powers of concentration in a program of self-help, using self-induced trances to reinforce the positive goals. Successful patients achieve a sense of respect, worth, and accomplishment because the cure comes from within themselves rather than from some external authority or from the negative effects of fear.

558. The answer is D. *(Kolb, ed 9. pp 775-776.)* Dreams are thought to display the same mental mechanisms used in the waking state. In dreams, the instinctual impulses are disguised by such processes as symbolization, condensation, and displacement. These processes, constituting the "dream work," lead to a manifest content representing the unacceptable impulses that comprise the latent content of the dream, impulses "scrubbed up," as it were. By free association, the manifest content leads to the latent content and hence an individual's basic conflicts. Dream analysis thus can help in discovering the forces that determine a patient's everyday responses. Dreams seem very much related to events in everyday life. The psychic residue of the day often appears in the dream, but altered in some way by attachment to, or the influence of, the unconscious.

559. The answer is E. *(Kaplan, ed 3. p 476.)* In a drug study, a double-blind design means that neither the evaluator nor the patient knows whether the patient receives the drug or placebo. This safeguard is necessary to eliminate what is known as the placebo effect, which depends on the expectations of the patient, and to protect investigators from their own biases either for or against the drug in question. Literally hundreds of new treatments, including the use of drugs, surgery, and biofeedback, initially have been reported as successful in uncontrolled studies that lacked the double-blind safeguard. When subjected to a double-blind study with scientifically acceptable criteria of judgment, in many instances such treatment modalities prove ineffective. Enthusiasm for the new, and frequently unverified, treatment invariably spreads like wildfire, whereas the proof of nonsuccess takes years to overcome the initial misinformation. Such has been the history of therapy. In evaluating all types of therapy, it is necessary to correct not only for the placebo effect but for the bias of physicians who need to prove their power, authority, and superiority by developing effective treatments. The double-blind provision protects therapists from mistaking their own needs for fact.

560. The answer is E. *(Wolberg, ed 3. p 766.)* In the use of biofeedback to retrain for muscle tension, the electrodes are placed in a band that is strapped around the muscle or muscle groups chosen for retraining. One of the most commonly used muscles is the frontalis, because its relaxation also is generally accompanied by relaxation of other muscles of the body. The state of muscular tension is made known to the patient by an audible feedback mechanism. Through muscle relaxation exercises, the therapist teaches the patient to relax, thus reducing the feedback sound level until it finally disappears. The act of thinking also causes tension in the muscles of the head, and the therapist can help patients reduce anxiety by "turning off" their thoughts.

561. The answer is B. *(Kolb, ed 9. pp 96-97.)* In confronting life's myriad experiences, the self constantly must deal with internal oppositional forces. On the one hand, the self absorbs into its habitual response system the values of family and social groups. On the other hand, that same self experiences various impulses and cravings that conflict with the sanctions and prohibitions established by conscience and society. These forces create, as it were, two different sets of personal goals. When presented with a situation in which the two forces pursue opposing solutions, a person may experience tension. This tension is felt as anxiety, evoking a severely painful affect. The various mental defense mechanisms are basically unconscious attempts to ward off feelings of anxiety and other painful reactions such as guilt, shame, or extreme anger. Although fear and anxiety are in some respects similar, the term "fear" is applied to a person's reaction to dangers from the environment, such as the feeling that is aroused by being chased by a bear. Anxiety is the term applied to a person's reaction to internal conflict, such as the feeling experienced when one steals to obtain money for life's luxuries despite the warnings of conscience.

562. The answer is A. *(Kolb, ed 9. p 771.)* Psychoanalysts generally regard free association as the basic method for disclosing psychodynamics. In using this technique, the therapist encourages the patient to verbalize all thoughts that occur in their exact sequence. The uncensored, uninhibited material that results theoretically will reveal the unconscious conflicts that underly the patient's symptoms. The therapist should not intrude by asking questions or inserting frequent interpretations. The goal is for patients to discover the interrelationships of their thoughts and their psychodynamic meaning. Presumably, this process leads to insights that allow patients to handle maturely any conflicts and anxieties that may arise.

563. The answer is C. *(Kaplan, ed 3. p 1187.)* Research by Brown, Birley, and Wing (1972) and by Vaughn and Leff (1976) has shown that family factors, in addition to drug maintenance, are critical to maintaining a schizophrenic patient in a remitted state. If patients are subjected to negative critical emotions for 35 or more hours a week, they are likely to become symptomatic again even if regularly receiving neuroleptic medication. Traumatic life events are also likely to trigger repeated breakdowns.

564. The answer is D (4). *(Kolb, ed 9. pp 794-798.)* Although few hard-and-fast principles have developed for group psychotherapy, a few general rules have emerged relating to the selection of patients and the composition of groups. Group therapy appears to be most successful when its members are composed of individuals of the same sex and of similar age and academic background. Group therapy can work well with children or the mentally retarded. Although some heterogeneity among members is desirable, patients with very divergent problems do not seem to function well in groups; for example, mixing alcoholic with paraphiliac persons or with individuals who have marital or family problems would be undesirable. Acutely psychotic, paranoid, and manic patients would be too disruptive to a group containing better-integrated members. The illnesses in these highly disturbed patients are often expressed too autonomously to permit constructive interaction among the group members.

565. The answer is A (1, 2, 3). *(Kolb, ed 9. p 982.)* In general, the courts respect the confidentiality of the patient-psychiatrist relationship even more than that of other physician-patient relationships. The doctrine holds for all patients, whether they are treated in private practice or state institutions. However, in some jurisdictions the law does not define or protect confidentiality; psychiatrists must be familiar with the circumstances in their own locality. If patients so wish, they may waive the right of confidentiality when it appears that a psychiatrist may have information beneficial to their case. Before a patient accepts such a waiver, the psychiatrist must review the implications of the decision with the patient, allowing the patient to exercise the waiver from the vantage point of informed consent.

566. The answer is A (1, 2, 3). *(Kaplan, ed 3. pp 183, 2356.)* Current data indicate that deficiencies of some vitamins may lead to mental illness. Deficiencies of the B group of vitamins may cause well-delineated syndromes, such as pernicious anemia resulting from B_{12} deficiency, Wernicke-Korsakoff syndrome and beri-beri resulting from thiamine deficiency, and pellagra resulting from niacin deficiency. Pyridoxine deficiency may cause seizures and mental retardation. It fails to follow, however, that because some overt vitamin deficiency states correlate with specific mental illnesses, all or even a few other mental illnesses are the result of vitamin deficiency. Until the megavitamin and orthomolecular advocates present evidence that meets the generally accepted scientific criteria for efficacy, their theories must be considered controversial. Indeed, megadoses of many vitamins, for example A and D, are clearly harmful. Thus, megavitamin therapy is not free of danger.

567. The answer is E (all). *(Kaplan, ed 3. pp 2846-2852.)* Langsley lists ten problems that beset the community mental health centers in action. The first one listed, neglect of the chronically ill, is cited as the major criticism. Mental health centers have failed to set up sufficient services for patients discharged from hospitals, who form the bulk of the chronically ill. Also underserved are children, the geriatric population, rural people, and minority groups. Staffing problems are common, finding expression in conflicts among various personnel about role responsibilities; psychiatrists are particularly unhappy over the failure of centers to treat the seriously ill and at being relegated to writing prescriptions. Because staff members have been fearful of being inundated by requests for services, mental health centers commonly have been less than vigorous in promoting their services to the community. Thus, too few people know of the services to which they are entitled. Other problems listed by Langsley include clashes between governing factions that can destroy important programs, financial problems, unrealistic rigidity in defining catchment areas, inability to prevent mental illness, and provision of second-class service.

568. The answer is D (4). *(Kaplan, ed 3. pp 2169-2170.)* Much misinformation exists about hypnosis. Hypnosis is not a form of sleep. It is a state of enhanced or focused concentration different from sleep in both clinical characteristics and also in EEG pattern. In general, mentally healthy individuals who have the ability to maintain their concentration on a task are more easily hypnotized than mentally ill subjects, including those who are weak and passive. A high level of hypnotizability thus more appropriately reflects mental health than mental illness. The removal of symptoms by hypnosis has not been proven to result in substitution of another, more serious symptom, as was widely believed in the past.

569. The answer is E (all). *(Wolberg, ed 3. pp 18-22.)* Spontaneous psychiatric cures probably are fairly common; one or several factors may be responsible in any given individual although the exact mechanism is unknown. The pain of intrapsychic conflict may stimulate the sufferer to reactivate and strengthen repressive mechanisms or to develop a different philosophy of living. The environment may change fortuitously, removing precipitating stresses or even reconditioning the sufferer. The latter situation probably can occur only if the new environment does not recreate the punishing and defeating aspects of the old. Probably those individuals who demonstrate the most lasting and extensive spontaneous change are those who have the least character pathology or whose neuroses have failed to solidify.

570. The answer is E (all). *(Kaplan, ed 3. pp 1645-1649.)* Established features of caffeinism include restlessness and anxiety, palpitation and tachycardia, and insomnia. Excess use of caffeine is higher in mentally ill than in psychiatrically healthy populations, but cause and effect remain to be established. Withdrawal headaches, which may occur in many patients who discontinue caffeine abruptly, are generalized and throbbing. Such headaches appear about 18 hours after the cessation of caffeine ingestion and respond to the ingestion of caffeine. Caffeine also may have adverse effects in psychiatric patients taking lithium or monoamine oxidase inhibitors. High caffeine intake correlates with other evidence of a "drug-prone" personality, such as the use of other drugs like nicotine, alcohol, sedatives, and minor tranquilizers.

571. The answer is A (1, 2, 3). *(Kolb, ed 9. p 567.)* In anaclitic therapy, therapists encourage patients to regress to an infantile stage. The therapist, either personally or with aids and environmental manipulations, tries to meet a patient's dependency needs. This technique may work to establish therapeutic contact before long-term psychotherapy can be completed. In the hospital setting, hired mother-substitutes can effectively promote the therapy. Anaclitic therapy works in infantile depression, but its appropriateness in older patients is less clear. Still, all therapy in a sense is anaclitic because some dependency is fostered by the very nature of the therapeutic relationship between the ostensibly authoritarian, all-knowing and all-powerful professional and the apparently helpless patient. Symbolically, even the prescribing of oral medication has anaclitic implications.

572. The answer is C (2, 4). *(Slaby, pp 110-112.)* A physician treating a woman who says she has been raped should first inquire about the details of the incident. For example, a woman may describe her husband's urgent request for sex when she is unreceptive as "rape"; others may describe an aggressive male gesture without penetration as "rape." While the psychiatrist often must determine whether or not sexual contact has occurred, only the court can determine if this contact constitutes a rape. Nevertheless, in all cases of suspected rape the physician must follow certain procedures. To be prepared for a court subpoena, the physician must take a written history using the patient's exact words, record the results of the physical examination, and save all clothing. No exact diagnosis should be recorded. After the patient's written consent is obtained, a vaginal smear should be obtained from which the police laboratory may determine the presence of acid phosphatase and the blood antigen of the semen. Appropriate tests for gonorrhea and syphilis should be performed, and treatment for these conditions started immediately. Pregnancy prevention is also an important part of the emergency treatment regimen. Psychiatric counseling of the rape victim — which should begin immediately in the emergency room — should encourage ventilation of feelings, a return to regular routine, and follow-up psychiatric care if needed. Any underlying psychiatric condition should be treated only after the crisis surrounding the rape and the patient's feelings about it have been dealt with.

573. The answer is A (1, 2, 3). *(Kaplan, ed 3. pp 1787-1788.)* In many ways, the Masters and Johnson techniques for therapy of sexual dysfunction depend on the traditional medical model of history-taking and examination, but the actual therapy more closely resembles behavioral modification techniques. The therapy centers on the couple as a dysfunctional unit. Initially, the partners verbalize their concerns about their sexual problems, and then they begin a stage of sensate focus. During this stage, sexual intercourse is forbidden, and the partners learn to touch and enjoy touching each other's bodies, with the exception of the breasts or the genital region. Verbal communication is urged to increase the "pleasuring." The couple next will include the genital areas in the touching and fondling. Later, intercourse is permitted and attempted. During the periods of touching, fondling, and sexual contact, the partners should refrain from "spectatoring," by which is meant judging the adequacy and quality of their own sexual performance as a spectator might. Spectatoring fosters performance anxieties. The making of analytical judgments is antithetical to sensate focus and the release of autonomic functions necessary for sexual arousal and performance. The essential approach to this type of treatment is to provide the means to allow sexual contact to develop spontaneously, because sexual arousal and performance are autonomic reflexes, with which anxiety and cerebration interfere.

574. The answer is E (all). *(Wolberg, ed 3. pp 66-67.)* Many complex problems are involved in adequately researching the results of psychotherapy — for example, choosing and measuring behavioral phenomena that reflect change in the patient, bias of the observers (which include the patient and therapist), and difficulties in selecting appropriate control groups. In order to conduct a useful research study, a competent statistician must be included from the inception of the program to assure an operationally stated hypothesis, determine the kinds of data to be gathered, establish adequate reliability of observers, and outline the employment and proper interpretation of appropriate statistical methods. It is only by careful attention to the complexities of such research that valid conclusions can be reached. To date, research into psychotherapy has had little influence on clinical practice because of the contradictory results of various studies.

575. The answer is C (2, 4). *(Usdin, pp 537-560.)* Individual psychotherapy techniques can be divided into three basic types: psychoanalytic therapy (often called psychoanalysis), exploratory or intensive psychotherapy, and supportive psychotherapy. While psychoanalysis and intensive psychotherapy have much in common, such as free association, empathetic responsiveness of the therapist, and development of patient insight, they also differ in some ways. In psychoanalysis, the therapist sits on a chair placed behind the patient, who reclines on a couch. In intensive psychotherapy, the therapist and patient sit face-to-face. Psychoanalytic sessions are likely to occur more frequently and over a greater period of time, e.g., four to five times weekly versus one to three times weekly, and for several years versus approximately one year. Psychoanalysts, like intensive psychotherapists, avoid making important decisions for their patients, who are expected to make their own. The fundamental difference between these types of therapy is that the development of a transference neurosis is encouraged in psychoanalysis and discouraged in intensive psychotherapy. Much of the later stage of psychoanalysis is devoted to the resolution of the transference neurosis, whereas the intensive psychotherapist tries to resolve any transference feelings as they arise. The role of the supportive therapist is to direct and encourage the patient and to de-emphasize deeper patient insight and discussion of the therapist-patient relationship. Supportive therapy as a sole or main technique generally is used for chronically and severely disabled patients who are unable to utilize the nondirective, insight-producing techniques associated with psychoanalysis and psychotherapy.

576. The answer is D (4). *(Kaplan, ed 3. pp 1762-1769.)* There is no agreement among the many studies of the endocrinology and families of homosexuals and heterosexuals concerning the biological or psychodynamic origins of homosexuality. The endocrine studies have failed to produce consistent results on replication. The studies of the families of homosexuals fail to produce clear evidence of causal factors. Such studies are unable to separate the reaction of the child to the parent from the possibility that the parent reacted to something in the child. When reading Rorschach test results blindly, experts failed to distinguish homosexuals from heterosexuals at better than chance expectations. Most surveys of the incidence of homosexuality place the incidence among females as substantially less than in males. Once again, the social factors that might alter the expression of homosexuality in females cannot be separated from the biological ones. If homosexuality itself is not defined as a mental illness, the frequency, degree, and types of established mental illnesses differ little between homosexuals and hererosexuals.

577. The answer is B (1, 3). *(Kaplan, ed 3. p 2227.)* According to Peter Martin, marital therapy is indicated when it is requested by a couple with interpersonal difficulties who are committed to remaining married, when other forms of therapy fail to help the emotional problems of either partner, and for individuals with symptoms clearly due to marital upheavals. Marital therapy is generally unsuccessful for those individuals with certain personality disorders (paranoid or narcissistic), for those with secrets they don't wish revealed, and for those who are firmly committed to divorce. It is often difficult to decide during an initial interview whether marital therapy is suitable for any particular couple. This matter must be frequently reassessed during the course of therapy.

578. The answer is A (1, 2, 3). *(Usdin, pp 7-9.)* A chief complaint of patients about their medical care is "My doctor doesn't listen to me." Most patients appreciate and give a more complete history to physicians—whether male or female—whom they perceive as warm and caring than to physicians who appear remote and "professional." Physicians who appear warm and caring convey their concern by meeting the patient's gaze, listening attentively, and letting their patients know that their opinions and observations are important. The patient relates a more accurate history, in most cases, if the doctor is understanding and empathizes with the feelings of alienation, fears of death, and confusion that afflict every ill person. Physicians should make evident their awareness of the patient's fear of physical and emotional pain, thereby demonstrating a capacity for tenderness that should be part of every physician's technical skill. The physician must recognize that the patient may react adversely not only to fears regarding the illness itself, but also to particular traits in the physician. A minority of patients may be made anxious by an overly warm approach. Physicians mindful of their own tendencies to be too reserved or too aggressively "warm" will modify their approach if they perceive that it is making a patient uncomfortable.

579. The answer is C (2, 4). *(Usdin, pp 16-19.)* Above all, medical practitioners must understand their own behavior and how they react to "difficult" patients. Such self-knowledge can keep a physician from responding inappropriately to patients' provocative, inappropriate, or symptomatic behaviors. For example, physicians who know that they tend to be authoritarian and angry if patients insist on a degree of autonomy in dealing with their own illnesses are in a position to cope with their own anger and accept the patient with greater equanimity. In any case, most attempts to hide feelings are unsuccessful. One can deal appropriately or inappropriately with feelings, but trying to mask them without understanding them generally leads to confused relationships. All people, physicians included, are vulnerable to certain kinds of "difficult" behavior in others and respond unfavorably, despite attempts to understand themselves better. For example, if a physician persists in responding with counterhostility to hostile patients, often the best practice is to refer these patients to another doctor. Physicians who cannot control their own sexual behavior with flirtatious patients must refer such patients to another practitioner. The physician should learn how to explore in a sensitive and respectful way those behaviors of patients that interfere with treatment in order to help them understand and control their feelings. Behaviors that are noninterfering can be accepted with equanimity even though they may differ from the physician's concept of a "good" patient. Patients whose behaviors are symptoms of an underlying psychiatric disorder or who call forth unmanageable or destructive feelings in the physician should be referred to other professionals who, by training or temperament, can manage them more successfully.

580. The answer is A (1, 2, 3). *(Kaplan, ed 3. pp 1790-1791.)* Hypersexuality in the form of the need for sexual satisfaction at inappropriate times and places and with excess frequency has been reported in both males and females with Huntington's chorea. During the manic phase of manic-depressive illness, affected males and females may show promiscuity and excessive interest in sexual matters. The females may express interest in becoming pregnant and even display pseudocyesis. The Kleine-Levin syndrome, which manifests most commonly in young males, may be associated with excessive and inappropriate sexuality. Two psychosurgical procedures, prefrontal lobotomy and amygdalotomy, do not appear to result in hypersexuality.

581. The answer is E (all). *(Usdin, p 6.)* Cassell has pointed out that physical illness brings certain psychological accompaniments to every person. These may include a sense of disconnection from one's personal world, which may range from mild feelings of alienation to great hopelessness; an awareness of one's vulnerability, evidenced at times by severe denial of physical symptoms; a lack of rational thinking about the illness; and a feeling of lack of control over one's life. All these reactions may become intertwined with the illness and should be understood by physicians so that treatment can be more effectively administered. Sensitivity to and proper management of the range of adverse psychological reactions of normal persons to illness are among a physician's most important responsibilities.

582. The answer is D (4). *(Usdin, pp 276-277.)* Patients with personality disorders have a reputation for resistance to treatment and, once engaged in therapy, being a challenge to therapists. Many such patients are unresponsive to any form of individual therapy except the supportive type in crises. However, many other patients can respond, especially if therapists can establish themselves as trustworthy. The therapist also must display openness, honesty, and a respectful attitude toward these often provocative and alienating patients. Only a trial of psychotherapy can sort out responsive from the unresponsive patients. The use of ECT is not recommended. Pharmacotherapy is not only useless but often misused in this generally drug-dependent population. Long-term individual supportive and milieu therapy can help, even with some severely ill, hospitalized patients.

583. The answer is A (1, 2, 3). *(Kolb, ed 9. pp 18-20.)* The psychobiological theory of Adolf Meyer (1866-1950) attempted in a general way to unify the many biological, psychological, and experimental factors that probably influence personality development. The generality of the theory, however, led to scientific sterility and testable hypotheses rarely were generated. The general systems theory may perhaps be more fruitful in delineating the methods by which the various aspects of science could be applied to the study of human psychobiology. The critical subsystems are: (1) information processing mediated by the brain, which handles messages from within and from outside the individual; (2) matter-energy processing, and (3) the reproduction subsystem comprising the internal environment of the living system. The general systems theory has proved to be of little scientific value in explaining the development of personality.

584. The answer is C (2, 4). *(Usdin, pp 459-474.)* Suicide statistics are notorious for their unreliability; many cases of suicide are unreported. The number of unreported suicides varies according to the attitudes of the various national, religious, and socioeconomic groups involved. Insurance agencies or religious groups that withhold benefits if a group member commits suicide contribute to this situation. Some nations have poor facilities for recording suicides, or deliberately discourage the reporting of suicide deaths. Nevertheless, certain facts about the epidemiology of suicide do, in part, reflect actual conditions. Suicide rates, especially among young people, appear to be increasing throughout many parts of the world. There is no clear, positive relationship between hardship conditions and suicide rates of any given population. For example, Greece, Mexico, and Spain all have consistently low suicide rates, but have large populations of low-income people living under hardship conditions. Denmark, West Germany, and Sweden, with much higher per capita incomes, have some of the highest suicide rates in the world. Hungary, with the highest suicide rate of any nation (39.9/100,000), would appear on the surface to have a less affluent population than the city of West Berlin, which has an even higher rate. In the United States, blacks, who have higher unemployment rates than whites, have consistently lower suicide rates. In the United States, individual states vary considerably in their suicide rates, but this variation lacks any apparent correlation to hardship conditions such as hostile climate or low per capita income. The reported rates of suicide vary from 7.5/100,000 in New Jersey to 26.7/100,000 in Nevada. The western states generally have higher suicide rates than the eastern states. Perhaps the diversity of reporting policies among the various states largely contributes to the discrepancies in reported suicide rates. Although many social and economic factors affect suicide rates, methods of reporting vary so widely among various groups that only gross trends can be detected. Currently, therefore, much of the information about causes of suicide must be derived from individual studies of patients rather than from epidemiology statistics.

585. The answer is C (2, 4). *(Gilman, ed 6. p 545.)* No specific personality pattern is known to predispose an individual to addiction, but those who become addicted tend to be more impulsive and antisocial. No amount of intelligence or knowledge of the dangers inherent in drug abuse protects against addiction, as evidenced by the high incidence of addiction among medical and paramedical personnel. The use of heroin has spread from cities to smaller communities, and it is estimated that between 2-3 percent of individuals 18-25 years of age have tried heroin at least once.

586. The answer is C (2, 4). *(Usdin, pp 235-236.)* The individual characterized by a hysterical personality generally has poor mechanisms for coping with stresses, and thus shows a high level of dependency on other persons. While hysterical individuals may engage in seductive acts and approval-seeking behavior, they do so without insight or awareness of these traits.

Because they do so much taking and so little giving, their interpersonal relationships lack closeness, depth, and conviction. Some of their mechanisms for soliciting attention are dramatization, overreaction, and intrusion in the affairs of others. The individual with a hysterical personality is prone to develop conversion reactions and dissociative states.

587. The answer is A (1, 2, 3). *(Kolb, ed 9. p 512.)* Patients with the Munchausen syndrome repeatedly visit doctors or seek admission to hospitals, usually with a complaint of an emergency nature such as bleeding, pain, or loss of consciousness. These patients are basically hostile, evasive individuals who seem to have a strong need to dupe the medical profession. They masochistically accept painful diagnostic procedures and unnecessary surgery. They learn much medical jargon and utilize it in describing their fictitious illnesses. After admission to a hospital, their hostility emerges and they may provoke some incident that leads to their signing out against medical advice. These patients have a severe characterological flaw that may involve dozens of hospitalizations. Psychiatric therapy generally fails to benefit such individuals.

588. The answer is E (all). *(Usdin, pp 625-626.)* The battered wife syndrome, while common, frequently is difficult to uncover. The physician may not ask questions about anger and self-control as part of a regular examination, and may fail to recognize the significance of repeated bruises or "falls." Battered women tend to conceal their situation, perhaps as part of their depression and denial. In spite of being physically abused, such women tend to cling to their abuser for realistic as well as psychodynamic reasons. They may lack the financial or emotional resources to effect a separation. Moreover, the abusive male, who tends to be sociopathic, may intersperse the beatings with protestations of affection and concern.

589. The answer is A (1, 2, 3). *(Usdin, pp 232-234.)* According to psychoanalytic theory, phobias arise in response to impulses or desires that are forbidden by the conscience. In the normal person, such conflicts were resolved during childhood development. In the phobic person, nearness of an object, person, or event that could revive a forbidden impulse may precipitate panic reactions. The phobic object, which is symbolic of the conflict, is thus stringently avoided in an effort to keep the forbidden impulses under control and anxiety at bay. The three most common sources of phobias are impulses of a sexual, aggressive, or acquisitive nature. Phobias due to acquisitive impulses develop when the desired object can be obtained only by means forbidden by the conscience, e.g., a large diamond desired by a housemaid who could attain one only by stealing. Altruistic impulses are generally regarded as a mature mental mechanism and would not, in themselves, be a source of phobias.

590. The answer is D (4). *(Hoekelman, p 951.)* The most important diagnostic feature of breath-holding spells is a history of some distinct provocative event that causes frustration, anger, or fear just prior to the onset of an attack. The attack then customarily follows a definite, stereotyped sequence consisting of expiratory apnea, cyanosis, opisthotonic rigidity, and then sudden return of breathing. Afterward, affected children generally appear groggy and sleepy for a period of time. These spells most commonly begin in late infancy and disappear by the middle of the first decade. These children do not show an increased incidence of mental illness as they mature. Psychotherapy is of no help to individuals suffering from such spells.

591. The answer is D (4). *(Kaplan, ed 3. pp 2388, 2676-2677.)* Dance therapy has found wide application in psychiatry. It can be used with all types of patients, including those who are mentally retarded and senile. No prior dance training is required. The basic theory is that patients' movements reflect their current psychic states. The therapist does not try to criticize, correct, or train the patient according to precepts of dance technique. Instead, the patient is encouraged to develop free, rhythmic movements that are presumed to aid in affective expression, to give the patient a better body image, and to foster better interaction and communication.

592. The answer is B (1, 3). *(Kaplan, ed 3. pp 2149-2150.)* In contingency contracting, therapists attempt to change patients' feelings and attitudes by first changing their behavior. As applied to marital counseling, the technique requires the marital partners to make behavioral changes in their own home—i.e., in the natural environment in which the unwanted behavior occurs. The couple makes explicit contracts about behavior. Each spouse specifies the behavior he or she wishes changed in the other, and therapist and participants agree on the immediate goals or behavioral changes that constitute the contract. The couple periodically reports its progress to the therapist; further goals may then be contracted. The idea behind such counseling is to replace negative contingencies with positive ones and encourage a system of mutual reward rather than mutual punishment. The couple should honor the contract, which specifies acceptable behaviors, rather than arbitrarily changing their actions.

593. The answer is E (all). *(Kaplan, ed 3. pp 2143-2152.)* In the treatment of a person who stutters, a behaviorist would instruct those persons around the patient to ignore the stuttering but pay rapt attention to fluent speech, with the intention of reversing the contingencies of reinforcement to effect a change toward speech fluency and away from stuttering—a process known as extinction. Desensitization involves gradual exposure of the patient to the circumstances that produce the undesired behavior, thereby deconditioning the anxiety. The anxiety-producing event is imaginatively reproduced. Reciprocal inhibition is a gradual approach to an event feared by the patient, planned and paired with a preceding iatrogenic state of lessened anxiety. To achieve a low anxiety state, patients are taught to relax their muscles, a process that can be accelerated by intravenous administration of methohexital (Brevital). Flooding may be approached gradually, as in systematic desensitization, but without being paired with deep relaxation.

594. The answer is C (2, 4). *(Kaplan, ed 3. pp 2161-2163.)* According to Carl Rogers, in client-centered psychotherapy therapists seek to establish a warm, caring relationship with clients, communicating directly the feelings they experience. Throughout the sessions, therapists foster an unconditional regard for the client and attempt to recognize what they themselves are experiencing. This rule does not insist that the therapist communicate every insignificant passing thought, but does necessitate the sharing of persistent and recurrent genuine feelings at the appropriate time.

595. The answer is B (1, 3). *(Kaplan, ed 3. p 2389.)* Jogging, for many people, provides an avenue to improved mental and physical health. Its advocates claim a feeling of health, vigor, and well-being that extends to other daily activities. They believe it produces a feeling of physical competence and a better body image. Joggers report, as a regular experience, euphoric feelings that lead to a sense of tranquility, peace, and satisfaction generated by the healthy working of the body, rather than by the ingestion of drugs. Jogging, which requires a minimum of decision making and attention (in contrast, say, to tennis or basketball), frees the mind for fantasy. Nevertheless, joggers have their own special injuries such as sprained ankles, nipple burns in women, and the ever present danger of automobiles or criminal assault.

596. The answer is B (1, 3). *(Kaplan, ed 3. pp 1954-1955.)* The tendency of persons to be involved in accidents, particularly car accidents, is associated with the use of alcohol and an unconscious sense of guilt and need for atonement. Both alcoholism and the guilt-atonement duality have implications of self-punishment, as does the occurrence of the accident itself. Recent studies have failed to confirm an increase in accidents during the later, "negative" phase of the biorhythm cycle. Biorhythm theories, in general, have gained little acceptance owing to their lack of substantiation by carefully controlled scientific studies. Individuals involved in auto accidents tend to display aggressive, acting-out, impulsive behavior rather than a contemplative personality.

597-601. The answers are: 597-E, 598-D, 599-C, 600-B, 601-A. *(Kaplan, ed 3. pp 722-724, 2122-2123.)* A keystone of psychoanalysis is the recognition and management of resistances. Basically, resistances arise when some distressing material in a person's unconscious threatens to become conscious.

Conscious resistance takes the form of deliberate censorship of material during free association, material that patients feel will cause the analyst to think poorly of them, or that will engender within themselves feelings of shame, guilt, or embarrassment.

The ego may expend much energy in repression resistances, which keep instinctual impulses from reaching conscious recognition. Repression resistance describes the efforts of the ego to prevent disclosures being made during the analytic process. If analysts can aid their patients to overcome the repression resistances, the ego will finally accept or reject the repressed instinctual material, thereby disposing of a permanent threat and the need to expend energy previously required to maintain the repression.

Patients with transference resistance transfer to the therapist significant feelings generated by some previously encountered person for whom the therapist acts as a symbol. Transference resistance has the particular quality of both reflecting and expressing the patient's struggle with early experience and feeling. Although the transference can be positive, it frequently takes a negative form that may be evidenced by silence, sarcasm, or by a veiled or overtly hostile question or remark. Therapists must recognize these kinds of response as clinical transference phenomena and be careful not to respond in kind. The patient presented in question 598 had been struggling to cope with feelings about his father, but the patient was unable to connect his veiled criticisms of his father with their instinctual origins—an example of repression resistance. He then transferred the resistance to recognizing his feelings about his father to the analyst, whom he criticized for being silent. Such resistances appearing as transference can be dealt with very productively by the analyst. A transference resistance can become a transference attachment. Otherwise, the negative aspects of the transference resistance may dominate and seriously impede the therapeutic relationship.

Id resistance refers to the inability to change some ingrained behavioral pattern, often in the form of a compulsion, which derives from a particular instinctual drive that is very powerful. The washing of hands as a manifestation of unacceptable sexual impulses, exhibited by the patient presented in question 599, is such an example. The resistance is to unlearning the ingrained, maladaptive pattern of behavior that serves to mask, as it were, the unacceptable impulses from which the behavior originates.

In superego resistance (exhibited by the patient presented in question 600), patients on the verge of achieving some seemingly cherished goal find themselves too guilt-ridden about the achievement to accept it. Such promptings of the conscience prevent these patients from taking any step in either their lives or their psychoanalysis that would benefit them. This is the fear-of-success syndrome. The resistance is to the disclosure of the infantile strivings that make the goals attractive.

Patients with secondary gain resistance (like the woman presented in question 601) cling to certain of the practical advantages accruing from the illness, such as the attention, comfort, and services provided by spouses and relatives. The ability to relinquish all of the advantages of the illness is seldom achieved. Secondary gain is most conspicuous and difficult to deal with in compensation cases; frequently, it is better for the mental health of the patient if a monetary settlement can be reached as quickly as possible.

602-605. The answers are: 602-D, 603-A, 604-C, 605-B. *(Kaplan, ed 3. pp 740-797.)* Six people are commonly thought of as belonging to the cultural and interpersonal "school" of psychoanalytic thought, and all are widely acclaimed as effective and innovative therapists. Alfred Adler (1870-1937) was a member of Freud's circle from 1902-1911. When Adler disputed Freud's theory of innate aggressive drive, he became disassociated from Freud. Best known for his theory of the "inferiority complex" and striving for superiority as motivating human behavior, Adler also introduced a number of other widely held theories regarding the basic social nature of humans and the necessity for taking responsibility for one's own behavior. In his therapeutic practice, he finally came to stress that patients must increase their social interest in order to increase their self-esteem.

Karen Horney (1885-1952) was trained in psychoanalysis by Karl Abraham and his school in Berlin and came to the United States, where her creativity was encouraged. In her famous book *The Neurotic Personality of our Time*, she presented evidence to demonstrate that culture and environmental events are potent etiological factors in the production of neurosis. Horney based her therapy primarily on the reduction of "blockages" or resistances in order to free patients from a "compulsive," stereotyped approach to life.

The name of Harry Stack Sullivan (1892-1949) is practically synonymous with the "interpersonal" approach to psychiatry and human behavior. Trained in the United States, he underwent classical analysis but early in his career rejected classical psychoanalysis on both theoretical and pragmatic grounds. Sullivan's guiding principle in therapy was to preserve and increase a patient's self-esteem. He also regarded each psychiatric interview, no matter how short, as an opportunity for therapy.

Of all the workers who materially tried to change the field of psychoanalysis, Sandor Rado (1890-1971) never broke from it. He endeavored to increase the scientific underpinning of psychoanalysis and keep it within the fold of medicine. Rado defined an emotionally healthy person as self-reliant and capable of experiencing affection, pride, friendliness, optimism, and joy. Accordingly, his therapy was aimed at enhancing these characteristics in his patients in addition to developing their independence.

Jules Masserman was trained in psychoanalysis by Franz Alexander and in psychobiology by Adolf Meyer. His research and clinical careers have been devoted to an amalgamation of biological and psychological concepts. He has used laboratory methods to investigate methods of psychotherapy and has evolved an eclectic approach that invokes all ethical procedures in helping patients find a better life style and life view.

Transactional analysis was developed by Eric Berne in the 1950s after he decided traditional psychoanalysis took too long to effect change in patients. He was originally influenced by Paul Federn and the Vienna Psychoanalytic Society, but parted ways in a friendly spirit from classical analysis. Berne developed not only script analysis but also a total theory of personality in which he took ideas from California group therapists. Frederick Perls's gestalt techniques were particularly useful to Berne in delineating ego states and interpersonal games. In his therapy, Berne tried to demystify the complexities of human behavior by reducing problem behavior to its simplest form, thereby helping patients to see destructive forms of human interaction (games). The final phase of therapy was to help patients interrupt their "games."

The above six pioneers, through their writings and speeches, have influenced not only several generations of psychiatric trainees but the general public as well. Adlerian groups exist throughout the world, and Berne fostered a creativity in his followers that has enabled transactional analysis to grow in the decade since his death.

Diagnostic Procedures

DIRECTIONS: Each question below contains five suggested answers. Choose the **one best** response to each question.

606. Lesions affecting the visual fields usually result in loss of perceptual functions in which of the following sequences?

(A) Color, form, and movement
(B) Form, color, and movement
(C) Form, movement, and color
(D) Movement, color, and form
(E) Movement, form, and color

607. In persons with normal hearing, tests for efficiency of air and bone conduction of sound (Rinne test) demonstrate that

(A) air conduction is better than bone conduction
(B) bone conduction is better than air conduction
(C) bone and air conduction are equal
(D) bone conduction is better in children; air conduction is better in adults
(E) air conduction is better in children; bone conduction is better in adults

608. The brain tumor LEAST likely to be detected by a psychiatric interview, neurologic examination, and psychologic testing is a

(A) right parietal lobe glioma
(B) left posterior parasylvian area (parieto-occipito-temporal confluence)
(C) posterior frontal glioma, right or left
(D) butterfly glioma of the corpus callosum
(E) large pituitary adenoma

609. In an ophthalmoscopic examination, opacification of the cornea is best visualized by using a lens having a strength of

(A) − 10
(B) − 5
(C) + 5
(D) + 15
(E) none of the above

610. Cold caloric irrigation of the left ear produces nystagmus and causes the person's eyes to deviate

(A) slowly to the left and kick back quickly to the right
(B) quickly to the left and kick back slowly to the right
(C) quickly to the right and kick back slowly to the left
(D) slowly to the right and kick back quickly to the left
(E) with equal speed in both directions

611. In conducting an ophthalmoscopic examination of a patient's left eye, the examiner, who is facing the patient, should look through the instrument with

(A) the right eye
(B) the left eye
(C) either the right or left eye
(D) the dominant eye only
(E) the nondominant eye only

612. The best conclusion about the adult who produced the drawings shown below is that their originator

FIGURES PRESENTED   **PATIENT'S COPIES**

 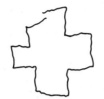

(A) lacks formal education
(B) refused to cooperate in the examination
(C) has hemiparesis
(D) has a right parietal lobe lesion
(E) has diffuse cerebral disease

DIRECTIONS: Each question below contains four suggested answers of which **one** or **more** is correct. Choose the answer

A	if	1, 2, and 3	are correct
B	if	1 and 3	are correct
C	if	2 and 4	are correct
D	if	4	is correct
E	if	1, 2, 3, and 4	are correct

613. A normal or minimally abnormal EEG is common in organic psychosis associated with

(1) petit mal status
(2) lysergic acid diethylamide intoxication
(3) Alzheimer's presenile dementia
(4) Wernicke-Korsakoff syndrome

614. In a normal EEG, the alpha rhythm has which of the following characteristics?

(1) It is frequently lower in amplitude on the left than on the right
(2) It blocks with opening of the eyes
(3) It disappears during sleep
(4) It is enhanced by concentrated thought

615. Traditional mental status tests for "organicity" that have been shown to be of little value in distinguishing functional from organic brain disease include

(1) orientation to time, person, and place
(2) subtraction of serial sevens
(3) recall of three unrelated objects
(4) digit repetition

616. The dexamethasone suppression test is most likely to be useful in which of the following situations?

(1) Distinguishing most cases of "endogenous" depression from other forms of depression
(2) Evaluating the efficacy of somatic treatment
(3) Differentiating between primary anxiety disorder with depressive features and primary depressive disorder with anxiety features
(4) Helping to make a decision for or against somatic treatment in depressed patients with accompanying character disorder

617. Of the Wechsler Adult Intelligence Scale subtests for measuring behavior and intellectual function, those in which patients with organic brain disease show the least deterioration include

(1) vocabulary
(2) picture completion
(3) object assembly
(4) arithmetic

618. Seizures that may occur with some frequency without a concomitant discharge during a routine EEG include

(1) myoclonic seizures
(2) generalized motor seizures (grand mal)
(3) psychomotor seizures
(4) classical petit mal absences

619. Correct statements concerning directive interviewing include which of the following?

(1) Physicians strive to obtain long, descriptive answers from patients
(2) This technique nearly always offends patients and should usually be avoided
(3) The focus of the interview is direct at the beginning and later tends to become diffuse
(4) Interviewers assume a dominant role and tend to discourage unsolicited comments by patients

DIRECTIONS: The groups of questions below consist of lettered choices followed by several numbered items. For each numbered item select the **one** lettered choice with which it is **most** closely associated. Each lettered choice may be used once, more than once, or not at all.

Questions 620-623

For each definition appearing below, choose the statistical term that is most appropriate.

(A) Mean
(B) Median
(C) Standard deviation
(D) t distribution
(E) Normal distribution

620. A bell-shaped frequency distribution curve such as would be generated by plotting the height of a large number of people

621. The arithmetic sum of the observations divided by the number of observations

622. A bell-shaped curve with the tails containing more area than a z distribution

623. The square root of the variance

Questions 624-627

Match the following.

(A) Peabody
(B) Rorschach
(C) Halstead-Reitan
(D) Bender
(E) Wechsler

624. A test originally designed to disclose the structure, dynamics, and boundaries of the personality and that also may produce inferences about intelligence

625. A test originally designed to test visual-motor abilities in children and that also can serve as a test for memory and as a projective test

626. A test battery originally designed to disclose the effects of brain lesions on mental, motor, and sensory performance

627. A test battery originally designed to evaluate cognitive, verbal, and performance abilities and that also can disclose patterns of organic deficit and can be used projectively

Questions 628-631

For each definition appearing below, choose the type of validity that it most accurately describes.

(A) Construct validity
(B) Predictive validity
(C) Correlative validity
(D) Concurrent validity
(E) Content validity

628. The extent to which the items in a rating scale sample the universe of behaviors of interest to the observer; e.g., in a rating scale for depression, how well the items of the rating scale reflect behaviors actually found in depression

629. Relation between test results and another criterion evaluated at about the same time; e.g., a comparison of self-rating depression scale results with ratings made on the basis of clinical judgment

630. Ability of a measuring instrument to forecast another measurement by a different criterion at a later time; e.g., comparison of results of a self-rating depression scale

631. Demonstration that certain explanatory constructs such as depression or anxiety, for example, account for some portion of variability of the ratings

Questions 632-635

Match each group of sounds listed below with the mechanism or type of articulation that it tests.

(A) Palatal closure (palatals or plosives)
(B) Tongue elevation (lingual)
(C) Lip closure (labial)
(D) Sibilants or fricatives
(E) Voiceless consonants

632. P, B, M, or W

633. Sh, Puh, T, and K

634. L, T, or D

635. "See the gray geese"

Diagnostic Procedures
Answers

606. The answer is A. *(Adams, ed 2. p 171.)* The usual order of loss of function in lesions affecting the visual fields is color, form, and movement. Movement is the most resistant function and will remain the longest. The same object that may not be perceived when motionless may be perceived when moving. Complete visual field examination requires evaluation of each of these functions. The size and color of the visual target also influence the sensitivity of visual field testing. Usually, in neurologic diseases that affect the visual fields, red is the first color to become imperceptible.

607. The answer is A. *(DeMyer, ed 3. pp 278-279.)* Air conduction is better than bone conduction in normal persons of all ages. Thus, the efficiency of the usual channel for sound perception through the ear is better than the artificial channel of bone stimulation, which occurs only in a test situation and not in nature. If bone conduction is better than air conduction, a problem exists in the external canal, eardrum, or ossicles. The relative efficiency of bone-versus-air conduction may be tested by placing a vibrating tuning fork on the patient's mastoid process. The patient indicates the instant that the sound disappears. The examiner then places the fork in the air beside the patient's ear, and the individual with normal hearing should still perceive some sound.

608. The answer is D. *(Adams, ed 2. pp 319-320, 445-446. Kaplan, ed 3. pp 274-280.)* Tumors of the cerebral hemispheres that affect the motor or sensory pathways are the most likely to produce signs detectable on the standard neurologic, psychiatric, and psychologic tests. Right posterior parietal lesions manifest by contralateral sensory loss and anosognosia. Right or left posterior frontal lesions manifest by hemiparesis, while intrasellar, parasellar, and occipital lobe lesions are likely to cause visual field defects. Left posterior parasylvian lesions may cause aphasia or components of Gerstmann's syndrome. However, a butterfly glioma, which crosses the corpus callosum, may cause only personality changes early in its course, without causing any of the classical deficits to which the neurologic examination, most psychological tests, and the psychiatric interview are sensitive. Sphenoid ridge or falx meningiomas and lesions of the frontal or temporal poles also may produce mental changes with few or no signs detectable by the classical methods of clinical investigation.

609. The answer is D. *(Adams, ed 2. p 166.)* To inspect the surface of the cornea for corneal deposits or opacifications, an emmetropic examiner would use a strong positive lens in the +15.00 range. Corneal inspection is especially important in patients taking long-term medications such as phenothiazines, which may cause corneal and other ocular changes. Routine checkups of these patients should include corneal inspection with the proper lens to bring the corneal surface into focus. By using successively weaker (less positive) lenses, an examiner can make a series of "tomographic" cuts through the media of the eye until the retina is visualized.

610. The answer is A. *(DeMyer, ed 3. pp 285-289.)* After cold caloric irrigation of the left ear, the eyes deviate slowly to the left and kick back quickly to the right to show a jerk-type of nystagmus. By convention, this would be called nystagmus to the right because nystagmus is named for the quick component; but the deviation phase, the slow phase, is the vestibular component. Irrigation of the left ear with hot water would produce exactly the opposite direction of nystagmus. The eyes would deviate slowly to the right and show the quick, kickback phase to the left. In conventional clinical testing, either hot or cold water is irrigated in one ear then the other, and the duration and amplitude of nystagmus from the two sides are compared. Normally, the results should be about equal for both eyes.

611. The answer is B. *(DeMyer, ed 3. p 118.)* In facing a patient for ophthalmoscopy, the examiner should use the right eye to examine the patient's right eye and the left eye to examine the patient's left eye. If the examiner peers through the ophthalmoscope with the right eye to examine the patient's left eye, for example, the examiner must tilt into an uncomfortable position or rub noses with the patient. Although the examiner may at first find it easier to use only the dominant eye, most persons can learn to use either eye with facility.

612. The answer is D. *(DeMyer, ed 3. pp 339-341.)* The patient described in the question made acceptable drawings of the right half of each figure, but failed to complete the left halves. The ability of the patient to adequately draw half of the picture shows that the deficit on the left side is not due to lack of formal education, paralysis of the limbs, or lack of cooperation. A patient with a right parietal lobe lesion characteristically can complete the right half of drawings but errs in trying to complete the left half. The patient ignores stimuli from the left half of space and has constructional apraxia for the left half of drawings. Patients with diffuse cerebral disease may display other types of constructional or drawing apraxia, but they will not show the specific defect limited to the left side.

613. The answer is C (2, 4). *(Adams, ed 2. p 24.)* Some organic psychoses characteristically cause little or no change in the EEG. The EEG can identify the cause for the psychosis in such disorders as petit mal status by showing the continuing epileptiform discharges. It can assist in diagnosing an organic psychosis by displaying nonspecific changes such as generalized slowing, or it may remain normal even in a patient affected with an alcohol withdrawal syndrome or who suffers from intoxication by hallucinogens. Thus, an organic psychosis may be accompanied by either a normal or an abnormal EEG. A normal EEG in the presence of an organic psychosis is compatible with a metabolic derangement such as alcoholism or some types of drug intoxications. Even in some organic encephalopathies such as Pick's disease, the EEG may remain normal despite evidence of brain atrophy and frank dementia.

614. The answer is A (1, 2, 3). *(Adams, ed 2. pp 18-21.)* Normal alpha rhythm frequently is lower on the left, blocks with eye opening, and disappears during sleep. It also disappears during concentrated thought and is most prominent with the subject in repose. These characteristics help to identify normal alpha rhythm in the EEG and to distinguish it from other rhythms and from abnormal rhythms that imitate it, as occur in alpha coma. Thus, the frequency and amplitude of a rhythm must be correlated with the factors that may influence it to be certain of its identity.

615. The answer is C (2, 4). *(Lazare, p 206.)* Several of the traditional tests used to determine "organicity" lack strong discriminative ability. Failure in tests of orientation to time, person, and place and recall of three unrelated objects do give strong support to the diagnosis of an organic disease. Subtraction of serial sevens and digit repetition do not adequately separate organic and functional deficits. On the subtraction of serial sevens test, introduced originally by Kraepelin, many normal individuals make errors. This is as much a test of attention span as of brain deficit.

616. The answer is C (2, 4). *(Carroll, Lancet 8163:331-332, 1980.)* The overnight dexamethasone suppression test involves oral administration of dexamethasone just before midnight and subsequent measurement of plasma cortisol levels from blood samples drawn at 8 A.M., 4 P.M., and midnight. According to B.J. Carroll et al., only about 40 to 50 percent of patients with "endogenous" depression show an abnormal response to the test (i.e., no suppression of cortisol), as indicated by plasma cortisol values greater than 6 $\mu g/100$ ml in any of the three postdexamethasone blood samples. False positive results are found in only about one percent of comparison populations, including individuals with other forms of depression. These findings indicate that in view of the high percentage of false negative results, the test would not be useful in distinguishing between most cases of "endogenous" depression and other forms of depression. Nor would the test help to differentiate "neurotic" or "anxious" depression from other forms of psychiatric illness. Carroll et al. point out that the dexamethasone suppression test is most likely to be useful in patients exhibiting an important "neurotic" or "characterological" component in which there is a difference of opinion about whether a trial period of somatic therapy is warranted. When treatment response is positive, the test response becomes normal; therefore, the test can be used to follow somatic treatment in test-positive individuals.

617. The answer is A (1, 2, 3). *(Adams, ed 2. p 295.)* The Wechsler Adult Intelligence Scale subtests vary in their sensitivity to brain impairment. Those scores that depend most heavily on premorbid levels of language and language-related skills are in general better preserved in patients with organic brain disease. On other subtests, however, such as arithmetic, digit-span, digit-symbol, and block design, such individuals will score relatively poorly. Thus, comparison of subtest scores provides more information than a simple record of performance, verbal IQ, and full-scale IQ.

618. The answer is B (1, 3). *(Adams, ed 2. pp 22-23.)* The EEG shows a concomitant epileptiform discharge during most, but not all, seizures. In trying to distinguish between organic and functional seizures, the EEG is not an infallible aid. Myoclonic seizures, psychomotor seizures with deep temporal foci, and some focal sensory or motor seizures can occur without concomitant EEG changes. On the other hand, generalized motor seizures and classical petit mal seizures virtually always show concomitant EEG changes. With myoclonic epilepsy, the seizures often occur without a concomitant EEG discharge even when the record shows multiple spikes. The appearance of the spikes and of the seizures show no direct correlation. Myoclonic seizures may even arise at spinal levels and are not reflected in the EEG. On the other hand, a patient who is simulating a grand mal seizure will lack the usual EEG concomitant of the seizure, thereby providing evidence against an organic origin of that particular seizure.

619. The answer is D (4). *(Usdin, pp 7-14.)* Directive interviewing has an honorable history in all types of medical practice. When used sensitively, physicians can obtain a good idea of the onset and course of symptoms without discomforting their patients. The usual technique requires that the doctor assume a dominant role and ask direct questions that become progressively more focused. This approach generally encourages patients to respond rather briefly without digressing into topics not expressly brought up by the doctor. When a doctor is trying to obtain a psychiatric history or learn about emotional components of an illness, directive interviewing often is unsuitable. In these situations, collaborative exploration usually is the technique of choice. The doctor encourages the patient's spontaneous flow of ideas and feelings, not so much by direct questioning as by making reflective remarks, restating the patient's ideas, or making a general request for more information.

620-623. The answers are: 620-E, 621-A, 622-D, 623-C. *(Kaplan, ed 3. pp 615-625.)* No physician can read the clinical or experimental literature critically without at least a minimum knowledge of experimental design and statistics. Many statistical analyses compare the mean of some variable in an experimental group to the mean of a control group. The mean, or arithmetic average, is defined as the total value of the observations added together, divided by the number of observations, or $\overline{X} = \frac{\Sigma X}{N}$, where $\overline{X}$ is the mean, X is an individual observation, and N is the number of observations. The mean is usually the most useful measure of the central tendency or grouping of the data.

Other measures of central tendency are the median and the mode. The median is the score midpoint between the highest and lowest value. The mode is the most frequently occurring value. The mean, median, and mode will be identical or virtually so for a large number of observations that follow a normal bell-shaped distribution. A bell-shaped curve, for example, would be the curve produced by plotting the heights of a very large number of individuals along the horizontal (X) axis and the frequency of each height along the vertical (Y) axis.

To describe the numerical characteristics of a population requires knowledge of the variation of the data. The values used for this purpose are the range, variance, and standard deviation. The range is the difference between the highest and lowest values in the data. The variance is the average squared deviation of the individual values from the mean. Each value is subtracted from the mean, squared, and then the products are added together and divided by the number of observations, as shown by the following formula for the variance (s) of a sample: $s^2 = \frac{\Sigma(x - \overline{x})^2}{n - 1}$.

The square root (square root of the mean square deviation) of the variance is the standard deviation: $s = \sqrt{\frac{\Sigma(x - \overline{x})^2}{n - 1}}$. The advantage of squaring all deviations from the mean is that all negative values when squared are converted to positive values, which can then be added together and divided by N to get an average deviation of the values from the mean.

A *t*-distribution resembles a bell-shaped normal distribution but has more area in the two tails of the curve. The *t*-distribution reflects the fact that for small samples (30 or fewer) the standard deviation, on the average, will be larger than for an infinite population. Therefore, in order to achieve statistical significance with small numbers of subjects, the difference between the control and experimental groups has to be greater than is the case with large numbers of subjects.

624-627. The answers are: 624-B, 625-D, 626-C, 627-E. *(Kaplan, ed 3. pp 931-955.)* Among the widely used psychological tests with clinical application are those devised by Rorschach, Wechsler, Bender, and by Halstead and Reitan. As originally designed, each test was meant to serve some specific purpose, such as intelligence testing, assessment of personality structure, or evaluation of sensory perception. Some of the tests also assess motor function. Although designed to serve a specific goal, each test allows the interpreter to draw certain conclusions about a patient's mental capacity, psychodynamics, and the organic integrity of the patient's brain. Clinicians must have knowledge of the validity and sensitivity of the tests for each of these various aspects of brain function.

Wechsler tests are available in two forms, one for adults and another for children. Results of these tests are widely used by clinicians to derive IQ scores and to make inferences about the organic integrity of the brain, although in this regard the tests' limitations need fuller appreciation. While some examiners use the Wechsler test results projectively to assess personality structure, either the Rorschach or Bender tests, or the Minnesota Multiphasic Personality Index, are much more commonly used for this purpose. The IQ score is derived as a Full-Scale score, a Verbal score, and Performance score. Certain brain lesions will be reflected in the test scores, but a normal Wechsler score does not exclude organic disorders of the brain. In general, patients with right hemisphere lesions score poorly on the Performance scales, and those with left hemisphere lesions score poorly on the Verbal scales. As arbitrarily incorporated in the scaling, the Verbal and Performance IQs in normal subjects should be about the same. Any large discrepancy suggests an organic disorder, but Wechsler test results alone can neither establish nor exclude an organic lesion. The results have to be integrated with the information from a patient's history, physical examination, neuroradiological studies, EEG, or autopsy findings before a diagnosis can be made.

Lauretta Bender adopted the Gestalt figures of Wertheimer to test the visual-motor skills of children as a function of their maturation and to study the effects of brain lesions and retardation. The patient copies nine designs, which are then scored for accuracy, rotation, relation to each other, excesses or deletions, size, and pressure of lines. Generally, children younger than three cannot perform the test, whereas most normal 10-12-year-old children can. Because the examiner gives few instructions, patients are compelled to call upon their own resources. While some overlap exists between subjects who are normal and those who have brain damage, brain damaged subjects, in general, perform less well than normal subjects. Usually, patients with right parietal lobe lesions perform least well, whereas patients with lesions in other locations may produce essentially normal results. By asking a subject to produce the designs without looking at the originals, the examiner can test the patient's memory. By interpreting the distortions in the patient's drawings, the examiner may make inferences about the personality dynamics of the patient.

The Rorschach test requires the subject to respond to ten cards with inkblot figures, some of which are multicolored. What patients perceive from the relatively formless figures expresses their personality. A major criticism of the test is that the personality of the interpreter cannot always be separated from that of the patient. The examiner scores a patient's responses according to location determinants and content. The location refers to the areas of the figure to which the patient responds, as well as to whether the response involves the figure partially or as a whole. A large number of responses to the figure as a whole is associated with high intelligence and organizational ability. The content score indicates the breadth and range of the patient's interests and includes whether the patient responds in human, animal, sexual, or natural terms. The determinants of each response indicate the factors that made the patient produce the particular response—such as the form, shading, color, and sense of apparent movement. For example, an over-emphasis on form would suggest an inhibited rigid personality; a lack of form might suggest inadequate control, inability to comply, or poor organizational ability. (The Murray Thematic Apperception test has applications similar to the Rorschach. The Sentence Completion Test also has similar projective uses, but is thought to tap data at a more conscious level than the other projective tests like the Rorschach and the Murray.)

The Halstead-Reitan battery was devised because the psychological instruments available in the 1940s, such as the Wechsler, Rorschach, and Bender tests, too often failed to disclose abnormalities in patients with confirmed brain lesions. Halstead, at the University of Chicago, and Reitan, at Indiana University School of Medicine, worked with patients from neurological and neurosurgical services who had confirmed brain lesions. They devised new tests and new interpretations of old tests based on empirical correlations of test results with clinical, neuroradiologic, and postmortem findings. The resultant battery includes the new versions of the Wechsler, the Halstead category tests, and a variety of motor and sensory tests. Originally designed to evaluate adults, a battery is now available for children as young as five years of age. The battery requires several hours to administer, but includes the widest variety of tests and yields the most complete assessment of brain function of any neuropsychological instrument now available. The work has put to final rest a holy grail of psychologists, which was to develop a **single** test for brain damage. The complexity and range of brain functions cannot be tested on one dimension. Clinical conclusions based on converging lines of evidence from many sources are far more secure than conclusions relying on a single pathognomonic finding, which, when present, relieves the clinician of having to struggle with the diagnosis. The Halstead-Reitan battery, with its many cognitive, performance, and sensory tasks—some taken from the standard neurological examination—recognizes this principle.

628-631. The answers are: 628-E, 629-D, 630-B, 631-A. *(Kaplan, ed 3. pp 2401-2404.)* Behavior-rating instruments are usually examined for several types of validity. Validity is defined as the extent of the usefulness of the measuring instrument for a specific purpose of the user, who is generally engaged in research. Before the validity of any scale can be determined, its reliability must be estimated. Reliability, defined as the consistency of the instrument in differentiating one subject from the other, is most efficiently determined by applying correlational measures to ratings established by different judges. In subjects who rate themselves, reliability is determined by comparing scores of two halves of the instrument. No rating instrument can have validity without adequate reliability.

While all forms of validity are interrelated, there are differences and it is possible for a rating scale to have one form of validity and lack another. Before researchers decide to use a particular scale, they must determine whether it has content validity—i.e., does the scale in fact measure the behavior that the researcher intends to measure.

A second important type of validity, concurrent validity, is determined by comparing test results with some independent criterion of measurement. For example, the scores of a self-rated depression scale could be compared with the clinical judgment of a psychiatrist following an interview. The measurement of change in a patient's clinical condition over a period of time following treatment is also a form of concurrent validity.

In predictive validity, a determination is made as to how well a measuring instrument can predict another measurement by another means at a later time. Some scales are designed to have predictive ability, such as those that foretell the follow-up status of schizophrenic patients. The difference between concurrent and predictive validity involves differences in the time periods when the criterion measures are obtained; i.e., concurrent validity measures are performed at the same time, and predictive measures at different times.

Construct validity refers to the extent that an instrument measures an explanatory construct. A researcher must make predictions that certain types of scores will be obtained if the test adequately measures the researcher's construct. If the researcher is interested in inferred and unobservable processes, the construct validity is important.

Several rating scales, in addition to clinical judgment, are commonly used by investigators in evaluating treatment procedures in psychiatric patients to allow adequate determinations of validity.

632-635. The answers are: 632-C, 633-E, 634-B, 635-A. *(DeMyer, ed 3. pp 160-163.)* The medical interview provides physicians with the opportunity to listen to and explore a patient's speech production. The sounds P, B, and M are labials. They require strong lip action—lip closure in particular—for their adequate articulation. Patients with unilateral or bilateral facial palsies have difficulty producing the labials, as do patients with extrapyramidal rigidities.

Sh, Puh, T, and K variously require tongue, lip, and palatal articulations. What they have in common is the fact that they are voiceless consonants. Their articulation, while commonly accompanied by phonation, does not require it. A patient with hysterical aphonia may produce all these sounds and may whisper, proving that the articulation mechanisms remain intact.

L, T, and D are lingual sounds. Lingual sounds require that the tip of the tongue elevate to the roof of the mouth for their production. Patients with tongue palsies have difficulty producing these sounds.

"See the gray geese" tests palatal action in the production of the vowel sounds A and E, and the plosive G. These sounds require competent palatal closure in order to direct a strong puff of air into the mouth. Other plosives are Kuh and Puh.

Knowledge of the various mechanisms and types of articulation enable the clinician to diagnose the common forms of neurologic disturbance of speech expressed in control of the mouth, lips, and throat. Speech disturbances at the neuromuscular levels have to be distinguished from the forms of dysarthria caused by lesions of the cerebrum and cerebellum. Higher level speech disturbances include plateau speech as displayed in parkinsonism, scanning speech resulting from cerebellar lesions, pseudobulbar speech associated with bilateral upper motor neuron lesions, the aphasias, and stuttering. Thus, analysis of speech disorders requires an orderly search through the central and peripheral mechanisms involved. The thought processes of language, cerebral-cerebellar control, phonation and articulation, as well as the neural control of breathing, all may produce patterns of disordered speech characteristic of the mechanisms involved.

Miscellaneous

DIRECTIONS: Each question below contains five suggested answers. Choose the **one best** response to each question.

636. During the colonial period of the United States (from about 1647 until 1790), the prevailing attitudes or practices concerning the management of mentally ill persons are reflected most accurately in which of the following statements?

(A) The concepts of Roger Williams took hold early in the 18th century
(B) The ideas of the Tukes and of Philippe Pinel were influential and widely practiced in the mid-18th century
(C) All insane people were considered to be witches, and most were tortured and burned at the stake
(D) Most insane persons were jailed, sold into slavery, or ignored
(E) Most mentally ill individuals were cared for in large municipal institutions

637. The prevalence of a disease is defined as the

(A) number of cases per 100,000 of the population
(B) number of cases in a certain area at a certain time
(C) number of newly diagnosed cases per year
(D) median number of cases found during a unit of time
(E) ratio of new cases to live born infants

638. As used in reporting clinical studies, the term "statistically significant" means that

(A) it has been proved that the events studied have a cause and effect relationship
(B) the likelihood that the results obtained could have occurred by chance is acceptably small
(C) the studies have established a scientific truth and need not be replicated for purposes of additional validation
(D) the observed result has clinical significance
(E) the original design of the study was valid

639. Current knowledge about sensory-perceptual differences between psychiatric and nonpsychiatric patients is adequately described by which of the following statements?

(A) A recent technological advance is on the verge of revealing important new data
(B) It has been proved that lack of motivation is the chief cause of any demonstrated differences
(C) Patient reports alone suggest such differences, but these are not reliable
(D) If differences exist, they are small and difficult to demonstrate
(E) None of the above

640. Prediction of those individuals who are most likely to prove dangerous is best achieved on the basis of

(A) the standard psychiatric interview
(B) the Legal Dangerousness Scale
(C) formulation of a patient's psychodynamics
(D) electroencephalography
(E) judicial opinion

641. The Social Security Administration, in judging a person's eligibility for disabled worker benefits, uses which of the following sets of guidelines for determining if a mental disorder impairs the individual's ability to work?

(A) Two licensed practitioners, one of whom must be a board certified psychiatrist or psychologist, must submit a diagnosis of a major mental disorder, e.g., schizophrenia or manic-depressive psychosis

(B) Any hospitalization for at least one month for any type of psychiatric disorder as defined in *DSM-III* constitutes disability. Disability payments cease upon release from the hospital, except for cases of undue hardship.

(C) Psychiatric disorders are divided into four groups, each having a set of clinical findings, of which at least one must be present, and a set of functional restrictions, all of which must be present

(D) While medical and psychological reports of practitioners are considered, the major evidence comes from personal interviews by a Social Security representative with both the applicant and a family member

(E) The applicant must have been hospitalized for at least 2 weeks in a psychiatric hospital or ward, during which time the treating psychiatrist will evaluate the patient's capacity to work either full- or part-time

DIRECTIONS: Each question below contains four suggested answers of which **one** or **more** is correct. Choose the answer

A	if	1, 2, and 3	are correct
B	if	1 and 3	are correct
C	if	2 and 4	are correct
D	if	4	is correct
E	if	1, 2, 3, and 4	are correct

642. Psychiatrists who accept high-level administrative posts may find their clinical training to be a liability because they

(1) appreciate the interpersonal relations of staff members and factions of the organization
(2) make immediate decisions that may hurt or cause anxiety among particular staff members
(3) recognize the resistance of staff members to the authoritarian symbolism of the institution
(4) accept and implement broad principles that may disrupt individuals or groups within the organization

643. The child psychiatrist, in preparing reports for the juvenile court, should follow which of the following procedures?

(1) Be as inclusive as possible so that the judge can have a full picture of the problem
(2) Avoid medical and psychological terms
(3) Summarize for the court all reports from other agencies
(4) End the report with treatment recommendations for both the child and family

644. Objectionable modes of physical restraint and treatment of mentally ill persons in the late 18th century were eliminated with the material assistance of

(1) Grand Duke Peter Leopold of Florence
(2) Vincenzo Chiarugi of Italy
(3) William Tuke of England
(4) Philippe Pinel of France

645. Mental illness among blacks and whites is accurately described by which of the following statements?

(1) The number of blacks admitted to mental hospitals or psychiatric units is proportionately higher than that of whites
(2) The incidence of Alzheimer's disease is much greater among blacks than whites
(3) Psychoneuroses are less commonly diagnosed in blacks than whites, and psychosis and alcoholism much more commonly diagnosed
(4) Genetic factors explain the differences in mental illness between whites and blacks

646. Real differences between community psychiatry and traditional clinical psychiatry probably are reflected in which of the following statements?

(1) Community psychiatry is more committed to the general population than to individual patients
(2) There are differences in the organizational approach to providing services
(3) Community psychiatry implies more responsibility for providing for all of the mental health needs of a given population
(4) Despite similarities in specific treatment modalities, community psychiatry uses more neuroleptic medications

647. The testamentary capacity of patients to make a will is determined by ascertaining that

(1) they understand that they are engaged in making a will
(2) they are aware of the nature and extent of their property
(3) they comprehend who are their beneficiaries
(4) their emotional reactions to family members are duly recorded

648. Interest in the ethics of the psychiatric profession was renewed as a consequence of the

(1) refusal of a California psychiatrist to reveal the details of psychotherapy of his patient, who sued an assailant for causing his psychiatric difficulties (1969)

(2) failure of a United States senator to make public disclosure, prior to his nomination (1972) as a vice-presidential candidate, of psychiatric treatment he had received earlier in his career

(3) burglarizing of a psychiatrist's office to obtain the records of a patient who was to be tried for treason (1973)

(4) formulation by the United States Supreme Court of a new set of rules of evidence clarifying the nature of doctor-patient confidentiality to be used in Federal courts (1973)

649. The "right to treatment" doctrine for committed patients empowers the state to

(1) place a patient in the least restrictive environment

(2) define appropriate treatment

(3) specify physical facilities and staffing requirements for treatment

(4) confine nondangerous mentally ill persons without providing treatment

650. Correct statements applying to the civil rights of a patient adjudged neither insane nor incompetent, but committed to virtually any mental hospital in the United States, include which of the following?

(1) Commitment to a mental hospital requires a court hearing

(2) The patient loses the right to initiate legal proceedings

(3) Relatives or other interested parties may petition for the commitment

(4) The patient automatically loses the right to vote, marry or divorce, and to buy and sell or dispose of property

DIRECTIONS: The groups of questions below consist of lettered choices followed by several numbered items. For each numbered item select the **one** lettered choice with which it is **most** closely associated. Each lettered choice may be used once, more than once, or not at all.

Questions 651-655

Match the following.

(A) *Mens rea*
(B) *Lex talionis*
(C) *Non compos mentis*
(D) *Habeas corpus*
(E) *Parens patriae*

651. The right to challenge the lawfulness of detention

652. Lack of capacity to exercise sound judgment

653. The guilty mind

654. Retributive justice

655. The right of the state to hold in custody a dangerous individual

Questions 656-660

For each contribution to the historical development of psychodynamic ideas that follows, choose the worker with whom it is most commonly associated.

(A) Hippolyte-Marie Bernheim
(B) Pierre Janet
(C) Alfred Adler
(D) Carl Jung
(E) Karen Horney

656. Devised the word association test for uncovering unconscious personality conflicts

657. Evolved ideas that led to the concept of "dissociation"

658. First to emphasize cultural determination of neurosis, including "masculine protest" as a reaction of women to their inferior social status

659. Among the first psychiatrists to suggest a psychological approach to studying schizophrenia

660. Probably first to use the term "psychoneurosis" in connection with hysteria

Miscellaneous Answers

636. The answer is D. *(Kaplan, ed 3. pp 4-98.)* The prevailing attitude in the American colonies toward insane people was that they should be punished. This attitude led to various inhumane practices. One of the most infamous was the series of witch trials in Salem, Massachusetts, in 1692, leading to the deaths of 23 people, mainly by hanging. Even though a year later all survivors accused of witchcraft were released, superstitious and punitive attitudes lingered until the end of the 18th century. Most insane people were either jailed, boarded out in private homes where they were exploited, sold as slaves, or left to fend for themselves. The American colonies' first general hospital, the Pennsylvania Hospital in Philadelphia, which opened in the mid-18th century, was also the first to accept mentally ill persons as in-patients. However, it was not until the 1790s that the enlightened ideas of Roger Williams, founder of Rhode Island colony, William Tuke, an English Quaker, and Philippe Pinel, a French physician, began to gain widespread support, thereby leading to significant reform in the care of emotionally disturbed persons during the 19th century.

637. The answer is B. *(Kaplan, ed 3. p 628.)* The prevalence of a disease refers to the number of cases existing in a certain geographical area at a certain time. The unit of time and the geographic area may vary with the use for which the prevalence figure is derived. Prevalence differs from incidence, which is defined as the number of new cases that occur during a **period** of time. Incidence and prevalence statistics have different uses. A short-lived, seasonal disease might have a zero prevalence on a given day for a given area, whereas a chronic disease, even though much less common, might have a greater prevalence.

638. The answer is B. *(Kaplan, ed 3. pp 618-620.)* The term "statistically significant" means that the likelihood that a given result could have occurred by chance has been estimated mathematically and is found to be acceptably small. When the results of treated and untreated groups of patients are compared, chance will cause some difference in the results. Statisticians have developed methods to estimate the likelihood that any given difference between groups could occur by chance. If it is likely that the difference could have occurred by chance, then the likelihood of a relationship between cause and effect is reduced—not eliminated, but reduced. If it is unlikely that the difference could have occurred by chance, then a relationship between cause and effect is more likely. A statistically significant result proves neither the truth of the original proposition, nor the validity of the original design or conception, nor the clinical significance or importance of the results. One of the requirements for scientific proof, even if a study appears to be soundly designed and to have statistically significant results, is that the study be replicated.

639. The answer is D. *(Kaplan, ed 3. pp 344-345.)* One reason for researchers' extreme interest in sensory and perceptual functions is the frequent verbal reports by psychiatric patients of disturbances in these functions. However, researchers have had difficulty in convincingly demonstrating the existence of such disturbances. There are several reasons for this phenomenon. First, any sensory and perceptual differences between psychiatric and nonpsychiatric patients probably are small, and the instruments used for detection would need to be extremely sensitive. Second, when significant differences have been reported, an explanation often proffered is that psychiatric patients have not been as well motivated as the nonpsychiatric controls. However, researchers also have not convincingly demonstrated the validity of this response bias. Even though patient reports remain as the chief evidence of sensory disturbance, these reports should be taken seriously and continuing efforts made to improve research techniques. While techniques to measure sensory and perceptual phenomena have grown steadily, particularly methods for computing average transient evoked brain waves by computer analysis, a breakthrough in knowledge is not imminent. Much solid work is needed to control for artifacts and to detect response bias.

640. The answer is B. *(Kolb, ed 9. pp 872-874.)* The problem of predicting how dangerous an individual may become remains unsolved. Dangerousness is defined as violent, assaultive behavior against other persons. Standard psychiatric and neurologic methods of investigation fail to provide information of strong predictive value. In fact, medical experts cannot be said to predict dangerousness any better than other individuals. What is more, the accuracy in predicting which of those individuals already in custody for a serious offense will become dangerous may well be no better than chance. A high score on the Legal Dangerousness Scale seems to have the best predictive value. Items such as severity of the previous crime, previous arrests and convictions, and juvenile delinquency are factors that are scored on this scale.

641. The answer is C. *(American Medical Association, pp 52-56.)* Eligibility for cash benefits to disabled persons who are unable to work is determined by the special Disability Determination Unit of the Social Security Administration, whose representatives never see the applicant but require medical documentation of symptoms and laboratory findings. Neither the presence of symptoms alone nor the applicant's statement of inability to work is sufficient evidence for the award of claims. The definition of disability is "inability to engage in any substantial gainful activity" because of mental or physical illness "which can be expected to result in death or has lasted or can be expected to last for a continuous period of not less than 12 months." To determine disability because of mental illness, the Social Security Administration considers that diagnosis alone is insufficient as an estimate of the severity of the illness. Criteria of severity have been arranged into four groups: chronic brain syndromes, functional psychoses, functional nonpsychoses, and mental retardation. Consideration is given to the degree of limitation in a patient's daily activity, the patient's range of interests, ability to care for personal needs, and relationship to others. Because patients frequently are confined to, and released from, institutions for reasons other than severity of illness, duration and severity of impairment are based on documented medical and laboratory evidence from all available sources.

642. The answer is C (2, 4). *(Kaplan, ed 3. pp 3094-3095.)* Psychiatrists, by virtue of their clinical training, offer both assets and liabilities in the carrying out of high-level administrative responsibilities. Those qualities that generally are helpful include an ability to understand the dynamics of relations between staff members, a willingness to show patience with resistant colleagues and to bring conflicts into the open, and a potential for settling disputes. On the other hand, psychiatrists may overlook broad institutional problems because of overinvolvement either in personal difficulties afflicting individuals or in the problems of small groups. Thus, out of solicitude for individual feelings, the psychiatrist-administrator may fail to make decisions necessary for efficient functioning of the institution. The psychiatrist's clinical sensitivities may forestall decisions that, in Hirschowitz's words, "require swift political action."

643. The answer is C (2, 4). *(Barker, ed 3. pp 204-209.)* Child psychiatrists should follow several basic principles in helping the courts to understand both the child and family appearing before them. Thus, physicians should prepare reports in clear, short sentences that avoid ambiguities and employ terms understood by the laity. The report should be sufficiently informative to assist a court in reaching a practical and just decision. Information from other agencies and examiners should not be repeated, except for special reasons. In addition to supplying a diagnosis, recommendations for treating both child and parents are helpful to a judge, because most children appearing in juvenile court do not have a "major psychiatric condition."

644. The answer is E (all). *(Kaplan, ed 3. pp 4-98.)* Philippe Pinel (1745-1826), superintendent of the Bicêtre and Salpêtrière in Paris, achieved renown for dramatically freeing mental patients from physical bondage during the Reign of Terror. Two other individuals, Vincenzo Chiarugi (1759-1820) of the Hospital Bonifacio in Florence, Italy, and William Tuke (1732-1822), founder of the Retreat near York, England, accomplished the same feat in their hospitals. However, Dr. Pinel's fame soon outstripped theirs. These three men did not work in a vacuum. The politics of Florence, led by the Grand Duke Peter Leopold (1747-1792), fostered many social reforms, including the passage in 1774 of the insanity law to protect mental patients. The Grand Duke himself was responsible for building the Hospital Bonifacio and for appointing Dr. Chiarugi as medical director. In England, as early as 1671 the Society of Friends advocated reform in the treatment of mental patients. All of the Tukes, i.e., grandfather William, son Henry, and grandson Samuel, were Quakers and spent their lives in administering the York Retreat. They were aided throughout by the Society of Friends. In France, although Josephe Daquin (1733-1815) in 1791 pushed for humane treatment of the insane, he was not in a position of power and did not become widely known. Consequently, Pinel, in contrast to Chiarugi and William Tuke, worked alone during the political instability and violence of the Reign of Terror, receiving much acclaim for his courage.

645. The answer is B (1, 3). *(Kolb, ed 9. pp 171-172.)* Scant accurate data are available for comparing the incidence of mental illness in whites and blacks. While it is known that the rate of admission of blacks to psychiatric hospitals exceeds that of whites, it is not known whether the criteria for diagnosis and the conditions of delivery of medical care cause the apparent difference or whether the data reflect a real difference. In the absence of scientifically valid population studies, it cannot be stated whether psychoneuroses or psychoses have a greater incidence in one group or another, in spite of the fact that psychoses and alcoholism are diagnosed proportionately more often in blacks than whites. Unless these cultural factors can be controlled, any conclusion about a genetic basis for differences in mental health, or about diseases like Alzheimer's disease that have a genetic component, would be invalid.

646. The answer is A (1, 2, 3). *(Kaplan, ed 3. pp 2841-2842.)* Clinical psychiatry as practiced before the advent of community psychiatry employed all the techniques of treatment that are practiced in community psychiatry today. The fundamental differences between the two approaches probably relate more to organization of delivery of services and to the primary commitments of each. Traditional psychiatry's primary purpose is to treat the individual patient, whereas community psychiatry movement is committed to treatment of a whole population—which is not to imply neglect of the individual. Rather, community psychiatry was conceived to provide all needed mental health services, including prevention, throughout its catchment area.

647. The answer is E (all). *(Kolb, ed 9. pp 880-881.)* Generally, psychiatrists must follow three criteria to determine the testamentary capacity of patients to make a will. Patients must fully recognize (1) that they are making a will, (2) what property they have to dispose of, and (3) the persons or institutions to whom they wish to distribute their legacy. Thus, in conducting interviews for this purpose, psychiatrists should require that a patient describe the nature of a will, recite the character and extent of the property, and name the beneficiaries. In addition, a psychiatrist should observe the emotional reactions of a patient to family members in an attempt to discern whether a family member is exercising undue influence, or whether the patient is experiencing paranoid delusions that would unfairly exclude a family member. The psychiatrist then reports these observations to the legal authorities.

648. The answer is E (all). *(Kaplan, ed 3. pp 3216-3217.)* Although ethics in the practice of psychiatry has always been a matter of concern to psychiatrists, the last decade has witnessed a decided resurgence of interest in the subject. Several events that were brought to national attention by the public media contributed largely to this renewed interest. Among these events were the resignation in 1972 of Senator Eagleton as a vice-presidential nominee for failure to reveal his previous psychiatric treatment, and in 1973 the break-in of the office of the psychiatrist of Daniel Ellsberg, who was accused of treason for theft of the "Pentagon papers." Even more effective, if less dramatic, in protecting the rights of patients was the United States Supreme Court's ruling in 1973 that patients have the right to refuse to disclose, and the right to prevent any other person from disclosing, confidential communications made in the course of their psychiatric diagnosis or treatment. Psychiatric and medical ethics is a complex subject whose focus continues to change with changing international, national, and local issues. Nevertheless, the profession needs to exercise vigilance in its reevaluation of ethical perspectives and its recommitment to ethical ideals.

649. The answer is A (1, 2, 3). *(Kolb, ed 9. p 878.)* The "right to treatment" doctrine came into existence in the early 1960s. It holds that if the state has the right to commit individuals to a mental institution, it may not deprive them of the right to treatment and must, therefore, provide treatment. In states that have adopted the doctrine, the tendency has been for the court to define the treatment, thus encroaching, to some extent, upon the domain of the medical profession. The legislation supporting an individual's right to be treated generally defines the physical facilities and staffing necessary to provide treatment. In defining such facilities, the law also may require the least restrictive environment for the individual who is committed. A corollary of the "right to treatment" doctrine is that a nondangerous mentally ill or mentally defective patient who does not need, or cannot be benefited by, treatment should not be committed. Such legislation should have a profound effect on state institutions and commitment policies.

650. The answer is B (1, 3). *(Kolb, ed 9. pp 874-877.)* Involuntary commitment of an individual to a mental hospital requires a court hearing. The hearing may be initiated by relatives or other interested parties. The patient loses neither the right to initiate legal proceedings nor the right to have a hearing on the legality of the commitment or imprisonment. Patients retain their legal rights—and those civil rights not impaired by mental illness—if they are adjudged neither insane nor incompetent. If judged insane or incompetent, patients lose such civil rights as the right to marry, divorce, make a will, and dispose of property. The determination of competency to exercise civil rights may be separated from the commitment process per se, but in some states commitment necessarily implies a judgment of incompetency. In the case of individuals who are declared insane or incompetent to manage their affairs, the court will appoint a legal guardian to protect their interest until competency is declared by another hearing.

651-655. The answers are: 651-D, 652-C, 653-A, 654-B, 655-E. *(DeMyer, ed 3. pp 229, 240. Kolb, ed 9. p 870.)* The traditional approach to crime and punishment holds that individuals are endowed with free will and therefore are responsible for their behavior, and that the threat of punishment deters antisocial behavior. According to these concepts, a person who by free will chooses to commit antisocial acts should receive punishment as a deterrence against such acts in the future, as well as a deterrence to persons who might otherwise be tempted to commit similar acts. When an antisocial act has been judged the result of free will, the doctrine of *lex talionis* applies. This doctrine, enunciated in the code of Hammurabi, justifies the taking of "an eye for an eye or a tooth for a tooth." Offenders are punished in kind for their misdeeds. Traditional doctrine holds that the degree of punishment depends on the state of mind of the person, which supposedly can be determined by the court's evaluation of legal and psychiatric evidence. It is, of course, possible to challenge every one of these assumptions. Nevertheless, some legal machinery is required to protect society.

The doctrine of *parens patriae* holds that the state may intervene and hold in custody persons deemed dangerous to themselves or others. This doctrine leads to commitment procedures for those individuals judged incompetent, insane, or dangerous to self or others.

All societies recognize that mental illness and dementia may ameliorate the doctrine of responsibility. The doctrine of *non compos mentis* recognizes that patients thus affected may lack the capacity to exercise free will, and therefore are less responsible for their behavior.

The concept of *mens rea,* the guilty mind, applies to a person accused of an antisocial act who is capable of having committed the act with deliberation and malice aforethought. If the accused individual is judged not to have the guilty mind, the punishment is correspondingly ameliorated. The psychiatrist's role has been to advise the court of the mental state of the accused individual. The court then decides on the weight to be accorded this information in setting the sentence, either for a prison term or detention in a mental institution.

The right of *habeas corpus* refers to the right of any detained person to have a hearing to determine the legality of the detainment. At a hearing, a judge will decide on the legality of the procedures involved in confining the person. This right applies to prisoners as well as to patients in mental institutions.

656-660. The answers are: 656-D, 657-B, 658-C, 659-D, 660-A. *(Kolb, ed 9. pp 11-17.)* Modern psychodynamic theory originated with scientists who were mainly concerned with biology and neurology, such as Charles Darwin and later John Hughlings Jackson (1835-1911), who nevertheless wrote that the study of dreams and jokes would elucidate psychological pathology. Sigmund Freud (1856-1939), also a neurologist, was well acquainted with the work of these individuals and later wove their ideas into his own theories. Freud also studied the ideas of Anton Mesmer (1734-1815), who treated disease by "mesmerizing" patients, and those of three famous and influential French physicians who contributed to the study of hypnotism and hysteria—Jean Martin Charcot (1825-1893), Hippolyte-Marie Bernheim (1840-1919), and Pierre Janet (1815-1947). The latter two workers developed concepts that are still valid. Bernheim divested hypnosis of much of its mystery, and probably was the first to identify hysteria and related conditions by the term "psychoneuroses." Janet believed that through a process of "dissociation," certain parts of consciousness acquired a separate existence in hysterical conditions such as multiple personalities and fugue states.

Both Alfred Adler (1870-1937) and Carl Jung (1875-1961) were early students of Freud, but broke with him in disputing the relative importance of infant sexuality in psychodynamics and formation of the personality. Many of Adler's writings concerning neuroses resulting from social pressures seem extremely modern, especially his idea that "masculine protest" in women stemmed from their inferior social position. Jung divided the unconscious into two divisions, one "collective" or "racial" and the other "personal." Some of his other ideas seem quite modern, especially the theories that word association tests are good avenues for exploring unconscious conflicts, and that parents with neuroses can cause behavior disorders in their children.

Other pioneers in psychodynamics, such as Anna Freud, Heinz Hartman, and Karen Horney, elaborated and expanded freudian theory. Another influential psychodynamist, Adolf Meyer (1866-1950), strayed far from freudian concepts and emphasized the pluralistic origins of personality. The most recent development in freudian psychodynamics is an attempt to synthesize psychoanalytic theories with those of the behavioralists such as Ivan Pavlov and B. F. Skinner.

Neurology Questions for Psychiatrists

DIRECTIONS: Each question below contains five suggested answers. Choose the **one best** response to each question.

661. The white appearance of the normal physiologic cup of the optic disk may be attributed to the fact that the

(A) optic nerve fibers are myelinated
(B) lamina cribrosa is exposed centrally
(C) lamina cribrosa bulges forward
(D) optic disk has drusen at that site
(E) cup normally undergoes ossification

662. Complete interruption of the right optic tract would produce

(A) bitemporal hemianopia
(B) right homonymous hemianopia
(C) left homonymous hemianopia
(D) right homonymous quadrantanopia
(E) left homonymous quadrantanopia

663. The second-order neuron for the dorsal column pathway is located

(A) at the level of entry of the primary axon into the cord
(B) within 1-2 segments of the level of entry of the primary axon
(C) at the medullocervical junction
(D) in the reticular formation
(E) in the thalamus

664. The site at which even a small lesion will produce complete loss of consciousness with minimal effects on other functions is the

(A) medullary tegmentum
(B) caudal pontine tegmentum
(C) midbrain tegmentum
(D) diencephalon
(E) cerebral cortex

665. An adult patient examined for schizophrenic symptoms is found to have mild ptosis of one eyelid. The eyelid elevates when the patient looks up. The patient has no ocular complaints and the remainder of the physical examination is normal. The best management would be to

(A) do an angiogram because of the possibility of a carotid aneurysm
(B) obtain a CAT scan to exclude a mass lesion compressing the IIIrd nerve
(C) do a sweat test for hemifacial anhidrosis
(D) request the patient to provide a childhood photograph
(E) request an ophthalmology consultation

666. The ocular muscle that has **only** a primary action and no secondary or tertiary action is the

(A) superior oblique
(B) inferior oblique
(C) superior rectus
(D) inferior rectus
(E) lateral rectus

667. The optic nerve fibers arise from the retinal

(A) rods
(B) cones
(C) amacrine cells
(D) bipolar cells
(E) ganglion cells

244

668. As a generalization, the axons that arise from the catecholaminergic nuclei of the brain stem are said to be

(A) poorly myelinated or unmyelinated
(B) richly myelinated
(C) about equally myelinated and unmyelinated
(D) myelinated depending on whether ascending or descending
(E) myelinated only if excitatory

669. The combination of dyscalculia, right-left disorientation, and dysgraphia suggests a lesion of the

(A) right posterior parasylvian region
(B) left posterior parasylvian region
(C) right anterior parietal region
(D) left anterior parietal region
(E) right inferior frontal region

670. In testing a patient for minimal or mild hemiparesis, an examiner should pay most attention to which of the following muscles?

(A) The strongest muscles, such as the quadriceps femoris and triceps
(B) The bilaterally acting muscles, such as the trunk muscles
(C) The pectoral and latissimus dorsi muscles
(D) Flexors of the elbows and hips and dorsiflexors of wrists and feet
(E) The sphincter muscles

671. To reinforce a hypoactive quadriceps femoris muscle stretch reflex, an examiner requests the patient to

(A) think about an emotionally stimulating event
(B) count slowly to ten
(C) close the eyes
(D) grasp one hand with the other and pull
(E) walk briskly around the room

672. If an examiner shines light in one eye of a normal person, which of the following pupillary responses occurs?

(A) Both pupils constrict equally
(B) Only the ipsilateral pupil constricts
(C) Only the contralateral pupil constricts
(D) The ipsilateral pupil constricts more than the contralateral one
(E) The contralateral pupil constricts more than the ipsilateral one

673. In bedside testing of a patient for range of ocular movements and for ocular malalignment, an examiner's moving finger (the target) should be placed

(A) as close as possible to the patient's face
(B) no more than 10-15 cm from the patient's face
(C) about 40 cm from the patient's face
(D) at least 200 cm from the patient's face
(E) at "infinity"

674. Ptosis associated with Horner's syndrome (sympathetic denervation) will

(A) disappear or improve when the patient looks up
(B) appear unchanged when the patient looks up
(C) worsen when the patient looks up
(D) worsen when the patient looks down
(E) worsen when the patient looks to the side

675. Auscultation of the carotid artery in the neck of a normal adult usually discloses

(A) heart sounds only
(B) breath sounds only
(C) heart and breath sounds
(D) moderately loud bruits, but no heart or breath sounds
(E) no sounds

676. When fully elevated, the normal soft palate assumes which of the following positions?

(A) It occludes the posterior choanae
(B) It contacts the epiglottis
(C) It contacts the posterior wall of the pharynx
(D) It contacts the roof of the pharynx
(E) It covers the laryngeal opening

677. If a patient displays complete paralysis of some muscles of an extremity with normal power in adjacent muscles of the same extremity, it is most likely that the patient has a

(A) lower motor neuron lesion
(B) upper motor neuron lesion
(C) combined upper and lower motor neuron lesion
(D) motor cortex lesion
(E) myopathy

678. Slow, writing, sustained movements of the trunk are usually classed as

(A) chorea
(B) athetosis
(C) ballismus
(D) dystonia
(E) tics

679. Closing the eyelids as tightly as possible normally results in

(A) a very weak eye closure that is easily overcome by an examiner's fingers
(B) eye closure that is strong enough to require considerable finger strength by an examiner to overcome
(C) much stronger eye closure on the side of the dominant hand
(D) normal myotonic after-contraction of the eyelid that narrows the palpebral fissure
(E) an eyeball that remains partially visible

680. To elicit clonus, an examiner does which of the following?

(A) Quickly jerks a part of the body that is at rest
(B) Slowly jerks a part of the body that is at rest
(C) Quickly jerks a part of the body that is under voluntary tension
(D) Slowly jerks a part of the body that is under voluntary tension
(E) None of the above

681. In the classical precentral motor cortex, the body parts are represented

(A) inversely
(B) upright
(C) only on the lateral aspect of the cerebrum
(D) only on the medial aspect of the cerebrum
(E) in random fashion

682. The swaying (Romberg) test is primarily a test of

(A) cerebellar function
(B) reticular formation function
(C) pyramidal tract function
(D) dorsal column function
(E) parasympathetic function

683. In testing the pupillary light reflex, an examiner should request the patient to

(A) look at a distant point
(B) look at the tip of the patient's own nose
(C) look downward
(D) look directly at the examiner's approaching flashlight
(E) partially close both eyes

684. A light ray striking the nasal side of the retina causes the person to experience a visual image as if it were coming from the

(A) nasal half of space
(B) temporal half of space
(C) midpoint of the horopter
(D) periphery of the horopter
(E) visual axis

685. When a normal person walks straight ahead, the medial margins of the heels fall

(A) more than 30 cm (12 inches) away from the midline
(B) 20-30 cm (8-12 inches) away from the midline
(C) 10-20 cm (4-8 inches) away from the midline
(D) 5-10 cm (2-4 inches) away from the midline
(E) essentially upon the midline

686. The most consistent and reliable sign of cerebellar dysfunction is

(A) unsteadiness of gait
(B) excessive swaying with eyes closed (positive Romberg test)
(C) nystagmus
(D) weakness
(E) dysphagia

687. The single most important part of the motor examination is

(A) elicitation of the plantar reflexes
(B) inspection for fasciculations
(C) strength testing
(D) muscle palpation
(E) watching a patient walk

688. To elicit the triceps surae muscle stretch reflex in a patient who is reclining, the examiner should

(A) straighten the patient's knee completely and apply slight downward pressure on the top of the foot
(B) straighten the patient's knee completely and apply slight upward pressure on the bottom of the patient's foot
(C) flex the patient's knee slightly and apply slight downward pressure on the dorsum of the patient's foot
(D) flex the patient's knee slightly and apply slight upward pressure on the bottom of the patient's foot
(E) request the patient to dorsiflex the foot

689. Which of the following statements about rigidity, in contrast to spasticity, is true?

(A) It is demonstrable only when an examiner quickly moves a patient's extremity
(B) It is demonstrable when an examiner slowly moves a patient's extremity
(C) It requires the exercise of slight voluntary tension by a patient in the extremity being tested
(D) It yields in a clasp-knife manner
(E) It affects mainly extensor muscles

690. In principle, a muscle displays greatest strength when acting from a position of

(A) full extension
(B) slight flexion
(C) half flexion
(D) full flexion
(E) either full flexion or full extension

691. Loss of position sense is first revealed in

(A) the thumb
(B) the index finger
(C) the fourth digit
(D) the little finger
(E) all digits equally

692. The reason for NOT striking a muscle directly to elicit a muscle stretch reflex is that

(A) no response will occur
(B) myoedema may result
(C) the pain for the patient is excessive
(D) a response is possible only by striking a tendon to stretch it
(E) the ensuing contraction could be due to percussion irritability

693. The rigidity of Parkinson's disease usually is expressed in which of the following muscles?

(A) Flexors only
(B) Extensors only
(C) Small muscles, mainly
(D) Large muscles, mainly
(E) Virtually all muscles, to some degree

694. Flaccid upper motor neuron paralysis is most likely to result from a lesion that is

(A) acute and small
(B) acute and large
(C) chronic and small
(D) chronic and large
(E) subacute

695. To elicit a muscle stretch reflex, an examiner grips the reflex hammer

(A) tightly, and strikes with a stiff wrist, using only elbow action
(B) loosely, and strikes with a stiff wrist
(C) loosely, and strikes with a loose, whiplash effect of the wrist
(D) near the striking end (rubber end) of the hammer
(E) with the handle firmly in the palm

696. To elicit the superficial abdominal muscle reflexes, an examiner

(A) instructs the patient to relax the abdominal muscles
(B) asks the patient to take a deep breath and hold it
(C) uses a cold metal object to stimulate the skin
(D) moves the stimulating object very slowly across the skin
(E) does none of the above

697. The receptor for the muscle stretch reflex is

(A) the pacinian corpuscle
(B) the muscle spindle
(C) the extrafusal muscle fiber
(D) located in the tendon
(E) located in the ligaments

698. In a patient with a true extensor toe sign, the toe usually begins to extend in response to a stimulating object

(A) immediately after placing the object on the foot
(B) after the object has moved part way along the foot
(C) only after the object reaches the base of the toes
(D) only after the object curves across the ball of the foot
(E) just as the object is removed

699. An operational, as contrasted to an interpretational, definition of rigidity is that it is the

(A) type of stiffness resulting from basal ganglia lesions
(B) expression of an imbalance between nigral and striatal output
(C) resistance resulting from oversensitivity of the muscle spindles
(D) muscle resistance resulting from underactivity of the dopaminergic pathway from the substantia nigra
(E) plastic resistance felt by an examiner when moving a patient's resting extremity

700. A basic function of the vestibular system is to

(A) counter-roll the eyes against the direction of head movement
(B) move the eyes in the direction of head movement
(C) elevate the eyes against the pull of gravity on the eyelids
(D) depress the eyes in response to gravity
(E) agitate the image on the retina to prevent visual fatigue

701. A frequent sign of meningeal irritation that is disclosed by an examiner's attempt to flex a patient's neck is

(A) tonic extension and supination of the upper extremities
(B) flexion and adduction of the lower extremities
(C) plantar flexion of the toes
(D) clonus of the legs
(E) systemic hypotension

702. Aphasic patients characteristically lose which of the following types of speech?

(A) Automatic, emotional, or expletive speech
(B) Propositional speech
(C) All forms of speech in equal degree
(D) Vowel sounds of speech
(E) Lingual sounds of speech

703. A patient with gait apraxia walks

(A) normally after once initiating the gait
(B) readily on toes or heels but not forward
(C) only on the toes or backward, but initiates the gait quickly
(D) by initiating the gait slowly, using tiny, shuffling steps
(E) by lifting the feet high and placing them irregularly

704. With the eyes in the primary position, in a normal person the free margin of the upper eyelid has which of the following relationships to the cornea?

(A) It lies slightly above the corneal limbus, exposing the sclera
(B) It covers the upper margin of the corneal limbus and iris
(C) It is just tangent to the corneal limbus
(D) It reaches to the pupillary margin
(E) None of the above

705. After sympathetic denervation, the pupil of the eye

(A) dilates because of unopposed tonus in the pupillodilator muscle
(B) dilates because of hypersensitivity of the pupillodilator muscle
(C) constricts because of hypersensitivity of the retina to light
(D) constricts because of denervation hypersensitivity of the pupilloconstrictor muscle
(E) constricts because of unopposed tonus in the pupilloconstrictor muscle

706. With the passage of a nerve impulse, some factor limits the peak magnitude of the reversal of the electrical potential across cell membranes. The factor thought to be of prime importance in setting this limit is

(A) exhaustion of ATP
(B) inhibition of energy production
(C) outflow of potassium ions from the cell
(D) increased permeability of the membrane to water
(E) sudden block in the membrane conductance to sodium

707. Atropine is believed to exert its major pharmacological action by

(A) blocking discharge of synaptic vesicles
(B) blocking acetylcholinesterase
(C) blocking active transport of choline
(D) stimulating production of choline acetyl transferase in the presynaptic endings
(E) combining with the receptor sites on the postsynaptic cell

708. The neurotransmitter of the nigrostriatal pathway is presumed to be

(A) mainly dopamine
(B) dopamine plus norepinephrine in about equal amounts
(C) norepinephrine and serotonin
(D) mainly serotonin
(E) serotonin plus γ-aminobutyric acid

709. The effect of interruption of one optic nerve will be to

(A) abolish the direct pupillary light reflex from that eye, but allow the consensual pupillary light response of the opposite to remain
(B) permit the direct pupillary response in that eye to occur, but abolish the consensual response of the opposite pupil
(C) abolish the direct and the consensual response from that eye, but allow the consensual response from the opposite eye to remain
(D) cause the ipsilateral pupil to be larger than the contralateral
(E) cause the ipsilateral pupil to be smaller than the contralateral

710. The blind spot in the normal visual fields is caused by

(A) the optic disk
(B) the macula
(C) the hyaloid canal
(D) a persistent artery in the lens
(E) a pigmented spot in the cornea

711. The widest field of vision of one eye is

(A) superior
(B) temporal
(C) nasal
(D) inferior
(E) none of the above—all are equal

DIRECTIONS: Each question below contains four suggested answers of which **one** or **more** is correct. Choose the answer

A	if	1, 2, and 3	are correct
B	if	1 and 3	are correct
C	if	2 and 4	are correct
D	if	4	is correct
E	if	1, 2, 3, and 4	are correct

712. The sensorium commune is correctly described as

(1) a component of the mental status examination
(2) the sense of who, where, and what one is
(3) the awareness of current circumstances and their bearing on the selection of appropriate behavior
(4) involving actual measurement of a patient's IQ

713. Early signs of dystonia musculorum deformans include

(1) spasmodic torticollis
(2) inturning of a foot
(3) loping gait
(4) tortipelvis

714. Features of Broca's (expressive) aphasia include

(1) sparse, telegraphic speech
(2) absence of prepositions, articles, and conjunctions in speech
(3) dysprosody
(4) frequent association with dyslexia and visual field defects

715. A 20-year-old patient notices a gradual reduction in visual acuity over several years. The neurologic examination discloses macular degeneration with acuity in the range of 20/300. The patient also would very likely have lost

(1) form perception
(2) movement perception
(3) night vision
(4) color vision

716. Factors that act to increase the potassium content of cells include

(1) high resistance of the cell membrane to potassium as compared to sodium
(2) exchange of intracellular sodium ions for potassium ions by the sodium pump
(3) higher concentration of extracellular potassium as compared to intracellular
(4) electrical negativity of the interior of the cell

717. The Brown-Séquard syndrome of spinal cord hemisection is characterized by

(1) an enduring loss of sphincter control
(2) a contralateral loss of pain and temperature sensation
(3) an ipsilateral cerebellar ataxia
(4) an ipsilateral loss of position sense

718. Correct statements concerning the normal optic disk include which of the following?

(1) The palest sector is lateral
(2) The optic cup appears pink
(3) The pigment ring is most conspicuous laterally
(4) The large vessels pierce the disk peripherally to the optic cup

719. Complete unilateral deafness indicates a unilateral lesion of the

(1) auditory cortex
(2) medial geniculate body
(3) lateral lemniscus
(4) VIIIth nerve

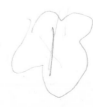

720. Criteria essential to establishing that a substance is a neurotransmitter include which of the following?

(1)   The substance must be present in the synaptic terminals
(2)   The substance should be released at the synaptic terminals when the axon is stimulated
(3)   The synthetic and degradative enzymes should be demonstrable in the perikaryon or synaptic region
(4)   The substance should be absent at sites other than the synapse and should have no other metabolic role

721. Proof of the importance of glucose as a substrate for the CNS comes from which of the following?

(1)   A respiratory quotient (RQ) of about 1
(2)   Removal of large amounts of glutamate, lactate, and pyruvate from the cerebral blood (large arteriovenous difference)
(3)   Very quick reversal of signs and symptoms of moderate hypoglycemia by administration of glucose
(4)   The large amount of glycogen stored in normal neurons

722. A tumor confined to the internal auditory canal would be very likely to cause

(1)   facial palsy
(2)   tinnitus
(3)   vestibular dysfunction
(4)   diplopia

723. The sodium pump in muscle may be described as

(1)   expelling sodium from the cell
(2)   being an ATP-dependent mechanism
(3)   acting against the diffusion gradient of sodium
(4)   maintaining an equal sodium concentration inside and outside the cell

724. Correct statements concerning axonal transmission, as compared to synaptic transmission, include which of the following?

(1)   It responds at a much greater rate of stimulation
(2)   It has a much more rapid response
(3)   It follows an all-or-none principle
(4)   It proceeds orthodromically and antidromically

725. In general, the entry of centrally active drugs into the brain may be said to

(1)   increase in proportion to the number of nitrogen atoms in the drug
(2)   increase in proportion to its lipid solubility
(3)   depend on active transport
(4)   decrease if the drug is highly ionized

726. Features of Wernicke's aphasia include

(1)   poor comprehension of spoken language (auditory word agnosia)
(2)   dysgraphia
(3)   fluent, paraphasic speech
(4)   dyslexia (visual word agnosia)

727. An examiner's hand and arm strength will just about match or can barely overcome the strength of the average person's

(1)   plantar-flexed foot
(2)   fully extended elbow
(3)   extended neck
(4)   dorsiflexed wrist

728. Loss of position sense may occur due to lesions of the

(1)   peripheral nerves
(2)   dorsal roots or dorsal columns
(3)   medial lemniscus
(4)   parietal cortex

729. According to Jackson's concept, release phenomena that occur following an upper motor neuron lesion consist of

(1)   hyperactive stretch reflexes
(2)   paralysis
(3)   flexion reflex of the lower extremity
(4)   absence of abdominal reflexes

SUMMARY OF DIRECTIONS				
A	B	C	D	E
1, 2, 3 only	1, 3 only	2, 4 only	4 only	All are correct

730. Correct statements concerning the tremor of Parkinson's disease include which of the following?

(1) It fails to affect the jaw and tongue
(2) It appears at rest but is accentuated by emotional tension
(3) It persists during sleep
(4) It has a frequency of 5-6 cps

731. Correct statements concerning spasticity due to a cerebral lesion include which of the following?

(1) It bears a direct relationship to the remaining muscle strength
(2) It affects predominantly the arm flexors and the leg extensors
(3) It has no association with hyperactive stretch reflexes
(4) It exhibits the clasp-knife phenomenon

732. Correct statements concerning the nigrostriatal pathway include which of the following?

(1) It is known to have only inhibitory effects on the striatal neurons
(2) It is thought to act by dopaminergic transmission
(3) It has a diffuse projection from each substantia nigra to the striatum on both sides
(4) It consists of small, unmyelinated axons

733. The distribution of axons from the nucleus locus ceruleus includes the

(1) cerebral cortex
(2) diencephalon
(3) cerebellum
(4) spinal cord

734. Peripheral nerve and dermatomal distributions coincide in the

(1) head
(2) neck
(3) arm
(4) thorax

DIRECTIONS: The groups of questions below consist of lettered choices followed by several numbered items. For each numbered item select the **one** lettered choice with which it is **most** closely associated. Each lettered choice may be used once, more than once, or not at all.

Questions 735-738

For each brain stem site listed below, select the cranial nerve group that attaches to it.

(A) III, IV, VI, and XII
(B) V, VII, IX, and X
(C) VI, VII, and VIII
(D) I and II
(E) III and IV

735. Midbrain   E

736. Brain stem (medulla, pons, and midbrain) in the paramedian plane   A

737. Ventrolateral aspect of the brain stem (lateral to the paramedian plane)   B

738. Pontomedullary sulcus   C

Questions 739-742

Match each muscle with its nerve supply.

(A) IIIrd nerve
(B) Ocular sympathetic nerve
(C) VIIth nerve
(D) IVth nerve
(E) Maxillary division of Vth nerve

739. Orbicularis oculi   C

740. Levator palpebrae   A

741. Pupillodilator muscle   B

742. Ciliary muscle   A

Questions 743-746

For each definition of a speech disorder listed below, choose the term with which it is most closely associated.

(A) Dysphasia
(B) Dysprosody
(C) Dysphonia
(D) Dysarthria
(E) Dyslalia

743. A disorder in the production of voice sounds   C

744. A disorder in the articulation of the sounds of speech   D

745. A disorder in the rhythm, tone, or inflections of speech   B

746. A disorder in the understanding or expression of words as symbols for communication   A

Questions 747-750

For each neuropathologic finding listed below, choose the movement disorder with which it is usually associated.

(A) Hemiballismus
(B) Athetoid cerebral palsy
(C) Parkinson's disease
(D) Gait ataxia with little or no arm involvement
(E) Dystonia musculorum deformans

747. Atrophy of the anterior vermis   D

748. Status marmoratus of the basal ganglia and thalamus   B

749. Degeneration of the substantia nigra   C

750. Destruction of the contralateral subthalamic nucleus   A

Neurology Questions for Psychiatrists
Answers

661. The answer is B. *(DeMyer, ed 3. pp 118-120.)* The optic cup appears white because the nerve fiber layer with its capillaries stops at the internal margin of the cup, leaving the white lamina cribrosa of the sclera exposed centrally. An examiner can avoid mistaking a very large but normal optic cup for optic atrophy by looking carefully for the preserved, pink ring of nerve fibers and capillaries around the cup margin.

662. The answer is C. *(DeMyer, ed 3. pp 109-111.)* Interruption of the right optic tract causes left homonymous hemianopia. One optic tract contains the nondecussated axons from the lateral half of the ipsilateral retina and the decussated axons from the medial half of the contralateral retina. Thus, the axons in one tract unite homonymous visual fields, and their interruption results in a contralateral homonymous visual field defect. A complete lesion of the visual pathway between the origin of one optic tract and the calcarine cortex will cause a complete contralateral homonymous hemianopia. Therefore, the localization of the lesion depends on the associated neurologic findings rather than on the visual field defect per se.

663. The answer is C. *(DeMyer, ed 3. pp 306-307.)* The second-order neuron for the dorsal column pathway is located at the medullocervical junction in the nuclei gracilis and cuneatus. The axon of the second-order neuron then decussates. By knowing where the second-order neuron of a sensory pathway is located, one also knows where the decussation of the sensory pathway occurs. The decussation occurs at the level of the second-order neurons. This rule holds true for the general somatic sensory pathways. The medullocervical junction also is the site of another major decussation, the decussation of the pyramidal tract. Thus, this region contains a very important motor and sensory decussation.

664. The answer is C. *(DeMyer, ed 3. 360-364.)* The site at which even a small lesion will completely interrupt consciousness is the midbrain tegmentum. A small lesion located a few millimeters ventral to the aqueduct that destroys the tegmentum in a bilaterally symmetrical fashion will completely abolish consciousness with little effect on other functions. An individual so affected will continue to breathe and have adequate homeostasis to sustain life but will remain permanently unconscious if the lesion exceeds a certain size. The lesion is presumed to interrupt the activity of the ascending reticular activating system that is thought to mediate the conscious, waking state. Lesions of the medullary or caudal pontine tegmentum do not selectively abolish consciousness. Blood pressure and respiration may require artificial support, but the individual can retain consciousness. Bilaterally symmetrical lesions of the diencephalon will abolish consciousness but they must be much larger than the lesions that will abolish consciousness when situated in the midbrain. Similarly, severe bilateral cortical destruction will abolish consciousness, provided the lesion is extensive.

665. The answer is D. *(DeMyer, ed 3. p 105.)* In the differential diagnosis of ptosis, an examiner must include benign congenital ptosis. This not uncommon condition may constitute a false sign of neurologic disease. In the complete absence of any other symptoms or signs referable to the eyes or cranial nerves, a patient with ptosis should be requested to provide an old photograph. Identification of ptosis in the old photograph establishes that it is not a new abnormality and can be considered as a benign condition requiring no further diagnostic workup.

666. The answer is E. *(DeMyer, ed 3. pp 48-49.)* The origin and insertion of the lateral rectus muscle provide that it will only act to abduct the eye. Its action does not change with the position of the eye, unlike the superior and inferior recti and oblique muscles. Thus, the lateral rectus muscle, like its antagonist the medial rectus muscle, is said to have only a primary action and no secondary or tertiary actions. The nerve that innervates the lateral rectus muscle, the VIth cranial nerve, innervates no other muscle. However, the nerve that innervates the medial rectus muscle also innervates other eye muscles. With complete paralysis of a lateral rectus muscle, the eye cannot be abducted because the unopposed, tonic pull of the medial rectus will rotate the eyeball medially. In this position of full adduction, the other muscles that can potentially abduct the eye as one of their secondary actions will be unable to exert their secondary action. They will only act as abductors after the lateral rectus has begun abduction if the eye is already fully adducted.

667. The answer is E. *(Adams, ed 2. p 167.)* The optic nerve fibers arise from the ganglion cells. The rods and cones are the light receptors, which relay their excitation to bipolar and amacrine cells. These cells in turn influence the ganglion cells. The ganglion cell axons transmit the visual message to the brain by directing their axons toward the optic disk. To reach the disk, the axons travel over the surface of the retina, which is exposed to light. They are unmyelinated and transparent until they enter the optic nerve. If they were myelinated while in the retina, they would block light rays from reaching the rod and cone receptors. The optic nerve axons become myelinated just after they perforate the disk and enter the optic nerve. The cell that produces the myelin is the oligodendrocyte. Thus, the optic nerve is susceptible to the demyelinating diseases that involve the central nervous system.

668. The answer is A. *(Cooper, ed 3. p 163.)* The axons of the catecholaminergic neurons are deficient in myelin and, furthermore, accept silver stains poorly. For these reasons, their extensive distributions went unrecognized by the classical methods of neuroanatomy that depended on silver impregnation methods or other methods for detecting degeneration of myelinated fibers. Detection of the catecholamine-containing neurons or axons of the CNS depends on conversion of the catecholamine to a fluorescent substance, demonstration of the enzymes that synthesize catecholamine, or on autoradiography after injection of radioactive precursors.

669. The answer is B. *(DeMyer, ed 3. p 353.)* The combination of dyscalculia, right-left disorientation, and dysgraphia is characteristic of a lesion of the posterior parasylvian area on the left side. The addition of finger agnosia to these symptoms completes the tetrad of deficits known as Gerstmann's syndrome. A mirror image lesion on the right produces Babinski's anosognosia. Although the several components of the syndrome can occur with other lesions or in diffuse cerebral disease, the **combination** of features has localizing significance in most patients with a relatively well-preserved intellect. Not all of the four elements of Gerstmann's syndrome occur in every patient with a left posterior parasylvian area lesion.

670. The answer is D. *(DeMyer, ed 3. pp 180-188.)* In testing a patient for minimal weakness, an examiner should pay most attention to the deltoid and biceps muscles and the dorsiflexors of the wrist, hip, and foot. These muscles, in general, offer just about enough strength to counterbalance the strength of the examiner's hands and arms. If the examiner can overcome each of these muscles without exerting maximum strength, they are weak. However, the very strong muscles such as the arm triceps, the knee extensors, and foot plantar flexors can lose some strength and still will not yield to the opposing force of the examiner's arms and hands. Therefore, a slight loss of strength in these muscles may go undetected.

671. The answer is D. *(DeMyer, ed 3. pp 198-199.)* To reinforce a quadriceps femoris muscle stretch reflex, an examiner may try the maneuver of Jendrassik in which patients grasp their own hands and pull hard, while the examiner attempts to elicit the stretch reflex. The voluntary innervation of a part not being tested "overflows" to increase the excitability of the lower motor neurons of the quadriceps muscles, thus permitting the reflex to appear. Some normal individuals have such a high threshold for the muscle stretch reflex that reinforcement is necessary to demonstrate that the reflex arc is actually intact and that no pathologic condition exists.

672. The answer is A. *(DeMyer, ed 3. pp 99-102.)* In normal individuals, both pupils constrict equally when light is flashed in one. The central connections of the afferent retinal fibers disperse the pupillary reflex equally over both IIIrd cranial nerves. Any difference in the responses of the two pupils is evidence of a lesion somewhere in the reflex arc—i.e., between the retinal receptor and the pupilloconstrictor muscle in the iris. When the pupils react differently to light, an examiner must carefully inspect the retina and examine the visual fields, investigate for signs of midbrain lesions, and conduct a careful examination of the IIIrd cranial nerve and the sympathetic innervation of the iris.

673. The answer is C. *(DeMyer, ed 3. p 66.)* To test a patient's range of ocular movements, the examiner should place the target finger about 40-50 cm from the patient's face. If the examiner's finger is too close, the patient's eyes must converge, which alters ocular alignment and causes discomfort; if too far away, the procedure becomes awkward for the examiner. Ideally, however, in such an examination the patient should be looking at "infinity."

674. The answer is A. *(DeMyer, ed 3. pp 102-104.)* Ptosis resulting from sympathetic denervation is overcome by the relatively strong levator palpebrae muscle and will improve or disappear when the patient looks up. Ptosis due to a complete IIIrd nerve lesion, however, will not change when the patient looks up; if due to a partial IIIrd nerve lesion, ptosis will improve somewhat. Thus, having the patient look up is one step in differentiating between a IIIrd nerve lesion and sympathetic ptosis.

675. The answer is C. *(DeMyer, ed 3. p 9.)* On auscultation of the carotid artery in a normal person, an examiner hears both heart sounds and breath sounds. Bruits, unless transmitted from the heart, usually arise either from a stenotic region in the underlying vessel or from greatly increased flow, such as might occur in a vessel leading to an arteriovenous shunt. Bruits heard when auscultating the head but absent when auscultating the vessels arise in the head rather than in the heart or neck vessels. A bruit heard in the neck does not by itself establish the presence—much less the type—of vascular disease. Other methods of investigation such as Doppler flow studies or angiography are necessary for definitive diagnosis.

676. The answer is C. *(DeMyer, ed 3. pp 157-158.)* When fully elevated, the soft palate contacts the posterior pharyngeal wall. The posterior wall of the pharynx contains the adenoid tissue. The action of the soft palate seals off the nasopharynx from the oropharynx and detours food and liquids into the throat, or detours air out through the mouth when a person speaks. The muscle chiefly responsible for palatal elevation is the levator palatini muscle. Failure of the palate to contact the posterior pharyngeal wall causes speech difficulties involving plosives and the vowels *A* and *E*. The characteristic "palatal speech" may be caused by a cleft palate, myasthenia gravis or other myopathy, or by Xth nerve lesions that paralyze the levator palatini muscle.

677. The answer is A. *(DeMyer, ed 3. p 130.)* Complete paralysis of a set of muscles with preservation of adjacent muscles is evidence of a lower motor neuron lesion. Upper motor neuron lesions, in principle, do not cause paralysis of individual muscles, but, following the dictum of John Hughlings Jackson, they paralyze movements. This statement holds true whether the lesion affects the motor cortex, hemispheric white matter, internal capsule, brain stem, or spinal cord. Myopathies, while having predilections for certain muscle groups, do not, in principle, paralyze one set of muscles and spare an adjacent set. Instead, the myopathies tend to affect all muscles to some degree.

678. The answer is D. *(Adams, ed 2. pp 57-58.)* Slow, sustained, involuntary movements of the trunk are classed as dystonia. When the extremities are involved, observers may differ as to whether to classify the abnormal movements as athetoid or dystonic, but for a patient showing predominantly truncal movements, the term dystonia usually is applied. Dystonia is distinguished from athetosis not only by its anatomical distribution but also by its rate. Athetoid movements tend to be somewhat more rapid and involve the extremities. Both types of movement may be quite strong; a patient with tension athetosis, in particular, will be contorted and incapacitated by the strength of the involuntary movement.

679. The answer is B. *(DeMyer, ed 3. p 153.)* Eyelid closure is a fairly strong movement that normally requires considerable effort for an examiner to overcome. Normal closure leaves no part of an eyeball exposed. Clinically, the examiner is unable to differentiate between the strength of the dominant and nondominant side. Any after-contraction of the eyelid that narrows the palpebral fissure is pathologic and indicates either a myotonic muscle disorder or blepharospasm. Although myotonia occasionally can be demonstrated in the eyelids or even the ocular rotatory muscles, the disorder is not confined to eyelids and characteristically presents as a more generalized myotonic deficit, which can be demonstrated by percussion, by electromyography, and by having an affected individual produce maximal contractions of the muscles.

680. The answer is A. *(DeMyer, ed 3. pp 206-208.)* To elicit clonus, an examiner quickly jerks a part of the body that is at rest. The **quick** jerk is necessary to stretch the muscle spindles to set off the repetitive series of stretch reflexes that constitutes the clonus. With a slow jerk, the muscle spindles may fail to respond. Thus, to test for clonus properly, the initial stimulus must be a quick jerk. Before administering the jerk, the examiner should insure that the part of the patient's body under investigation is at rest and placed in a position that allows control of the amount of both tension and movement to be imparted. The examiner should deliver several jerks before concluding that the patient does not have clonus.

681. The answer is A. *(DeMyer, ed 3. p 129.)*   The classical motor cortex in the precentral gyrus represents the body parts inversely, with the face inferior and the legs superior and draped over the medial crest of the hemisphere. Thus, lesions of the lateral aspect of the motor area paralyze the face and arm, and lesions of the medial aspect paralyze the leg. This somatotopic arrangement persists through the white matter of the hemisphere into the brain stem. A somatotopic arrangement also exists in the secondary and supplementary motor areas of the cerebral cortex, but the movements obtained by electrical stimulation of these motor areas are less discrete and more generalized than those obtained by stimulation of the classical motor area.

682. The answer is D. *(DeMyer, ed 3. pp 312-313, 458.)*   The Romberg test is primarily a test of dorsal column function. Operationally, an examiner asks a patient to stand upright with heels together and eyes closed. The narrow base formed by the heels together stresses the patient's balance. With eyes closed, the patient must then rely on proprioceptive information provided by the dorsal columns to maintain balance. Frequently, this test is misinterpreted as a test for cerebellar dysfunction. Patients with a cerebellar lesion will balance equally well with eyes open or closed. Hysterical patients often sway violently during the Romberg test and either do not fall, which establishes the competency of the proprioceptive system, or fall in such a way as to avoid injury. Malingerers also may respond in this fashion. By diverting the patient's attention, the examiner may induce the patient with a functional disorder to perform well on the test. Standing with heels together, the patient is requested to hold the hands outstretched and to alternately touch the nose with one finger then the other. Immediately after the patient begins to do so, the examiner asks the patient to close his eyes. With his mind diverted to the finger-to-nose task, the functional patient automatically retains balance.

683. The answer is A. *(DeMyer, ed 3. pp 99-102.)*   In testing the pupillary light reflex, an examiner should request a patient to look at a distant point. This relaxes accommodation and any associated pupilloconstriction. If the patient looks at the approaching flashlight or the tip of the nose, the examiner cannot separate the pupilloconstriction of accommodation from that due to the light. Partial closure of the eyes also is liable to result in some accommodation. To avoid engaging one's own accommodation reflex the examiner should avoid squinting and should try to keep both eyes open when performing ophthalmoscopy. When testing the pupillary light reflexes, the examiner should use a dark room or at least avoid a brightly lit room. The ambient light may cause so much pupilloconstriction that little further response is obtained from a flashlight.

684. The answer is B. *(DeMyer, ed 3. pp 33-34.)*   A light ray striking the nasal side of the retina produces the experience of a visual image arising from the temporal half of space. Because of the physical optics of the eye, the image formed on the retina is inverted. The brain learns to associate stimulation of one half of the retina with light rays coming from the opposite half of space. This phenomenon of "projection" of the visual image permits a person to properly localize the origin of the light stimulus and the object from which it came. Knowledge of the inverted relationship between the retinal image formed by the physical optics of the eye and the physiologically superimposed visual image is necessary to an understanding of how to test visual function and the visual fields.

685. The answer is E. *(DeMyer, ed 3. pp 248-249.)*   When a normal person walks straight ahead, the medial margins of the heels fall essentially upon the midline. Any departure from this finding in a person of average or slight body build constitutes a broad-based gait. Individuals with huge frames and very large thighs will walk with their heels displaced somewhat from the midline. The true relation of the feet to the midline in walking surprises most persons, because in walking one is unaware of how neatly the feet track the midline. In the two extremes of life, the toddler and the aged person, however, the gait is broad-based. In the toddler, a broad-based gait compensates for an inchoate sense of balance, and in old age, for a declining sense of balance.

686. The answer is A. *(DeMyer, ed 3. p 261.)* The most consistent sign of cerebellar dysfunction is unsteadiness of gait. The Romberg test is a test of proprioception rather than cerebellar function. The relation of nystagmus to pure cerebellar lesions (lesions that do not affect the vestibular system or underlying pontomedullary structures) remains controversial. Although dysphagia occurs in cerebellar disease as a manifestation of the dystaxia, usually it is not a significant problem. Weakness occurs with cerebellar lesions, but generally only in the context of severe cerebellar signs affecting the extremities. Unsteadiness of gait is the most nearly universal sign of a clinically significant cerebellar lesion. Most lesions of the cerebellum, whether located in the vermis or hemispheres, will cause some unsteadiness of gait; one common cerebellar lesion, degeneration of the anterior vermis in alcoholic persons, expresses itself almost exclusively as unsteadiness of gait. It might be said that if a patient walks well, the cerebellum functions well.

687. The answer is E. *(DeMyer, ed 3. pp 180, 248-249, 343, 458.)* The single most important part of the motor examination is watching a patient walk, yet examiners frequently fail to do so. No other observation reveals so much so fast. In fact, if one is unable to diagnose the motor system defect from the gait, the diagnosis will be difficult to make at all. A wide variety of diseases of the central nervous system, peripheral nerves, muscles, or joints will manifest themselves in a disturbance of gait. One can almost — but not quite — say that if the gait is perfectly normal, the motor system is perfectly normal; if the motor system is perfectly normal, the sensory system is perfectly normal; if both motor and sensory systems are perfectly normal, the mentation is perfectly normal. (Watch any group of hospitalized retarded or mentally ill patients as they walk to the cafeteria. Hardly one will have a perfectly normal gait.) Gait testing, although not a complete neurologic and psychiatric examination, approaches this goal more nearly than any other single mode of examination.

688. The answer is D. *(DeMyer, ed 3. pp 197-198.)* To elicit the triceps surae reflex in a patient who is reclining, an examiner should flex the patient's knee slightly and apply slight upward pressure on the bottom of the patient's foot. Flexing the knee relaxes the triceps surae muscle, and dorsiflexing the foot slightly by pressure on the bottom restores the exact degree of tension required to elicit the reflex. By repeated experience, the examiner learns the "feel" of the required amount of tension. The patient's leg must be allowed to fall outward, the examiner assuming a position that affords free access for delivering a crisp blow with the reflex hammer on the Achilles tendon. The examiner uses the same position of the leg to elicit ankle clonus as to elicit the muscle stretch reflex.

689. The answer is B. *(DeMyer, ed 3. pp 209-210, 232.)* Rigidity is demonstrated by slowly moving an affected patient's extremities. Spasticity, which depends on engaging the muscle spindles quickly, requires a quick movement. Rigidity exhibits plastic resistance throughout the entire range of movement rather than the clasp-knife yielding that characterizes spasticity. Patients should be as relaxed as possible when being tested for either spasticity or rigidity. Voluntary tension interferes with the assessment of rigidity and spasticity; such assessment presupposes that the muscle is devoid of voluntary contraction. Encouraging the patient to relax for proper testing requires considerable skill and patience on the part of the examiner. Rigidity implies an extrapyramidal lesion — spasticity, a pyramidal lesion. Mixtures of spasticity and rigidity are common in some disorders that affect the motor system, such as cerebral palsy.

690. The answer is E. *(DeMyer, ed 3. pp 180-182.)* In principle, muscles show their greatest strength when acting from a fully shortened position. Thus, the biceps brachii shows little power with the elbow fully extended and maximum power with the elbow flexed. By understanding this fact, an examiner can place a weak muscle in a position to bring out its greatest strength or can place it at a disadvantage if it is too strong to test otherwise. An example of a muscle normally too strong for the examiner to overcome by hand and arm testing is the quadriceps femoris. When the leg is extended and the muscle shortened, the examiner cannot budge it with arm and hand strength. The muscle may have lost considerable strength, yet retains sufficient power to resist yielding. With a patient's leg fully flexed and the quadriceps lengthened, the examiner can test the power of the muscle.

691. The answer is C. *(DeMyer, ed 3. pp 309-310.)* Loss of position sense often can be demonstrated in digit four of the hand or foot, even if it remains intact or if there is only questionable impairment of the other digits. Therefore, an examiner should routinely test digit four. If position sense is intact in digit four, in all probability it is intact in the other digits, but intact position sense in the other digits does not preclude demonstrable loss in the fourth digit. Digit four has the least representation in the sensory and motor cortex of any of the digits, and it has the least efficient upper-motor neuron control. For example, finger-tapping speed is much slower in digit four than in the others. Because of its slight cortical representation, digit four loses position sense with smaller and subtler lesions than do the other digits.

692. The answer is E. *(DeMyer, ed 3. p 190.)* In order to elicit a muscle stretch reflex, an examiner does not strike a muscle directly because the ensuing muscle contraction may be due either to a muscle stretch reflex **or** to percussion irritability of the muscle. Direct percussion of a muscle will stretch some of the muscle spindles and may cause a stretch reflex to occur. Direct percussion also can elicit a contraction of the muscle because of the direct stimulation of the muscle fibers by the blow. The resultant muscle contraction appears the same, but in the first instance it is a neurally mediated reflex, and in the second it is an extraneural response dependent on mechanical irritability of the muscle fiber. If the examiner fails to elicit any muscle response when tapping a tendon, the muscle should be percussed directly. In neuropathies, such as the Landry-Guillain-Barré-Strohl syndrome, or in vinca alkaloid intoxication, the stretch reflexes are absent but direct percussion irritability of muscle remains.

693. The answer is E. *(Adams, ed 2. pp 54-55.)* Although parkinsonian rigidity occurs in virtually all muscles, it may be slightly more pronounced in the flexors; at least, in affected persons a flexion posture predominates. The muscles of the face, throat, trunk, and extremities all show resistance to movement or functional deficiencies such as plateau speech that, at least in part, can be explained by generalized muscular rigidity. By contrast, spasticity is manifested preferentially in the triceps surae, quadriceps, and adductor muscles of the lower extremities, and in the biceps and wrist and finger flexors of the upper extremities.

694. The answer is B. *(DeMyer, ed 3. p 212.)* Acute, large, destructive lesions that interrupt the upper motor neurons quickly and completely are more likely than the other lesions listed in the question to cause flaccid upper motor neuron paralysis. In the chronic stage of upper motor neuron lesions, spascitity is characteristic. The absence of tone in the acutely paralyzed extremities may lead a naive examiner to suspect a lower motor neuron paralysis. The examiner relies on the hemiplegic distribution of the paralysis, as well as the frequently present extensor toe signs, to make the correct diagnosis of an upper motor neuron lesion. Patients with slowly evolving interruption of upper motor neurons, as in gradual spinal cord compression, usually exhibit spasticity without going through a flaccid stage first, as would be the case with acute lesions.

695. The answer is C. *(DeMyer, ed 3. pp 193-194.)*   A reflex hammer is held loosely with the thumb and forefinger and struck with a loose, limp-wrist action. These provisions insure that the hammerhead achieves the maximum velocity. An examiner must deliver a high-velocity blow to stretch the muscle spindles rapidly in order to elicit the stretch reflex. The beginner's mistake is to strike with a tightly held hammer and stiff wrist. The resultant slow blow may fail to excite the muscle spindles. Unless the muscle spindles are stretched very rapidly, they accommodate and fail to transmit the afferent volley of impulses necessary to cause the muscle to contract. The examiner may then falsely conclude that the patient lacks muscle stretch reflexes.

696. The answer is A. *(DeMyer, ed 3. pp 226-227.)*   To elicit the superficial abdominal reflexes, an examiner instructs the patient to relax the abdomen. The reflex is weak and too much muscle tension may obscure it. A cold metal object may interfere with the reflex by causing abdominal muscle contraction. The examiner should move the stimulating object briskly across the skin to produce spatial and temporal summation. Upper motor neuron lesions abolish the abdominal reflexes, at least temporarily, but they may return in the chronic stage of the lesion and characteristically are present in children with spastic cerebral palsy.

697. The answer is B. *(DeMyer, ed 3. pp 191-193.)*   The receptor for the muscle stretch reflex is the muscle spindle. The spindle is a specialized bag of fibers that has its own afferent and efferent nerve supply. Unfortunately, clinicians are in the habit of calling the muscle stretch reflexes the "deep tendon" reflexes. This terminology leads to the notion that the receptor for the muscle stretch reflex is located in the tendon, rather than the muscle. The tendon serves only as a convenient way to stretch the muscle spindles in the muscle, i.e., to elicit a muscle stretch reflex.

698. The answer is B. *(DeMyer, ed 3. pp 219-220.)*   In a true extensor toe sign, the toe usually begins to extend after the stimulating object has moved partway along the foot. Although in some instances the toe will extend in response to almost any stimulus, usually the toe will extend only after the object has moved some distance, allowing spatial and temporal summation to occur. If the stimulating object encroaches on the base of the toes, the toe may move unpredictably and show a spurious extension that may be confused with a true extensor toe sign. The best way to distinguish a true toe sign from adventitious toe extension is to evaluate the relation of the toe response to the stimulus. The toe should begin to extend after the object has moved a short distance, remain extended as the stroke continues, and then slowly return to the resting position just after removal of the stimulus—and it should do so reproducibly. In other words, the response should be clearly linked to the stimulus. Thus, the relationship between the application and removal of the stimulus makes it possible to judge the significance of any toe movement observed.

699. The answer is E. *(DeMyer, ed 3. pp 40, 210.)*   An operational, as opposed to an interpretational, definition of rigidity is "The excessive plastic resistance felt by an examiner when moving a patient's resting extremity." The other definitions listed in the question are interpretations of the pathophysiology of rigidity. By understanding the difference between an operational and interpretational definition, examiners will avoid errors and premature conclusions. An operational definition describes the conditions necessary to reproduce, experience, observe, or recognize the phenomenon under question. Medicine in general, and psychiatry in particular, have been plagued by the failure to distinguish observation from interpretation; that is to say, the basic data from what it means. Each component of behavior studied by a clinician should have a definite, agreed upon operational definition.

700. The answer is A. *(DeMyer, ed 3. pp 396-397.)*   A basic function of the vestibular system is to counter-roll the eyes against the direction of head movement. Thus, under normal conditions, when the head turns to the right the vestibular system and neck proprioceptors tend to counter-roll the eyes to the left. In essence, the system acts to keep the eyes fixed straight ahead on the visual target in spite of changes in the position of the head. In an alert, conscious patient, fixation reflexes are also active. Vestibular counter-rolling appears in pure form in an unconscious patient who has no visual fixation. Then the eyes counter-roll; i.e., they remain straight ahead when the head turns. This response constitutes the oculocephalic or doll's eye reflex.

701. The answer is B. *(DeMyer, ed 3. p 392.)*   A sign of meningeal irritation, brought out when an examiner attempts to flex a patient's neck, is flexion and adduction of the lower extremities—so-called Brudzinski's sign. The exact mechanism of the sign is unclear. Flexion of the neck apparently elicits pain by stretching the spinal cord and nerve roots. Flexion of the lower extremities may relax some of the tension on the inflamed cord and roots. Whatever its explanation, Brudzinski's sign regularly occurs in patients who have irritation of the subarachnoid space due to inflammation or hemorrhage. As these pathologic processes resolve, Brudzinski's sign and the other signs of meningeal irritation disappear.

702. The answer is B. *(DeMyer, ed 3. p 351.)*   Aphasic patients, as Hughlings Jackson pointed out, characteristically lose propositional speech but retain automatic or emotional speech, particularly ejaculatory speech such as "ouch" or "damn." Propositional speech proposes something that was, is, or could be. One makes a proposition to buy a piece of property, or to invite an attractive person to one's quarters, or to conjecture about something that happened in the past. A proposition deals with something removed in time from the moment the proposition is made. Aphasic individuals lose the ability to speak in terms of proposals, but may retain the ability to express the emotional content of their present state of mind by use of expletives or automatic speech. Thus, after struggling and failing to produce the propositional sentence "I think it will rain tomorrow," the patient will say with complete clarity, "Damn, I can't do it."

703. The answer is D. *(Adams, ed 2. pp 80-85.)*   A patient with gait apraxia initiates the gait slowly and will stop during the process of walking. For example, a patient with gait apraxia will stop walking while attempting to speak. Thus, the patient either walks or talks but cannot do both simultaneously. The steps are tiny and broad-based, the feet shuffling along as if the soles were magnetized to the floor. The patient turns by planting one foot as a pivot and shuffling around it with the other foot. Gait apraxia, the *marche à petit pas* of the elderly, and the festinating gait of patients with basal ganglia disease merge into a clinical spectrum that requires better delineation.

704. The answer is B. *(DeMyer, ed 3. p 2.)*   With the eyes in the primary position, the free margin of the upper eyelid covers the upper arc of the corneal limbus and therefore part of the iris, but it does not reach the pupil. An examiner must be acquainted with this relationship in order to establish the presence of ptosis, exophthalmos, or enophthalmos, and to diagnose various lid anomalies such as blepharophimosis. The examiner should make a conscious effort to note the lid-limbus relationship during every physical examination. Any deviation in the relationship requires an explanation. If the lids are completely normal, but the relation of the lids to the iris margin is abnormal, the patient may have some type of heterotropia. For example, with hypertropia, the eyeball on one side is rotated up in relation to the other eye. The upper lid will then cover more of the iris of the hypertropic eye than of the normal eye.

705. The answer is E. *(DeMyer, ed 3. pp 97-100.)* After sympathetic denervation, the pupil of the eye constricts because of unopposed tonus in the pupilloconstrictor muscle. The pupilloconstrictor muscle is innervated by the parasympathetic nervous system. Normally the pupillodilator muscle is in tonic opposition to the constrictor muscle. Thus, the size of the pupil is the sum of the opposing forces. Either sympathetic denervation or parasympathetic denervation can occur independently, because the nerve fibers of the two systems reach the eye by different routes. Removal of one of these influences permits the other to predominate. The pupil can still change size to some extent, because excitatory **and** inhibitory effects can be expressed through either system.

706. The answer is C. *(Cooper, ed 3. pp 24-25.)* The factor thought to be of major significance in limiting the peak magnitude of the action potential is the migration of potassium out of the cell. As the cell membrane becomes depolarized, the conductance to sodium increases as the sodium ions tend to enter the cell to reach their equilibrium distribution. The outflow of potassium reduces the amount of cation in the cell and tends to maintain the negative polarity inside of the cell, as partly determined by the negativity of the intracellular proteins. The cell has ample energy to complete not only one, but numerous action potentials. The height of the action potential thus seems to be self-limiting on the basis of the ionic or electrical events rather than on primarily metabolic considerations.

707. The answer is E. *(Cooper, ed 3. pp 76-78.)* Atropine is presumed to exert its major pharmacologic action by combining with the receptor sites on the postsynaptic cell. It also may combine with sites on the presynaptic surface, where it may block some of the feedback inhibition of acetylcholine production and may enhance acetylcholine release and depletion in the cerebrum. Hemicholinium interferes with cholinergic transmission by blocking the active uptake of choline by the presynaptic ending. A steady supply of choline is necessary and rate-limiting in acetylcholine synthesis.

708. The answer is A. *(Adams, ed 2. p 49.)* The basal ganglia, and the striatum in particular, contain a rich concentration of a variety of putative neurotransmitters including dopamine, serotonin, acetylcholine, and γ-aminobutyric acid. The neurotransmitter identified with the nigrostriatal pathway is dopamine. The striatum contains high levels of dopamine in axon terminals as shown by the Falk-Hillarp fluorescence histochemical technique. The striatum also contains the enzymes for degradation of dopamine. Stimulation of the substantia nigra results in the release of dopamine; following lesions of the substantia nigra or its projection pathway to the striatum, the dopamine content of the striatum is consistently reduced. All these lines of evidence point to dopamine as the nigrostriatal neurotransmitter.

709. The answer is C. *(DeMyer, ed 3. pp 99-100.)* Interruption of one optic nerve will abolish the direct light reflex of that eye and the consensual response of the opposite eye. The consensual response of the pupil of the affected eye from the intact eye remains. Interruption of an optic nerve does not cause anisocoria; therefore, if a patient with an interrupted optic nerve also has anisocoria, some other cause for the anisocoria must exist. If the patient's pupil fails to react directly to light because of interruption of the optic nerve on that side, it will still constrict during accommodation. With IIIrd nerve interruption, the pupil will fail to react both during the direct light reflex and during accommodation.

710. The answer is A. *(DeMyer, ed 3. pp 113-115.)* The optic disk causes the blind spot in the visual field. The nerve fibers penetrate the sclera at the disk, but the disk has no receptor neurons. Therefore, light rays striking it produce no visual image. Apparently we fail to appreciate the presence of a blind spot in our visual fields under ordinary conditions of vision, but visual field testing will readily disclose it. The size of the blind spot will increase in papilledema as the edema inactivates the retina around the disk; it also enlarges in the presence of certain malformations or anomalies such as medullated nerve fibers. Retinal lesions, such as hemorrhages or areas of focal retinal destruction, also produce blind spots that can be mapped out by plotting the visual fields on a tangent screen.

711. The answer is B. *(DeMyer, ed 3. p 113.)* The widest field of vision is located on the temporal side. The true visual field, as plotted by full-range perimetry, shows that the periphery of the fields is not a true circle. The field expands on the temporal side, resembling a teardrop with the narrow part medially. The field maintains the same configuration whether the eye looks straight ahead or is deviated to the side. This fact shows that constriction of the medial fields is not caused by the nose, but depends on the structure of the eye itself.

712. The answer is A (1, 2, 3). *(DeMyer, ed 3. pp 329-334.)* The term sensorium commune refers to a person's sense of who, where, and what one is. This concept includes an awareness of current circumstances, both personal and environmental, and the use of this awareness to respond appropriately to all these circumstances. In short, sensorium commune refers to the common sense we all share about ourselves and about our proper relation to our circumstances. Thus, our common sense tells us not to walk off a cliff and to come in out of the rain. The exploration of a patient's common sense thus constitutes an integral part of the mental status examination. Common sense is unrelated to a patient's intellectual status as measured by IQ, assuming that the patient is neither mentally retarded nor demented. Consciousness itself is of course necessary for the awareness of self and environment that leads to appropriate behavioral responses. Therefore, determination of the level of consciousness is the first step in appraising the sensorium.

713. The answer is E (all). *(Adams, ed 2. p 814.)* Dystonia may be manifested in a variety of involuntary movements. Axial movements like torticollis or tortipelvis are common, as are various gait disturbances associated with inturning of the foot or the loping or so-called dromedary gait. The early signs frequently are so subtle and bizarre as to suggest a psychogenic disturbance. Clinicians seem particularly prone to misdiagnose dystonia when the main manifestation is the gait disorder. Patients with dystonia seem to have satisfactory control of their movements except in walking, when they may exhibit sudden loping movements, or contractions or flexions of the trunk, sufficiently bizarre in nature as to suggest hysteria. It often is helpful to examine all other available family members in such a case, looking for a *forme fruste* of dystonia. The presence of subtle torticollis, writer's cramp, or mild dystonic movements of the trunk or pelvis in a close relative helps to establish the diagnosis of an hereditary form of dystonia rather than a psychogenic disorder. Absence of a significant psychiatric disorder, and failure of the movement disorder to respond to suggestion or psychiatric treatment, also provide evidence in support of an organic disease.

714. The answer is A (1, 2, 3). *(Adams, ed 2. pp 327-329. DeMyer, ed 3. pp 350-352.)* The features of Broca's aphasia include sparse, telegraphic speech, absence of prepositions and conjunctions in speech, and dysprosody. Because of the usual location of the lesion in the posterior frontal convolution, victims of Broca's aphasia have no visual field defects. Dyslexia and visual field defects occur with lesions in the parieto-occipito-temporal region (posterior parasylvian region) and would therefore occur with Wernicke's aphasia rather than Broca's. Because of the sparseness of word production, Broca's aphasia is classified as nonfluent aphasia. Nonfluent word production lacks the rhythms and inflection of normal speech; thus, lacking the normal prosody, the speech deficit is termed dysprosody.

715. The answer is D (4). *(DeMyer, ed 3. p 107.)* Macular lesions destroy the cones that mediate visual acuity and color vision. The retina can be regarded as a dual organ with the central part (the macula) devoted to acuity and color vision and the periphery devoted to vision in dim light and to movement perception. Patients with peripheral pigmentary degenerations that spare the macula will complain of loss of night vision. Testing visual fields with colored objects may provide a subtler evaluation than use of a white object.

716. The answer is C (2, 4). *(Cooper, ed 3. pp 21-23.)* Factors that act to increase the concentration of intracellular potassium are the relatively free movement of potassium across cell membranes as compared to sodium, the sodium pump that exchanges an intracellular sodium ion for a potassium ion, and the electrical negativity of the cell interior. The concentration of potassium, being higher inside the cell than outside, tends to oppose entrance of potassium into the cell. Both ionic pump mechanisms and electrical gradients may be involved in controlling the transfer of ions through the cell membrane and in maintaining their relative concentrations.

717. The answer is C (2, 4). *(Adams, ed 2. p 114.)* Hemisection of the cord causes ipsilateral loss of dorsal column function, thus position sense, and contralateral loss of pain and temperature sensation from interruption of the crossed ascending pain and temperature pathway. Ipsilateral cord lesions do not usually cause enduring loss of sphincter control. Spinal cord hemisection could not produce cerebellar signs ipsilateral to the cord lesion, even if another lesion of the cerebellum were present. Interruption of the ipsilateral corticospinal tract by the hemisection would cause paralysis, precluding a test of cerebellar function.

718. The answer is B (1, 3). *(DeMyer, ed 3. pp 118-120.)* The normal optic disk is palest laterally and has the most conspicuous pigment deposition along the lateral boundary. The large vessels of the retina pierce the disk within the optic cup. The cup itself appears white. The clinician must be familiar with these normal anatomical features of the disk in order to identify lesions or congenital anomalies of that area. Other significant features of the disk that should be noted during the ophthalmoscopic examination include the size of the disk, the color of the nerve fiber layer and its degree of capillarity, the size of the vessels, and the distinctness of the disk margins.

719. The answer is D (4). *(DeMyer, ed 3. pp 277-278.)* Complete unilateral deafness indicates a lesion of the ipsilateral VIIIth nerve. Lesions at the remaining sites in the auditory pathway (the lateral lemniscus, geniculate body, and auditory cortex) do not cause complete unilateral deafness because the central pathways disperse the incoming auditory impulses bilaterally. Therefore, a unilateral lesion of the central pathways does not cause a complete loss of hearing in one ear. With the application of computer technology to the recording of brain stem auditory evoked responses (BAER test), clinicians may pinpoint the location of a lesion along the course of the central pathways; such localization is not possible by auditory testing at the bedside.

720. The answer is A (1, 2, 3). *(Cooper, ed 3. p 240.)* Criteria to establish a substance as a neurotransmitter include demonstration that the substance is produced by nervous tissue, and that it is stored, released, exerts its action, and is then inactivated in the synaptic region. The substance may be present elsewhere in the body and may have other metabolic roles. For example, one function of the catecholamine pathway is the production of the pigment melanin.

721. The answer is B (1, 3). *(Cooper, ed 3. pp 48-50.)* An RQ of about 1 means that the consumption of O_2 by the brain equals the production of CO_2. This fact is interpreted to mean that the primary substrate is glucose, and that the brain does not utilize fatty acids or amino acids as substrates for the primary production of ongoing energy. CNS is almost the only tissue with an RQ of 1. Under normal conditions, the only energy-producing substrate consistently removed in large quantities from arterial blood by the brain is glucose. Other substances like glutamate, lactate, and pyruvate show little arteriovenous difference. Glucose, unlike most other substrates, can very quickly reverse the symptoms of hypoglycemia. The blood level of glucose correlates closely with the severity of the symptoms of hypoglycemia. These facts establish the primacy and importance of glucose in brain metabolism. In spite of the primacy of glucose, the storage of glycogen in normal neurons is slight.

722. The answer is A (1, 2, 3). *(Adams, ed 2. pp 462-464.)* A tumor confined to the internal auditory canal would affect only the VIIth and VIIIth cranial nerves, producing a facial palsy and disturbances of both the vestibular and auditory components of the VIIth nerve. Such a tumor would not cause diplopia because none of the cranial nerves to the ocular muscles run through the internal auditory canal. If the tumor increases in size, however, it may expand into the adjacent cerebellopontine angle and compress the VIth nerve, causing diplopia. It may also impinge on the Vth, IXth, and Xth nerves, and on the brain stem and cerebellum.

723. The answer is A (1, 2, 3). *(Adams, ed 2. p 869.)* The sodium pump in muscle expels sodium from the cell against the diffusion gradient of sodium and is an ATP-dependent mechanism. Normally, the intracellular sodium concentration is less than the extracellular concentration. The sodium pump restores the ratio of intracellular to extracellular sodium after an action potential has passed, and maintains the sodium-potassium equilibrium when the cell is in the resting state. The action of the sodium pump is one of the fundamental mechanisms that maintains the polarity of nerve and muscle cell membranes.

724. The answer is E (all). *(Cooper, ed 3. pp 27-28.)* Axonal transmission, as compared to synaptic transmission, responds at a much greater rate—a maximum of 1500 times per second as compared to 100. Axonal transmission proceeds much more quickly, without the 0.1 to 0.2 msec delay in synaptic transmission. Axonal transmission follows an all-or-none principle, whereas synaptic transmission can be influenced by inhibitory or excitatory transmitters that alter excitability without transmitting an impulse. Temporal summation can cause the postsynaptic cell to continue to fire after cessation of impulses arriving from the presynaptic cell. In general, synaptic transmission proceeds only orthodromically, whereas in an axon, a nerve impulse proceeds orthodromically and antidromically after stimulation anywhere along its length. Furthermore, the axon is electrically excitable whereas the synapse is not. All of these differences provide evidence for an essentially electrical event for axonal transmission and an essentially chemical event for synaptic transmission.

725. The answer is C (2, 4). *(Cooper, ed 3. pp 18-20.)* As a general rule, the entry of a drug into the brain increases in proportion to its lipid solubility and decreases if the drug is highly ionized. The centrally acting drugs usually enter by passive diffusion rather than active transport. The amount of drug available to pass the blood-brain barrier depends on the drug's protein-binding affinity. Drugs that are tightly bound to protein will fail to pass through the capillary. Thus, the proportion of free, nonprotein-bound drug determines the amount that can enter the brain. The entry of the nonprotein-bound drug depends on its ionization and lipophilia; once the drug passes the blood-brain barrier and gains access to the extracellular space of the nervous system, it can diffuse freely through the extracellular fluid. It may also enter the cerebrospinal fluid, which, having a zero concentration initially, acts as a sink. After the drug passes the blood-brain barrier, no additional anatomic barriers to its free passage into the cerebrospinal fluid have been identified.

726. The answer is E (all). *(Adams, ed 2. pp 329-330.)* Wernicke's aphasia includes poor comprehension of spoken language (auditory word agnosia), fluent paraphasic speech, dyslexia (visual word agnosia), and dysgraphia. Current concepts of aphasia derive from Wernicke's proposals. He recognized that the brain has primary receptive areas for the various modalities like sound, sight, hearing, touch, and smell. "Association" cortex surrounds these primary receptive areas and receives fiber pathways from them. The association cortex elaborates the primary sensations into their symbolic significance. The association cortex in the posterior superior temporal lobe, around the primary auditory cortex, links sounds with the words they signify. Fiber pathways, now thought to be the arcuate fasciculus, connect the auditory association cortex with Broca's area in the posterior inferior frontal convolution, which directs the motor apparatus of speech. Presumably, the cortex of the left posterior parasylvian area, in its transition area to the occipital lobe, is essential for recognition of visual impulses as words, and lesions of this region result in dyslexia. This region also is the site of the lesion in Gerstmann's syndrome, one element of which is dysgraphia. Patients with Wernicke's aphasia have varying combinations of receptive aphasia and one or more elements of Gerstmann's syndrome.

727. The answer is D (4). *(DeMyer, ed 3. pp 180-183, 376.)* An examiner's hand and arm strength will just about match or barely overcome the average person's dorsiflexed wrist, but cannot overcome the plantar-flexed foot, fully extended elbow, or extended neck. With the foot plantar-flexed, or the neck, elbow, knee, or trunk fully extended, the muscles responsible for these movements act from their strongest, i.e., shortest, positions. When any of these antigravity muscles act from their strongest positions, the rule is that the examiner's arms and hands are not strong enough to overcome them. Indeed, the examiner's arm and hand strength just matches or barely overcomes the strength of the antagonists to the antigravity muscles when acting from their strongest position. Such is the case with the wrist or foot dorsiflexors, hip flexors, or the elbow flexors. Thus, the theory of antigravity (antigravity muscles of a quadruped) or nonantigravity muscles reminds the examiner which ones can be readily tested by arm and hand strength and whether to try to test them in their strongest or weakest positions.

728. The answer is E (all). *(DeMyer, ed 3. pp 309-312.)* Loss of position sense may occur with lesions of the peripheral nerve, dorsal roots or dorsal columns, medial lemniscus, or parietal cortex. It also can occur following lesions of the thalamus and internal capsule. Loss of position sense due to interruption of the pathway from periphery to the parietal cortex is called statanesthesia, to distinguish it from loss due to a cortical lesion, which would be an agnosia or statagnosia. In analyzing a patient for loss of position sense, the clinician should "think through" the entire pathway from periphery to cortex to consider the possible sites of the lesion.

729. The answer is B (1, 3). *(DeMyer, ed 3. p 205.)* Jackson distinguished release phenomena from deficit phenomena. Release phenomena are new behaviors, such as spasticity, clonus or flexion reflexes (including the Babinski sign) that appear after an upper motor neuron (UMN) lesion. Deficit phenomena are behaviors that **dis**appear after a UMN lesion, as exemplified by paralysis and absence of superficial abdominal reflexes. The mechanism of release phenomena remains a mystery. Although an intact UMN pathway "prevents" the appearance of release phenomena, it does not follow that the UMN pathway keeps release phenomena in check by an active inhibitory process. It was, however, to direct attention to the two changes that occur—a deficit of volitional activity and an increase in reflex activity—that Jackson coined the terms "deficit" and "release" phenomena.

730. The answer is C (2, 4). *(Adams, ed 2. pp 69-70.)* Parkinsonian tremor appears during rest but is accentuated by emotional tension. It slackens during times of emotional repose and disappears during sleep. Intensification of the tremor by stress and its disappearance during sleep may lure the unwary examiner into suspecting a psychogenic disorder, when in fact these features identify the tremor as parkinsonian and therefore organic. The resting tremor of parkinsonism stands in direct contrast to tremors in those diseases in which there is a tremor only when making a volitional movement and no tremor at rest. Patients with a rest tremor, as in parkinsonism, have a lesion of the substantia nigra, whereas patients with tremor only during volitional movements have a lesion of the cerebellum or its pathways.

731. The answer is C (2, 4). *(Adams, ed 2. p 40.)* In general, no necessary relationship exists between spasticity due to a cerebral lesion and a patient's remaining strength. After complete upper motor neuron paralysis, spasticity usually appears in parallel with the return of movement, but may vary in proportion to residual strength. Spasticity, hyperactive stretch reflexes, and the clasp-knife phenomenon characteristically are all present simultaneously. Sometimes, however, discrepancies occur, with the stretch reflexes being hyperactive even though the extremities appear flaccid. The relationship between spasticity and specific underlying pathophysiological mechanisms or neuroanatomical pathways remains to be established. Another sign that usually, but not invariably, accompanies spasticity is an extensor toe sign. It will appear during the flaccid stage of hemiplegia and persists during the spastic stage.

732. The answer is C (2, 4). *(Cooper, ed 3. pp 168-169.)* The nigrostriatal pathway is thought to act by dopaminergic transmission. Whether nigral activation affects the striatal neurons solely by inhibition is disputable, although it appears that inhibition is the probable result. The axons that run to the striatum from the substantia nigra are small and unmyelinated and have a strongly unilateral, topographic distribution. Thus, hemiparkinsonism can occur from a localized lesion of the substantia nigra on one side of the midbrain. Hemiparkinsonism has been observed to follow unilateral lesions of the substantia nigra. The lesion may be a granuloma, neoplasm, or sequela of trauma.

733. The answer is E (all). *(Cooper, ed 3. pp 163-167.)* The nucleus locus ceruleus apparently has the widest distribution of axons of any nucleus in the CNS. No other nucleus of such restricted location is known to send axons to every major part of the CNS. This distribution appears to imply that the nucleus locus ceruleus has a widespread role in modulating neural activity rather than simply conveying some specific point-to-point message, as in the retinogeniculo-calcarine pathway. In these specific sensory pathways, a single axon synapses on one—or only a few—postsynaptic cells. The message of the firing axon thus is transmitted to a very restricted target. In the catecholaminergic system, the axons may disperse to many postsynaptic neurons; in fact, the norepinephrinergic axons show the widest dispersion of any known neuronal systems.

734. The answer is D (4). *(DeMyer, ed 3. pp 70-74.)* Peripheral nerve and somite distributions coincide only in the thoracic region. Rearrangement of the somites by development of the head and limbs produces a situation in which the peripheral nerves carry either more or fewer fibers than those from one somite. In the thorax, the somites retain their simple segmental arrangement, and each peripheral nerve carries the fibers of one somite. The muscles and bones derived from the somites display a similar pattern. In the limbs, many of the muscles and bones of the postfetal individual result from amalgamations of contributions from two or more somites. Since each part derived from a somite retains its original somite nerve supply, the muscles and bones of the extremities receive innervation from more than one somite. The axons from the somite nerves are redistributed in the plexuses to form the peripheral nerves of the limbs.

735-738. The answers are: 735-E, 736-A, 737-B, 738-C. *(DeMyer, ed 3. pp 80-81.)* Clinicians must be familiar with the attachment sites of the cranial nerves to the brain stem in order to localize neurologic lesions. By learning them in sets, their anatomy becomes easy to remember. These memory sets consist of the somite set, branchial arch set, and the set of cranial nerves that attaches at the pontomedullary sulcus. The somite set of cranial nerves innervates the cranial muscle derived from somites. This set contains cranial nerves III, IV, VI, and XII. The nuclei of these nerves are all paramedian in location, the nerve fibers running a straight course through the brain stem and all exiting in the paramedian plane in line with the somite nerves of the spinal cord. The IVth cranial nerve exits dorsally, but it is still in the paramedian plane.

The second set of cranial nerves, the branchial arch set, innervates cranial muscles derived from the branchial arches. This set consists of cranial nerves V, VII, IX, and X. They are predominantly responsible for visceral functions such as chewing, breathing, swallowing, and phonating. The XI nerve may belong to this group, but it arises in the spinal cord rather than the brain stem. The nuclei of origin of the branchial nerves lie in the ventrolateral part of the brain stem tegmentum, and their fibers run a looped internal course rather than a straight course; for example, the VIIth nerve loops over the VIth nerve nucleus. All branchial nerves attach to the ventrolateral aspect of the brain stem rather than in the paramedian plane.

The third set of cranial nerves that is useful to learn as an aid in remembering attachment sites contains VI, VII, and VIII—a somite nerve, a branchial arch nerve, and a solely sensory nerve respectively. These three nerves all attach to the pontomedullary junction. In fact, they attach in ventrodorsal order (VI, VII, and VIII), the VIth nerve exiting most ventrally (in the paramedian plane); the VIIth nerve, and then the VIIIth nerve, exit most dorsally. By knowing the components of this set of cranial nerves—VI, VII, and VIII—and their attachment site at the pontomedullary sulcus, then one knows that IX, X, XI, and XII must attach caudal to the pontomedullary junction, hence to the medulla or spinal cord, and I-V must attach rostral to it. Thus, the pontomedullary junction serves as a very convenient watershed for remembering the attachment sites of all cranial nerves.

739-742. The answers are: 739-C, 740-A, 741-B, 742-A. *(DeMyer, ed 3. pp 97-98, 150-151).* The muscles of and around the eye receive their innervation from a number of different sources. The VIIth nerve innervates the orbicularis oculi muscle; the IIIrd nerve innervates the levator palpebrae and ciliary muscles (the ciliary muscle adjusts the thickness of the lens). The carotid sympathetic nerve innervates the pupillodilator muscle. The maxillary division of the Vth nerve is a sensory nerve and thus provides no motor fibers to the ocular muscles. Knowledge of the various sources of motor fibers to the eye is necessary for clinical analysis of abnormalities of ocular rotation and pupillary size, and disorders of the eyelid manifesting as ptosis or weakness of eye closure.

743-746. The answers are: 743-C, 744-D, 745-B, 746-A. *(Adams, ed 2. pp 331-336. DeMyer, ed 3. p 353.)* The terms dysphonia, dysarthria, dysprosody, and dysphasia designate the function of the speech apparatus at fault in the various disorders of speech. The distinctions they convey justify their use in clinical practice.

Dysphonia means a disorder in the production of voice sounds. The disorder may originate in the larynx itself (such as hoarseness due to a vocal cord tumor), or it may involve the nerves to the larynx or supranuclear control of that organ. Vagus nerve lesions produce a lower motor neuron type of dysphonia. Spastic dysphonia occurs in cerebral palsy and as an idiopathic disease in adults. Aphonia, especially if sudden in onset, implies hysteria, but the patient with Broca's aphasia due to a large hemispheric lesion also may exhibit aphonia. Hysterical persons usually can communicate perfectly well by whispering, whereas aphasic individuals cannot.

Dysarthria means a disorder in the articulation of speech sounds. The process of articulation requires action by the vocal cords, oropharynx, nasopharynx, teeth, palate, tongue, mandible, and lips. Any anatomic deviation of these parts or their nerve supply or muscles may cause dysarthria. Supranuclear lesions involving the corticobulbar tracts or lesions of the left posterior inferior frontal region may cause central dysarthria. Cerebellar or basal ganglia lesions also may produce dysarthria.

Dysprosody means a disorder in the rhythm, tone, or inflections of speech. Stuttering, singsong speech, the scanning speech of patients with cerebellar disease, or the plateau speech of those with parkinsonism constitute common examples of dysprosody. Autistic children characteristically display a flat, inappropriately inflected, dysprosodic speech.

Dysphasia means a disorder in the understanding or expression of words as symbols for communication. A patient with dysphasia has a disorder at the level of the cerebrum, most commonly in the parasylvian area of the left central hemisphere.

747-750. The answers are: 747-D, 748-B, 749-C, 750-A. *(Adams, ed 2. pp 66-67.)* Some movement disorders have a predictable lesion and others do not. Disorders with the best-established lesions include the association of alcoholism with gait dystaxia and degeneration of the anterior vermis, parkinsonism with degeneration of the substantia nigra, and hemiballismus with destruction of the contralateral subthalamic nucleus.

Other disorders, such as dystonia musculorum deformans, are not associated with lesions that are regularly demonstrable at autopsy. For many movement disorders such as rheumatic chorea, the pathoanatomic substrate is unclear. The lesions in this disease and many others are too subtle, diffuse, or nonspecific to allow a direct correlation with the clinical state of the patient. In other diseases with involuntary movements, the lesions may be striking enough but affect too many structures to permit the correlation of any particular lesion site with the clinical signs. The other confounding factor is that the effects of multiple or diffuse lesions may be additive or subtractive in respect to the expression of the movement disorder. Thus, given a particular lesion that may cause a movement disorder, another lesion elsewhere may tend to increase or decrease the clinical expression of the disorder.

Bibliography

Adams RD, Victor M: *Principles of Neurology,* 2nd ed. New York, McGraw-Hill, 1981.

Alexander MP, Struss DT, Benson DF: Capgras syndrome: a reproductive phenomenon. *Neurology* 29:334-339, 1979.

American Medical Association: *Disability Evaluation Under Social Security: A Handbook for Physicians.* Washington, U.S. Dept. Health, Education and Welfare, 1979.

American Psychiatric Association: *Diagnostic and Statistical Manual of Mental Disorders,* 3rd ed. Washington, American Psychiatric Association, 1980.

Barchas JD, et al (eds): *Psychopharmacology: From Theory to Practice.* New York, Oxford University Press, 1977.

Barker P: *Basic Child Psychiatry.* New York, Science House, 1971.

Bates B: *A Guide to Physical Examination.* Philadelphia, JB Lippincott, 1979.

Bell WE, McCormick WF: *Neurologic Infections in Children,* vol 12. Philadelphia, WB Saunders, 1975.

Benson DF, Blumer D: *Psychiatric Aspects of Neurologic Disease.* New York, Grune & Stratton, 1975.

Blackwood W, Corsellis JAN (eds): *Greenfield's Neuropathology,* 3rd ed. Chicago, Year Book Medical, 1976.

Blass JP: Disorders of pyruvate metabolism. *Neurology* 8:280-286, 1979.

Bondy PK, Rosenberg LE (eds): *Duncan's Diseases of Metabolism,* 7th ed. Philadelphia, WB Saunders, 1974.

Carpenter MB: *Core Text of Neuroanatomy,* 2nd ed. Baltimore, Williams & Wilkins, 1978.

Carroll BJ, Greden JF, Feinberg M: Neuroendocrine disturbances and the diagnosis of aetiology of endogenous depression. *Lancet* 8163:321-322, 1980.

Cole G, DeVilliers F, Proctor NSF, et al: Alexander's disease: case report including histopathological and electron microscopic features. *J Neurol Neurosurg Psychiatry* 42:619-624, 1979.

Cooper JR, Bloom FE, Roth RH: *The Biochemical Basis of Neuropharmacology,* 3rd ed. New York, Oxford University Press, 1978.

DeMyer M: *Parents and Children in Autism.* Washington, VH Winston & Sons, 1979.

DeMyer W: Megalencephaly in children: clinical syndromes, genetic patterns, and differential diagnosis from other causes of megalocephaly. *Neurology* 22:634-643, 1972.

DeMyer W: *Technique of the Neurologic Examination: A Programmed Text,* 3rd ed. New York, McGraw-Hill, 1980.

Gilman AG, et al (eds): *The Pharmacological Basis of Therapeutics,* 6th ed. New York, Macmillan, 1980.

Gilroy J, Meyer JS: *Medical Neurology,* 2nd ed. New York, Macmillan, 1975.

Goldensohn ES, Appel SH (eds): *Scientific Approaches to Clinical Neurology.* Philadelphia, Lea & Febiger, 1977.

Groves JR: Taking care of the hateful patient. *N Engl J Med* 298:883-887, 1978.

Hackett TP, Cassem NH: *Massachusetts General Hospital Handbook of General Psychiatry.* St. Louis, CV Mosby, 1978.

Hoekelman RA, et al (eds): *Principles of Pediatrics: Health Care of the Young.* New York, McGraw-Hill, 1978.

Horell JA: The neuroanatomy of amnesia: a critique of the hippocampal memory hypothesis. *Brain* 101:403-445, 1978.

Kaplan HI, Freedman AM, Sadock BJ: *Comprehensive Textbook of Psychiatry,* 3rd ed. Baltimore, Williams & Wilkins, 1980.

Kaplan OJ: *Psychopathology of Aging.* New York, Academic Press, 1979.

Kolb LC: *Modern Clinical Psychiatry,* 9th ed. Philadelphia, WB Saunders, 1977.

Lazare A (ed): *Outpatient Psychiatry: Diagnosis and Treatment.* Baltimore, Williams & Wilkins, 1979.

Lemire RJ, et al: *Normal and Abnormal Development of the Human Nervous System.* Hagerstown, Harper & Row, 1975.

Lippman S: Renal function monitoring of lithium. *Psychiatr Ann* 11:177-181, 1981.

Plum F, Posner JB: *The Diagnosis of Stupor and Coma,* 3rd ed. Philadelphia, FA Davis, 1980.

Reese WL, Gordon O, Goodniah PJ: The value and limitation of lithium in psychiatric disorders. *Psychiatr Ann* 11:143-153, 1981.

Reitan RM, Davison LA (eds): *Clinical Neuropsychology: Current Status and Applications.* Washington, VH Winston & Sons, 1974.

Robson P: Shuffling, hitching, scooting, or sliding: some observations in 30 otherwise normal childen. *Dev Med Child Neurol* 12:608-617, 1970.

Rosenzweig N, Pearsall FD (eds): *Sex Education for the Health Professional: A Curriculum Guide.* New York, Grune & Stratton, 1978.

Russell DS, Rubenstein LJ: *Pathology of Tumors of the Nervous System,* 4th ed. Baltimore, Williams & Wilkins, 1977.

Slaby AE, Lieb J, Tancredi LR: *Handbook of Psychiatric Emergencies.* New York, Medical Examination Publishing, 1975.

Spitzer RL: DSM III: the major achievements and an overview. *Am J Psychiatry* 137:151-164, 1980.

Stanbury JB, Wyngaarden JB, Frederickson DS: *The Metabolic Basis of Inherited Disease,* 4th ed. New York, McGraw-Hill, 1978.

Swaiman KF, Wright FS (eds): *The Practice of Pediatric Neurology.* St. Louis, CV Mosby, 1975.

Taveras JM, Wood EH: *Diagnostic Neuroradiology,* 2nd ed. Baltimore, Williams & Wilkins, 1976.

Usdin G, Lewis JM: *Psychiatry in General Medical Practice.* New York, McGraw-Hill, 1979.

Vinken PJ, Bruyn GW (eds): *Handbook of Clinical Neurology,* vol 20. New York, North Holland Publishing, 1977.

Wells CE (ed): *Dementia,* 2nd ed., vol 15. Philadelphia, FA Davis, 1977.

Wolberg LR: *The Technique of Psychotherapy,* 3rd ed. New York, Grune & Stratton, 1977.